MEDICATION
TEACHING AIDS

MEDICATION TEACHING AIDS

Springhouse Corporation
Springhouse, Pennsylvania

Staff

Executive Director, Editorial
Stanley Loeb

Senior Publisher
Matthew Cahill

Art Director
John Hubbard

Senior Editor
June Norris

Associate Clinical Director
Joanne DaCunha, RN, MSN

Clinical Editors
Joan E. Mason, RN, EDM (project editor); Marlene M. Ciranowicz, RN, MSN; Galene Sellers, LPN; Rosemarie Marinaro, RN, MSN

Drug Information Editor
George J. Blake, RPh, MS

Editors
Mary Lou Ambrose, Jane V. Cray, Kathie Goldberg, Barbara Hodgson, Kevin Law, Edith McMahon, Gale Sloan, Jean Wallace

Copy Editors
Cynthia Breuninger (supervisor), Traci A. Ginnona

Designers
Stephanie Peters (associate art director), Matie Patterson (senior designer)

Illustrators
John Gist, Robert Jackson

Cover
John Gist

Typography
David Kosten (director), Diane Paluba (manager), Elizabeth Bergman, Joyce Rossi Biletz, Phyllis Marron, Robin Mayer, Valerie Rosenberger

Manufacturing
Deborah Meiris (director), T.A. Landis, Anna Brindisi, Katrina Davis

Production Coordination
Pat McCloskey

Editorial Assistants
Maree DeRosa, Beverly Lane, Mary Madden

℞ A member of the Reed Elsevier plc group

Library of Congress Cataloging-in-Publication Data
Medication teaching aids.
   p. cm.
Includes bibliographical references and index.
1. Patient education—Handbooks, manuals, etc. 2. Drugs—Administration—Handbooks, manuals, etc.
I. Springhouse Corporation.
   [DNLM: 1. Drug Therapy—handbooks.
2. Drugs—administration & dosage—handbooks. 3. Patient Education—handbooks. WB 39 M4882 1994]
RT90.M42   1994
615.5'8'071—dc20
DNLM/DLC   93-19598
ISBN 0-87434-512-X   CIP

Contents

Foreword

By thoroughly teaching your patient about his medications, you can achieve several important aims. Most important, you can help him comply with therapy and recover sooner. After all, a patient who understands how to take his medication, what to do if he misses a dose, and what he must know about other drugs may require fewer doctor's visits, subsequent treatments, and hospitalizations. In addition, an informed patient may know how to respond if he experiences side effects, thereby possibly lessening their severity or avoiding them entirely.

The potential for improved patient teaching about medications is enormous. Consider that almost 30% of hospital admissions for older adults result from drug reactions. In cardiac care alone, one expert estimates that 125,000 deaths and 325,000 hospitalizations could be avoided annually through better patient compliance. Clearly, teaching patients about their medications can result in improved health and lower costs.

The federal government has sent a clear signal on patient education through the Omnibus Reconciliation Act of 1990. Part of this law requires that pharmacists offer counseling to Medicaid patients (most states are also including non-Medicaid patients in their regulations). This new focus on education has created a need for more patient-oriented information. Fortunately, this new book from the publisher of *Physician's Drug Handbook* and *Nursing94 Drug Handbook* convincingly meets this need.

Divided into three sections, *Medication Teaching Aids* begins with teaching aids that tell the patient how to perform more than 20 drug administration techniques—from how to take tablets, capsules, and liquid medications to how to perform complex procedures, such as infusion of clotting factors. Alphabetically arranged, the second and largest section of the book presents concisely written teaching aids for over 290 of the most commonly prescribed medications taken at home. The book's last section includes 20 teaching aids on supportive measures. These aids supplement the patient's drug therapy with important guidelines on comfort measures, dietary directions, health monitoring, and disease prevention.

Using large print, easily understood language, and illustrations, *Medication Teaching Aids* is designed with the patient in mind. What's more, for your convenience, a special binding allows the book to lie flat for convenient photocopying. When you give your patient one of these teaching aids, he can use the information to reinforce your teaching. He can also refer again and again to the teaching aid to refresh his memory about a step, a technique, or a piece of equipment used in his drug therapy.

All too often, patient education falls by the wayside as health care practitioners rush to meet the immediate demands of their practice. Fortunately, this book makes it easy for any nurse, pharmacist, or doctor to teach patients about their medications. *Medication Teaching Aids* is one resource you can't afford to pass up—and one that will provide a long-term return.

Jean Krajicek Bartek, RN, PhD, CARN
Assistant Professor
Department of Adult Health and Illness
University of Nebraska Medical Center
College of Nursing
Omaha

Administration techniques

When you measure and administer your patient's medication, you can be sure that he takes it properly. But what about when he goes home? Are you confident that he can continue correct drug administration on his own?

This section of *Medication Teaching Aids* can help you teach your patient to use proper administration techniques, enabling him to continue effective drug therapy at home. You can photocopy and give him the appropriate teaching aids and review the steps with him. For each administration technique, you'll find step-by-step explanations and illustrations that show your patient exactly how to proceed.

You may want to give the first teaching aid, "Taking your medication correctly," to all patients receiving drug therapy. It provides information to help your patient have a prescription filled, take and store medications, and avoid common problems. The next group of teaching aids covers *oral drugs* and describes how to take tablets, capsules, and liquid medications. Special tips on how to give these medications to a child are also given.

Taking inhaled drugs may seem complicated and confusing to your patient. The teaching aids for *respiratory drugs* can help boost your patient's confidence. They carefully describe each step for using and caring for metered-dose inhalers, inhalers with holding chambers, AeroVent inhalers, and aerosol equipment. Likewise, the teaching aids for *eye, ear, and nose drugs* provide step-by-step instructions on how to administer eye, ear, and nose drops, apply eye ointment, and use a nasal pump.

The teaching aids for *topical and other drugs* explain how to use medicated bath products, rectal suppositories, and vaginal medications. The last group, *injections*, can help you reinforce your instructions on giving injections. Your patient will gain assurance by studying the appropriate teaching aid on subcutaneous or intramuscular injections, use of an anaphylaxis kit, self-infusion of clotting factors, care of a central venous catheter, or use and care of an implanted port.

Taking your medication correctly

Dear Patient:

Your doctor has prescribed medication to help treat your condition. This medication will help you only if you take it correctly. Here's how.

Filling your prescription
• Have your prescription filled at the pharmacy you ordinarily use. That way, the pharmacist can keep a complete record of your medications. Tell him if you're allergic to any medications.
• If you need to refill your prescription, don't wait until the last minute. Refill it before you run out of medication.

Taking your medication
• Take your medication in a well-lit room. Double-check the label to make sure you're taking the right medication. If you don't understand the directions, call your pharmacist or doctor.
• If you forget to take a dose or several doses, don't take two or more doses together. Instead, ask your doctor or pharmacist for directions.
• Don't stop taking your medication unless your doctor tells you to. And don't save it for some other time.

Storing your medication
• Keep your medication in its original container or in a properly labeled prescription bottle. If you're taking more than one medication, don't store them together in a pillbox.
• Store your medication in a cool, dry place or as directed by your pharmacist. Don't keep it in the bathroom medicine cabinet, where heat and humidity may cause it to lose its effectiveness.
• If you have children, make sure your medication containers have childproof caps. Always keep the containers out of the reach of children.

Avoiding problems
• Keep the following information about each of your medications on index cards or on a chart: the drug's name, its purpose, its appearance, how to take it, when to take it, how much to take, and special precautions or side effects. Remember, most medications cause some side effects.
• If you have any questions about symptoms you're experiencing while taking your medication, call your doctor right away.
• If you're pregnant or breast-feeding, talk to your doctor before taking any medication or home remedy. Some medications may be harmful to the baby.
• Never take medication that doesn't look right or has passed the expiration date. The medication may not work. Even worse, it may harm you.
• Don't take nonprescription medications at the same time without first checking with your pharmacist. Another medication can change the way your prescribed medication works.
• Alcoholic beverages and some foods can change the way some medications work. Read the medication label. It may tell you what to avoid.
• Your medication has been prescribed just for you. Don't share it with family or friends. They could be hurt by it.

Additional instructions

_____

_____

Taking tablets, capsules, and liquid medications

Dear Patient:

Your doctor has prescribed medication to help treat your condition. Whether your medication comes in a solid form, such as tablets or capsules, or in a liquid form, such as a syrup, elixir, emulsion, or suspension, make sure you take it correctly. Here are some guidelines.

Taking tablets and capsules

First wash your hands. Then gather everything you need, such as the medication, a glass of water or juice and, if you plan to crush a tablet, a mortar and pestle or a commercial pill crusher. If you need to divide a scored tablet, get a knife. Now follow these steps.

1 Look at the medication container to make sure you have the right medication and the right dose.

2 Pour the prescribed number of tablets or capsules into the bottle cap. If too many pour out, drop the extra tablets or capsules back into the container without touching them. Now pour the medication from the cap into your hand.

3 Place the tablets or capsules as far back on your tongue as you can. You may do this with one tablet or capsule at a time or all of them at once.

4 Tip your head slightly *forward,* take a drink of water or juice, and swallow.

Special tips
• Take coated tablets and capsules with plenty of water or juice.

• Avoid touching the extra tablets or capsules you put back into the container. Doing so may contaminate the medication remaining in the bottle.
• If you have trouble swallowing a tablet or capsule, moisten your mouth with some water or juice before you take the tablet. It may also help to crush an uncoated tablet, open a soft capsule, or split a tablet.
• *Never* crush or open tablets or capsules that have a special coating. Doing so may affect the medication's effectiveness by changing the way your body absorbs the medication. If you're in doubt, ask your doctor or pharmacist if it's safe for you to crush or open your medication.
• Protect tablets and capsules from light, humidity, and air. If your medication changes color or has an unusual odor, discard it. Also discard all outdated medications.

Taking liquid medication
First wash your hands; then get the medication bottle and a medicine cup. Look at the container to make sure you have the right medication and to check the prescribed dosage. If the medication is in a suspension, shake it vigorously before proceeding.

1 Uncap the bottle and place the cap upside down on a clean surface.

2 Locate the marking for the prescribed dose on your medicine cup. Keeping your thumbnail on the mark, hold the cup at eye level and pour in the correct amount of medication. Swallow the medication after placing the bottle safely on a flat surface.

(continued)

Taking tablets, capsules, and liquid medications *(continued)*

3 Wipe the bottle's lip with a damp paper towel, taking care not to touch the inside of the bottle. Replace the bottle cap.

4 Rinse the medicine cup and store your medication properly.

Special tips
• When pouring liquid medication, keep the label next to your palm. This way, if any liquid spills or drips, it won't deface the label.
• If you pour out too much liquid, discard the excess. Don't return it to the bottle.
• If a liquid medication has an unpleasant taste, ask your doctor or pharmacist about diluting the medication with water or juice. Also consider sucking on ice to numb your taste buds or, if the dose is large enough, pouring the medication over ice and then drinking it through a straw. You may also wish to chill an oily liquid before taking it.
• To relieve a bitter taste after swallowing the medication, suck on a piece of sugarless hard candy or chew gum. Gargling or rinsing your mouth with water or mouthwash may also help.

Observing precautions
• Keep all medications out of the reach of children.
• For safety's sake, don't hesitate to ask your doctor or pharmacist about medications and directions you don't understand.
• Never share your medication with anyone else.

Additional instructions

_____

_____

_____

_____

_____

_____

_____

_____

_____

_____

_____

_____

_____

_____

_____

_____

_____

Giving children medication by mouth

Dear Parent or Caregiver:

Giving your child a medication doesn't have to be a problem for you or your child. With patience and care, you can make sure your child gets medication in a calm and careful way.

Take a positive approach
• Make sure you're giving the right medication and dose at the right time to the right child.
• Approach your child in a matter-of-fact but friendly manner to put him at ease. Act as though you expect his cooperation, and praise him when he cooperates.
• Give an older child choices, if possible, to give him a sense of control. For example, offer him a choice of beverage to take with (or after) his medication (unless the doctor tells you not to give the medication with certain beverages or foods).
• Taste a liquid medication (just a drop) before giving it to your child. This gives you an idea of how the medication will taste and whether you'll have to change the taste with flavoring. (Of course, don't taste a medication if you think you may be sensitive to it.)
• Explain the relation between illness and treatment to an older child. He may be more cooperative if he realizes that the medication will help him get better.
• Place a tablet or capsule near the back of your child's tongue, and give him plenty of water or flavored drink to help him swallow it. Then make sure he swallows it.
• Encourage your child to tip his head forward when swallowing a tablet or capsule. Throwing his head back increases the risk of inhaling the medication and choking.
• Give medication to an infant in a manner similar to feeding. Giving medication through a bottle's nipple, for example, takes advantage of the infant's natural sucking reflex. To make sure the infant gets the full dose, don't mix the medication with formula.
• Closely observe your child to see if the medication has the intended effect or any side effects.

Be honest and careful
• Never try to trick a child into taking medication. Doing so may make him resist you the next time he has to take it and may cause him to distrust you.
• Avoid telling a child that medication is candy. He may try to take more than the prescribed dose. Or he may not trust you when he learns it isn't candy.
• Don't promise that the medication will taste good if you've never tasted it or if you know it won't.
• Never threaten, insult, or embarrass your child if he doesn't cooperate. These actions can lead to resistance.
• Keep medication away from a place where your child or others could accidentally take it.
• Don't force your child to swallow his medication or try to hold his nose or mouth shut to promote swallowing. Doing so may cause choking.
• Don't try to give medication to a crying child; he could choke on it.

Additional instructions

_____

_____

Using an oral metered-dose inhaler

Dear Patient:

Inhaling your medication through a metered-dose inhaler (also called a *nebulizer*) will help you breathe more easily. Use the nebulizer exactly as your doctor directs at these times: _____ Here's how.

1 Remove the mouthpiece and cap from the bottle. Then remove the cap from the mouthpiece.

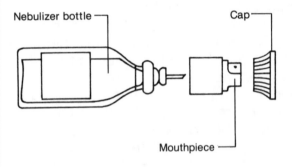

Nebulizer bottle

Cap

Mouthpiece

2 Turn the mouthpiece sideways. On one side of the flattened tip is a small hole. Fit the metal stem on the bottle into the hole to assemble the nebulizer.

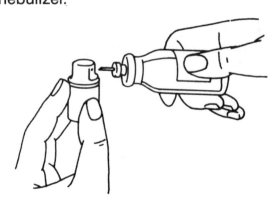

3 Exhale fully through pursed lips. Hold the inhaler upside down, as you see here. Close your lips and teeth loosely around the mouthpiece.

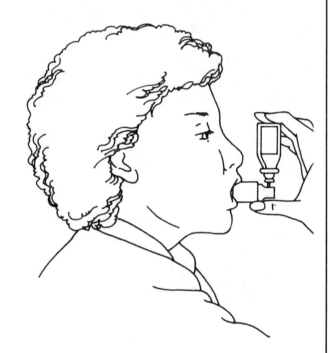

4 Tilt your head back slightly. Take a slow, deep breath. As you do, firmly push the bottle against the mouthpiece—one time only—to release one dose of medication. Continue inhaling until your lungs feel full.

(continued)

Using an oral metered-dose inhaler *(continued)*

To be sure you're taking the correct amount of medication, be careful to take only one inhalation at a time.

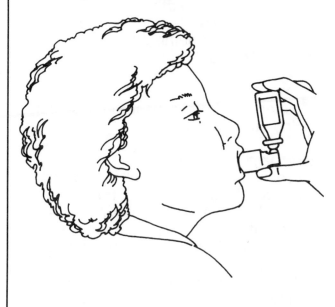

5 Take the mouthpiece away from your mouth, and hold your breath for several seconds.

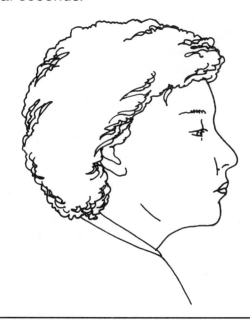

6 Purse your lips and exhale slowly. If your doctor wants you to take more than one dose, wait a few minutes and then repeat steps 3 through 6. Now rinse your mouth, gargle, and drink a few sips of fluid.

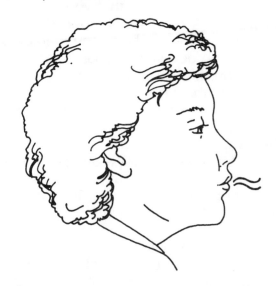

7 Remember to clean the inhaler once a day by taking it apart and rinsing the mouthpiece and cap under warm running water for 1 minute (or immersing them in alcohol). Shake off the excess fluid, let the parts dry, then reassemble them. This prevents clogging and sanitizes the mouthpiece.

Precautions

Remember to discard the inhalation solution if it turns brown or contains solid particles. Store your medication in its original container and put it in the refrigerator, if the label directs.

Important: Never overuse your oral inhaler. Follow your doctor's instructions exactly.

Using an oral inhaler with a holding chamber

Dear Patient:

Your doctor has prescribed an oral inhaler to help open your breathing passages. In this treatment, you'll inhale a medication called a bronchodilator through a small device that you put in your mouth. A holding chamber attached to the inhaler helps the medication to reach deeply into your lungs.

Common devices include the InspirEase System and the Aerochamber (some of these have a mask for easier use).

InspirEase System
This system has a holding chamber that collapses when you breathe in and inflates when you breathe out. To operate this inhaler, follow these steps.

1 Insert the inhaler into the mouthpiece and shake the inhaler. Then place the mouthpiece into the opening of the holding chamber, and twist the mouthpiece to lock it in place.

2 Extend the holding device, breathe out, and place the mouthpiece in your mouth.

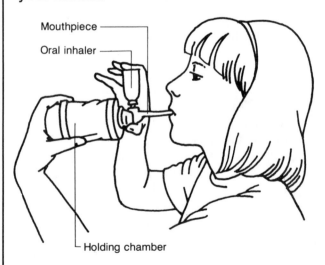

Mouthpiece

Oral inhaler

Holding chamber

3 Firmly press down once on the inhaler. Then breathe in slowly and deeply, collapsing the bag completely. If you breathe incorrectly, the bag will whistle. Hold your breath for 5 to 10 seconds, then breathe out slowly into the bag. Repeat breathing in and out.

4 Wait 5 minutes. Then shake the inhaler again and repeat the dose, following steps 2 and 3.

Aerochamber systems
These systems use a small cylinder called a valved chamber to trap medication. The device may also include a mask that helps deliver the medication more easily. Follow these steps for use.

1 Remove the cap from the inhaler and from the mouthpiece of the aerochamber. Then insert the inhaler mouthpiece into the wider rubber-sealed end of the aerochamber. Inspect for foreign objects, and check that all parts are secure.

2 Next, shake the device three or four times.

3 Breathe out normally, and close your lips over the mouthpiece.
If your device has a mask, place the mask firmly over your nose and mouth.
With either device, aim for a good seal. Leaks will reduce effectiveness.

4 Spray *only one puff* from the inhaler into the holding chamber. Take in one full breath slowly and deeply. If you hear a whistling sound, you're breathing too fast. Now hold your breath for 5 to 10 seconds.

(continued)

Using an oral inhaler with a holding chamber *(continued)*

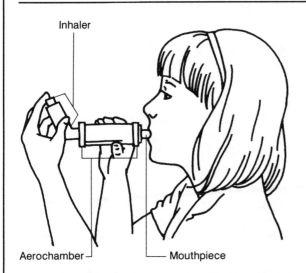

Inhaler

Aerochamber Mouthpiece

If your device has a mask, hold it firmly in place, and breathe in at least six times.

Caution: Spraying more than one puff into the holding chamber will give you the wrong dose of medication.

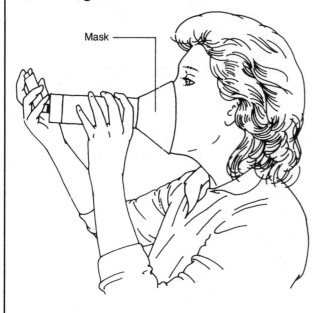

Mask

5 Repeat the steps directed by your doctor.

6 Remove the inhaler. Follow the manufacturer's directions for cleaning and storing it. Rinse any remaining medication from your face.

Additional instructions

_____

_____

_____

_____

_____

_____

_____

_____

_____

_____

_____

_____

_____

_____

_____

_____

_____

Using an AeroVent inhaler

Dear Caregiver:

The doctor has prescribed an AeroVent inhaler to treat the patient's respiratory problem. This device holds medication supplied by a metered-dose inhaler. It delivers the medication through a ventilator breathing circuit. Here are some guidelines for using the device.

Connecting the AeroVent to the circuit

Remove the AeroVent from its box. The device will join the ventilator circuit between the inspiratory tubing and the Y-connector that leads to the patient.

Now gently collapse the AeroVent holding chamber by compressing the device as you would an accordion. Push and rotate the springlike chamber slightly until the ends come together. Then press the bracketlike clasp down until it clicks into place.

Couple one end of the holding chamber to the Y-connector and one end to the ventilator tubing. *Caution:* Don't use too much force. If you do, you could damage the device or make it difficult to remove.

Be sure that the receptacle port (which will hold the inhaler) faces upward and away from the patient.

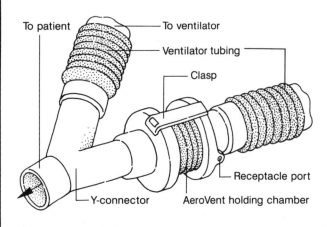

To patient
To ventilator
Ventilator tubing
Clasp
Receptacle port
Y-connector
AeroVent holding chamber

Opening the circuit

Before giving medication through the AeroVent, you'll need to expand the device. To begin, unlatch the external clasp and swing it open (180 degrees).

Grasp the coupled ends of the holding chamber. Then lightly rotate and stretch the device to the open position. Be careful not to damage the AeroVent by bending or rocking it.

Now reposition the receptacle, if needed, because it may be displaced when the chamber expands. To give medication correctly, the nozzle of the inhaler canister must point directly down. And the receptacle port must point up to receive the inhaler.

Giving medication

Shake the inhaler canister and insert its nozzle in the AeroVent receptacle port. Don't press on the inhaler yet.

When a ventilator exhalation ends, activate the inhaler by pressing on the canister's base as many times as the doctor prescribes. Don't press with too much force. This may jam the nozzle and damage the equipment.

After several uses, you may notice cloudiness in the chamber. Don't be alarmed. This results from collected moisture and medication particles.

Finishing your care

Once you've given the medication, remove the inhaler canister and collapse the AeroVent by gently pushing the ends together. Use a slight rotating motion until you compress the device securely. Now relatch the external clasp.

At all times, observe safety precautions. For example, replace a damaged AeroVent at once, and attach a new AeroVent when you change the tubing.

Caring for aerosol equipment

Dear Patient:

Your aerosol equipment includes a compressed air machine and disposable plastic parts—a mouthpiece, a mask, syringes, and medicine cups. All of this equipment must be kept clean. If it isn't, bacteria can enter your lungs along with the mist.

Cleaning the plastic parts
You don't need to clean the parts every time they're used, but you should rinse them in warm or cool water after each use. Allow them to air dry before storing them in a clean plastic bag or another clean container.

Clean the parts *daily,* following the doctor's recommendations or those of the equipment manufacturer. Or use the following procedure:
• Wash the plastic parts in warm water and a mild dishwashing detergent; then rinse. The air compressor doesn't require cleaning. *Never* submerge it in water.
• After rinsing, soak the parts for 30 minutes in a solution of 1 cup white vinegar and 3 cups warm water. Rinse well in cool water.

• Let the parts air dry before placing them in a clean storage container.

Maintaining the air compressor
Keeping the compressor in perfect working order promotes better treatments and extends the device's life. How often should you have the compressor serviced? That depends on the type of compressor and the manufacturer's recommendations.

Troubleshooting problems
If the machine isn't producing enough mist, the problem may be a simple one that you can solve yourself. For example, you might need to:
• change the air filter
• tighten the connections
• try a new aerosol cup.

If these measures fail, take the compressor to your medical equipment supplier to be checked. It may need internal cleaning. However, if the compressor is 8 to 10 years old, it probably needs to be replaced.

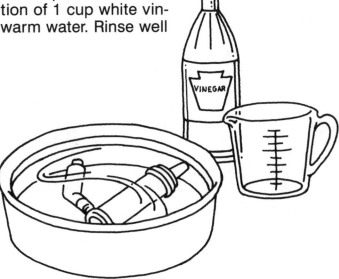

Giving yourself eyedrops

Dear Patient:

Your doctor has prescribed these eye-drops for you:

Medicine #1: _____
Use ___ drops ___ times a day in
your _____ eye.

Medicine #2: _____
Use ___ drops ___ times a day in
your _____ eye.

Here's how to put drops in your eye.

1 Begin by washing your hands thoroughly.

2 Hold the medication bottle up to the light and examine it. If the medication is discolored or contains sediment, don't use it. Instead, take it back to the pharmacy and have it checked.
   If the medication looks okay, warm it to room temperature by holding the bottle between your hands for 2 minutes.

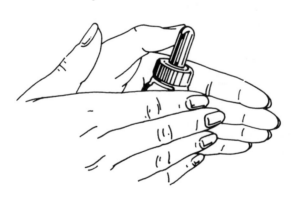

3 Moisten a rayon cosmetic puff or a tissue with water, and clean any secretions from around your eyes. Use a fresh rayon puff or tissue for each eye. Be sure to wipe outward in one motion, starting from the area nearest your nose.

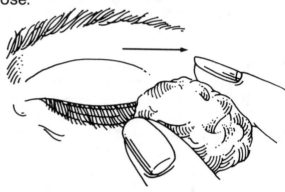

4 Stand or sit before a mirror, or lie on your back, whichever is most comfortable for you. Squeeze the bulb of the eyedropper and slowly release it to fill the dropper with medication.

5 Tilt your head back slightly and toward the eye you're treating. Pull down your lower eyelid.

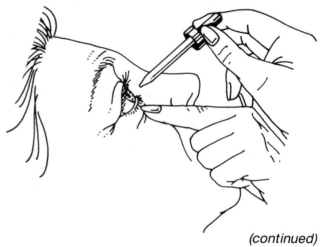

(continued)

Giving yourself eyedrops *(continued)*

6 Position the dropper over the conjunctival sac that you've exposed between your lower lid and the white of your eye. Steady your hand by resting two fingers against your cheek or nose.

7 Look up at the ceiling. Then squeeze the prescribed number of drops into the sac. Take care not to touch the dropper to your eye, eyelashes, or fingers. Wipe away excess medication with a clean tissue.

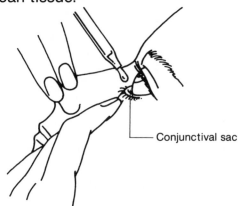

Conjunctival sac

8 Release the lower lid. Try to keep your eye open without blinking for at least 30 seconds. Apply gentle pressure to the corner of your eye at the bridge of your nose for 1 minute. This will prevent the medication from being absorbed through your tear ducts.

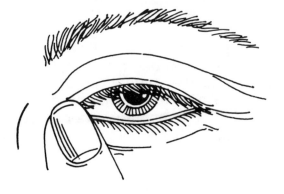

9 Repeat the procedure in the other eye, if the doctor orders.

10 Recap the bottle and store it away from light and heat.
If you're using more than one kind of drop, wait 5 minutes before you use the next one.
Important: Call your doctor immediately if you notice any of these side effects:

_____

_____

_____

_____

_____

_____

_____

_____

_____

_____

_____

_____

_____.

And remember, never put medication in your eyes unless the label reads "For Ophthalmic Use" or "For Use in Eyes."

Putting ointment in your eye

Dear Patient:

Your doctor has prescribed this eye ointment for you:

Name of medication: _____
Use this ointment _____times
a day in your _____eye.

Here's how to apply the ointment.

1 Wash your hands thoroughly. Then hold the ointment in your hand for several minutes to warm it before use.

2 Moisten a rayon cosmetic puff or a tissue with water, and clean any secretions from around your eye. Wipe outward in one motion, starting at the side near the nose. Remember to avoid touching the uninfected eye.

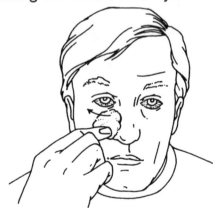

3 Stand or sit before a mirror, whichever feels most comfortable.

4 Gently pull down your lower eyelid and look up toward the ceiling. Squeeze a small amount of ointment (about ¼ inch to ½ inch) inside the conjunctival sac—the space between your lower eyelid and the white of your eyeball. Steady your hand by resting two fingers against your cheek or nose. Hold the tube close to its tip so that you don't accidentally poke your eye with the applicator tip.

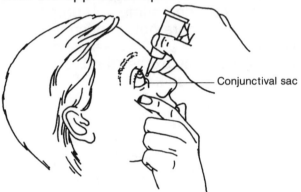

Conjunctival sac

5 Without touching the tube's tip with your eyelashes, close your eye to pinch off the ointment. Roll your eyeball in all directions with your eyes closed.

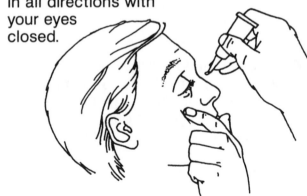

6 Recap the medication. If you're using more than one ointment, wait about 10 minutes before you use the next one. Don't worry if you have blurred vision temporarily after you use the ointment; this is normal.

Giving yourself eardrops

Dear Patient:

Your doctor has prescribed these eardrops:

_____.

Use them exactly as directed on the label. Here's how.

1 Wash your hands thoroughly and then check your medication. If it's discolored or contains sediment, notify your doctor and have your prescription refilled. If your eardrops are okay, proceed.

2 For comfort, warm the eardrops by holding the bottle in your hands for 2 minutes. Then shake the bottle, if directed, and open it.

3 Fill the dropper; then place the open bottle and dropper within easy reach.

4 Lie on your side to expose the ear you're treating.

5 To straighten your ear canal, gently pull the top of your ear up and back, as shown.

6 Position the dropper above your ear, taking care not to touch it to your ear. Squeeze the dropper's bulb to release 1 drop.

7 Wait until you feel the drop in your ear. Then, if directed, release another drop. Repeat these steps until you have given yourself the prescribed number of drops. To keep the drops from running out of your ear, remain on your side for about 10 minutes.

8 If you wish, you can plug your ear with cotton moistened with eardrops. Unless your doctor directs you to, don't use dry cotton. It will absorb your medication.

9 As your doctor directs, treat your other ear.

10 Recap the eardrop bottle, and store it away from light and extreme heat.

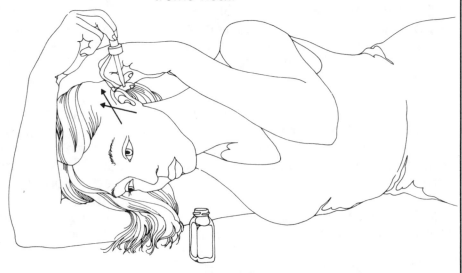

Giving eardrops to a child

Dear Parent or Caregiver:

To treat your child's ear problem, the doctor has prescribed eardrops. Use them exactly as directed on the label.

Getting ready

1 First wash your hands thoroughly. Then examine the medication. Does it look discolored or contain sediment? If it does, notify the doctor and have the prescription refilled. If it looks normal, you can proceed.

2 Warm the medication (for your child's comfort) by holding the bottle in your hands for about 2 minutes.

3 Then shake the bottle (if directed), open it, and fill the dropper by squeezing the bulb. Place the open bottle and dropper within easy reach.

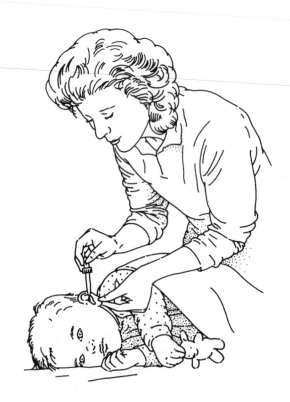

Giving eardrops

1 Have your child lie on his side to expose the ear you're treating. Now gently pull the earlobe down and back. This will straighten his ear canal.

2 Position the filled dropper above— but not touching—the opening of your child's ear canal. Gently squeeze the dropper's bulb once to release 1 drop.

Watch the drop slide into the ear canal. Or have your child tell you when he feels the drop enter his ear.

Then gently squeeze the dropper's bulb to release the number of drops prescribed.

3 Continue holding your child's ear as the eardrops disappear down the ear canal. Now massage the area in front of the ear. Ask your child to tell you when he no longer feels the drops moving in his ear. Then release his ear.

4 Tell your child to remain on his side and to avoid touching his ear for about 10 minutes. If your child is active, place an eardrop-moistened cotton plug in his ear to help keep the medication in his ear canal. Don't use dry cotton because it may absorb the medication.

If both ears require medication, repeat the procedure in your child's other ear. Finally, return the dropper to the medication bottle (or recap the dropper bottle).

Store the bottle away from light and extreme heat.

Using a metered-dose nasal pump

Dear Patient:

Your doctor has prescribed medication that you need to inhale through a metered-dose nasal pump. Take the medication at these times: _____.
Keep in mind that the pump delivers an exact amount of medication. Here's how to use the pump.

1 Remove the protective cap, and prime the pump as directed by the manufacturer. (Usually, pressing down about four times primes the pump. If refrigerated, the pump will stay primed for about 1 week. After that, you'll need to prime the pump again.)

2 To get the right dose, tilt the pump bottle so that the strawlike tube inside draws medication from the deepest part (as shown).

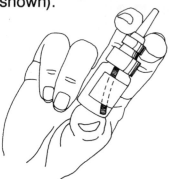

3 Insert the pump's applicator tip about half an inch into your nostril. Point the tip straight up your nose and toward the inner corner of your eye. (Don't angle the pump, or the medication may run into your throat.)

4 Without inhaling, squeeze the pump once, quickly and firmly. Try to use just enough force to coat the inside of your nostril, but not so much that you inject the medication into your sinuses. (Doing that will cause a headache.) Spray again if the package directions instruct you to, or repeat the procedure in the other nostril if your doctor directs you to do so.

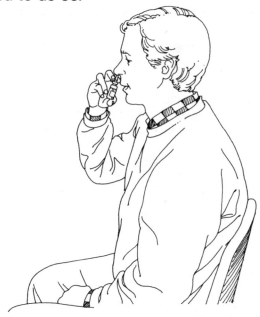

5 Keep your head still for several minutes so the medication has time to work. And don't blow your nose for a while.

6 Store the medication in the refrigerator.

Giving yourself nose drops

Dear Patient:

Your doctor has prescribed nose drops for you to use at home. Here is what you need to know.

Getting ready
Before you use your nose drops, look at the container to make sure you have the right medication and to check the prescribed dosage. Then follow these steps:
• Warm the medication container by holding it in your hands for about 2 minutes.
• With the dropper still in the bottle, squeeze the dropper bulb to load the dropper chamber with medication.

The method you use to instill the drops will vary, depending on the problem you're treating.

Treating the nasal passages
If your doctor has prescribed nose drops to treat your nasal passages, position the dropper as shown here. Doing so will help the drops flow down the back of your nose, not your throat. Then proceed.
• Squeeze the dropper bulb to insert the correct number of drops.
• Repeat the process in the other nostril, if indicated.
• Breathe through your mouth so that you don't sniff the drops into your sinuses or your lungs.

(continued)

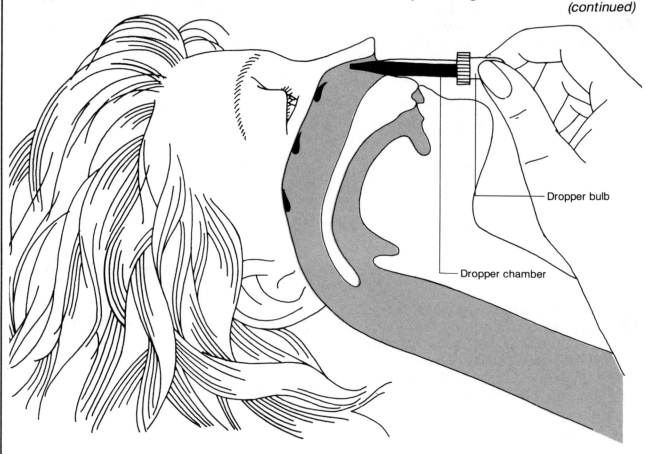

Dropper bulb

Dropper chamber

Giving yourself nose drops *(continued)*

Treating the ethmoid and sphenoid sinuses

To treat a problem in these areas, lie on your back with a pillow under your shoulders and your head tilted backward, as shown. Follow these steps:
• Position the dropper above one nostril, and squeeze the dropper bulb to release the prescribed number of drops.
• Breathe through your nose. This will help the medication move through your sinuses.

Treating the frontal and maxillary sinuses

To treat a problem in these areas, lie on your back with a pillow under your shoulders and your head tilted to one side, as shown. Then take these steps:
• Position the dropper above one nostril, and squeeze the dropper bulb to release the prescribed number of drops.
• Breathe through your nose. This will help the medication move through your sinuses.

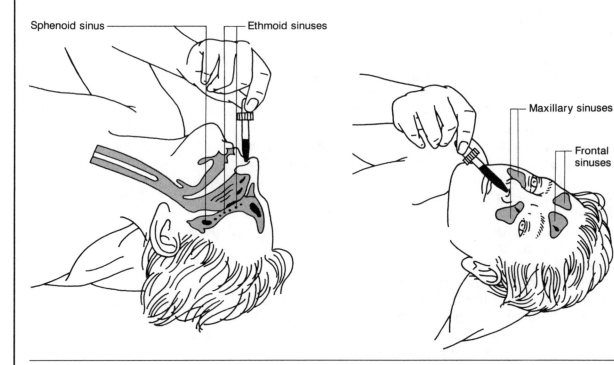

Taking precautions

• Follow your doctor's orders exactly. Don't overuse your nose drops.
• Because nose drops are easily contaminated, don't buy more than you'll use in a short time. Discard discolored nose drops and drops that contain sediment.
• Don't share your nose drops with anyone. Doing so may spread germs.

Additional instructions

_____

_____

_____

_____

Using medicated bath products

Dear Patient:

Your doctor has prescribed a medicated bath to help treat your skin problem. A medicated bath:
• cleans, softens, and lubricates your skin
• relieves itching
• softens scales and crusts (for easier removal).

Preparing the bath
Before beginning, make sure your bathroom is warm and draft-free. Then make sure the bathtub is clean.

Adding the medication
How you'll add medication to your bathwater will vary. Depending on the medication prescribed by your doctor, use one of these methods:
• If you're using a colloidal preparation, such as oatmeal, mix 1 measuring cup of oatmeal with a small amount of cool water to form a paste. Then begin filling the tub with warm water. Gradually swirl in the paste as the tub fills.
• If you're using an oil preparation, such as mineral oil (with a surfactant), fill the bathtub two-thirds full with warm water. Then add 2 ounces of the oil preparation to the bathwater. Stir the water to distribute the oil.
   Or you may find it more effective to mix ¼ teaspoon of bath oil with ¼ cup of water and then apply it to your skin as you would a lotion.
• If you're using a soda preparation, such as baking soda, first fill the bathtub to the correct level with warm water. Then add the powder, stirring until it dissolves.
• If you're using a starch preparation, such as cornstarch, first fill the bathtub

to the appropriate level with warm water. Meanwhile, slowly dissolve the powder in a small container of water. Then, when the water fills the tub to the prescribed level, add the starch solution.

Taking the bath
Before immersing yourself in the bathwater, be sure the temperature feels warm enough. Then get in the tub carefully, and bathe for about 20 minutes.

Finishing the bath
After you've finished bathing, be careful not to fall on the slippery tub surfaces as you get out of the tub. Pat yourself dry with a clean, soft towel, removing excess medication in the process. Keep in mind that a skin problem can cause you to lose body heat rapidly, so try not to become chilled. Once you're warm and dry, clean the tub so that it's ready for your next bath.

Additional instructions

_____

_____

_____

_____

_____

_____

_____

_____

Inserting a rectal suppository

Dear Patient:

Your doctor has prescribed a rectal suppository. You can learn to insert it quickly and easily in a few steps. Be cautious, though. Unless your doctor orders otherwise, don't use rectal suppositories or other laxatives routinely because you can become dependent on them.

Follow these steps.

1 Wash your hands. Then gather the items you'll need: the suppository, a disposable glove, and a tube of water-soluble lubricating gel.

2 Put the glove on your right hand (or on your left if you're left-handed). Now remove the foil wrapper on the suppository.

If you have trouble doing this, the suppository may be too soft to insert. Hold it under cold running water until it becomes firm, or put it in the freezer for a minute or two before inserting it—just don't let it get too cold and hard. Better yet, store your suppositories in the refrigerator.

3 Once you've removed the foil wrapper, put a generous dab of lubricating gel on the rounded end of the suppository. Hold the lubricated suppository in your gloved hand.

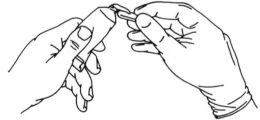

4 Now lie on your side with your knees raised toward your chest. Take a deep breath as you gently insert the suppository—rounded end first—into the anus with your gloved hand. Push the suppository in as far as your finger will go to keep the suppository from coming back out.

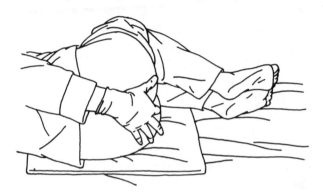

5 Once the suppository is in place, you'll feel an immediate urge to have a bowel movement. Resist the urge by lying still and breathing deeply a few times.

Try to retain the suppository for at least 20 minutes, so that your body has time to absorb it and get the maximum effect from the medication. After you have a bowel movement, discard the glove and wash your hands.

Additional instructions

_____

_____

_____

_____

Administering a vaginal medication

Dear Patient:

Your doctor has prescribed a vaginal medication for you. To insert the medication, follow these instructions.

1 Plan to insert the vaginal medication after bathing and just before bedtime to ensure that it will stay in the vagina for the appropriate amount of time.
   Collect the equipment you'll need: the prescribed medication (suppository, cream, ointment, tablet, or jelly), an applicator, water-soluble lubricating jelly, a towel, a hand mirror, paper towels, and a sanitary pad.

2 Empty your bladder, wash your hands, and place the towel on the bed. Sit on the towel, and open the medication wrapper or container.

3 Using the hand mirror, carefully inspect the area around the insertion site. If you see signs of increased irritation, don't insert the medication. Notify the doctor. He may change your medication.

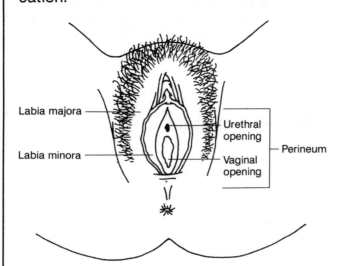

Labia majora

Labia minora

Urethral opening

Vaginal opening

Perineum

4 Place a vaginal suppository or tablet in the applicator, or fill the applicator with cream, ointment, or jelly.

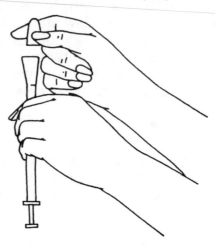

5 To make insertion easier, lubricate the suppository or applicator tip with water or water-soluble lubricating jelly.

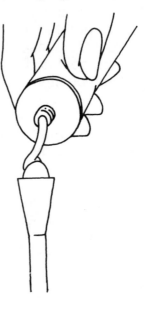

(continued)

Administering a vaginal medication *(continued)*

Now lie down on the bed with your knees flexed and legs spread apart.

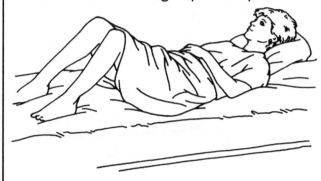

Spread apart your labia with one hand, and insert the applicator tip into the vagina with the other hand. Advance the applicator about 2 inches (5 cm), angling it slightly toward your tailbone.

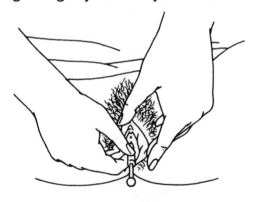

6 Push the plunger to insert the medication. Be aware that the medication may feel cold.

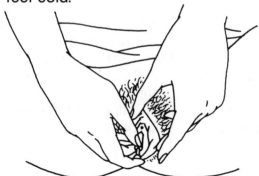

7 Remove the applicator and discard it—if it's disposable. If it's reusable, wash it thoroughly with soap and water, dry it with a paper towel, and return it to its container.

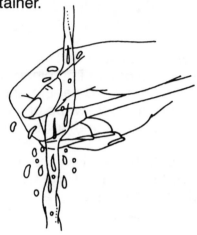

8 If your doctor prescribes it, apply a thin layer of cream, ointment, or jelly to the vulva (the area including the vagina, labia majora, and labia minora).

9 Remain lying down for about 30 minutes so that the medication won't run out of your vagina. (If you like, apply the sanitary pad to avoid staining your clothes or bed linens.)
Then check your vagina for signs of an allergic reaction. If the area seems unusually red or swollen, contact the doctor.

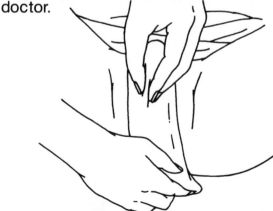

Giving yourself a subcutaneous injection

Dear Patient:

Before you can administer your injection, you must transfer the correct amount of medication from the bottle to the syringe. Follow these guidelines.

1 Wash your hands. Then assemble this equipment in a clean area: a sterile syringe and needle, the medication, and alcohol swabs or wipes (or rubbing alcohol and cotton balls).

2 Check the label on the medication bottle to be sure you have the right medication. For safety, also check the expiration date.

3 Clean the top of the medication bottle with an alcohol swab or wipe.

4 Select an appropriate injection site. Pull the skin taut; then, using a circular motion, clean the skin with an alcohol swab or wipe or a cotton ball soaked in alcohol.

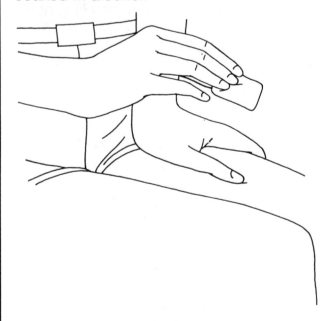

5 Remove the needle cover. *To prevent possible infection, don't touch the needle.* Touch only the barrel and plunger of the syringe. Pull back the plunger to the prescribed amount of medication. This draws air into the syringe.

Insert the needle into the rubber stopper on the medication bottle, and push in the plunger. This pushes air into the bottle and prevents a vacuum.

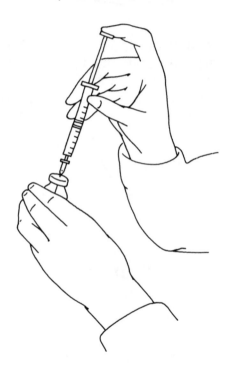

6 Hold the bottle and syringe together in one hand; then turn them upside down so that the bottle is on top. You can hold the bottle between your thumb and forefinger and the syringe between your ring finger and little finger, against your palm. Or you can hold

(continued)

Giving yourself a subcutaneous injection *(continued)*

the bottle between your forefinger and middle finger, while holding the syringe between your thumb and little finger.

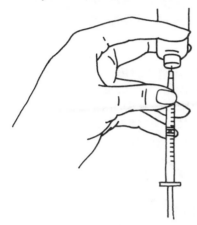

7 Pull back on the plunger until the top black portion of the barrel corresponds to the line that indicates you have withdrawn the correct medication dose. Then remove the needle from the bottle.

8 If air bubbles appear in the syringe after you fill it with medication, tap the syringe and push lightly on the plunger to remove them. Draw up more medication, if necessary.

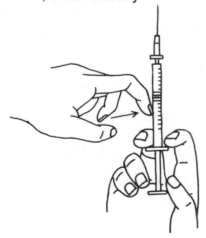

9 Using your thumb and forefinger, pinch the skin at the injection site. Then quickly plunge the needle (up to its hub) into the subcutaneous tissue at a 90-degree angle. Push the plunger down to inject the medication.

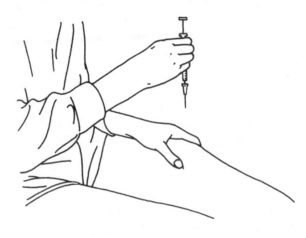

10 Place an alcohol swab or wipe over the injection site; then press down on it lightly as you withdraw the needle. Don't rub the injection site when withdrawing the needle.

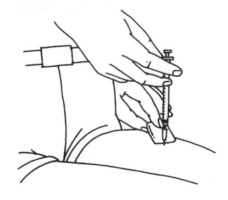

Snap the needle off the syringe, and properly dispose of both the needle and syringe.

Using an anaphylaxis kit

Dear Patient:

Because you could have a severe reaction to insect stings or certain foods or drugs, your doctor has prescribed an anaphylaxis kit for you to use in an emergency. The kit contains everything you need to treat an allergic reaction:
• a prefilled syringe containing two doses of epinephrine
• alcohol swabs
• a tourniquet
• antihistamine tablets.

   When needed, use the kit as follows. Also, notify the doctor immediately, or ask someone else to call him.

Getting ready
Take the prefilled syringe from the kit and remove the needle cap. Hold the syringe with the needle pointing up. Then push in the plunger until it stops. This will expel any air from the syringe.

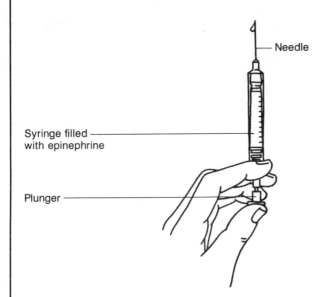

Needle

Syringe filled
with epinephrine

Plunger

Next, clean about 4 inches of the skin on your arm or thigh with an alcohol swab. (If you're right-handed, you should clean your left arm or thigh. If you're left-handed, clean your right arm or thigh.)

Inject the epinephrine
Rotate the plunger one-quarter turn to the right so that it's aligned with the slot. Insert the entire needle—like a dart—into the skin.

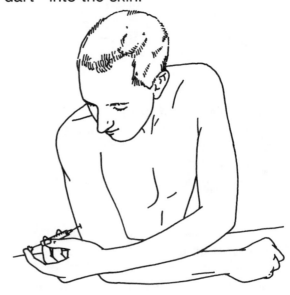

Push down on the plunger until it stops. It will inject 0.3 ml of the drug for an adult or a person over age 12. Withdraw the needle.
   Note: The dose and administration for babies and for children under age 12 must be directed by the doctor.

If you've been stung by an insect
Quickly remove the insect's stinger if you can see it. Use a dull object, such as a fingernail or tweezers, to pull it

(continued)

Using an anaphylaxis kit *(continued)*

straight out. Don't pinch, scrape, or squeeze the stinger. This may push it farther into the skin and release more poison. If you can't remove the stinger quickly, stop trying. Go on to the next step.

Apply the tourniquet
If you were stung on your *neck, face,* or *body,* skip this step and go on to the next one.

If you were stung on an *arm* or a *leg,* apply the tourniquet between the sting site and your heart. Tighten the tourniquet by pulling the string.

After 10 minutes, release the tourniquet by pulling on the metal ring.

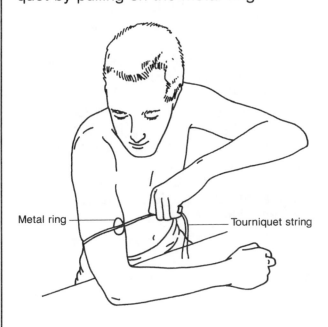

Metal ring —   — Tourniquet string

Take the antihistamine tablets
Chew and swallow the antihistamine tablets. (For children age 12 and under, follow the dosage and administration directions supplied by your doctor or provided in the kit.)

What to do next
Next, apply ice packs—if available—to the affected area. Avoid exertion, keep warm, and see a doctor or go to a hospital immediately.

Important: If you don't notice an improvement within 10 minutes, give yourself a second injection by following the directions in your anaphylaxis kit. If your syringe has a preset second dose, don't depress the plunger until you're ready to give the second injection. Proceed as before, following the instructions to inject the epinephrine.

Special instructions
• Keep your kit handy to ensure emergency treatment at all times.
• Ask your pharmacist for storage guidelines. Find out whether the kit can be stored in a car's glove compartment or whether you need to keep it in a cooler place.
• Periodically check the epinephrine in the preloaded syringe. A pinkish brown solution needs to be replaced.
• Make a note of the kit's expiration date. Then renew the kit just before that date.
• Dispose of the used needle and syringe safely and properly.

Additional instructions

_____

_____

_____

_____

_____

Learning self-infusion of clotting factors

Dear Patient:

These instructions will help you give yourself clotting factors at home.

Remember, if you're infusing clotting factors for a minor bleeding episode, keep a record of it. Write down when you did the infusion, why you needed it, and how much clotting factor you used. Be sure to take this information with you the next time you go to the doctor.

If you give yourself clotting factors for major bleeding, call your doctor afterward to tell him about it.

Use these directions to help you do what your nurse or doctor taught you. And to avoid infection, be sure to use only new needles and syringes every time you give yourself an infusion.

1 Gather your equipment. Make sure you have your clotting factor concentrate and sterile water, a syringe, a butterfly needle set, a tourniquet, alcohol wipes, gauze pads, and tape.

2 Thoroughly wash your hands with soap and water.

3 Remove the flip-top lids on the clotting factor concentrate bottle and the sterile water bottle. Use the alcohol wipes to clean the stoppers. Add sterile water from the water bottle to the powder in the concentrate bottle to make a liquid.

4 If you're using *nonvacuum bottles,* inject air into the sterile water bottle and withdraw the water. Inject water into the concentrate bottle. Direct the water against the bottle's side so that you don't make any bubbles or foam.

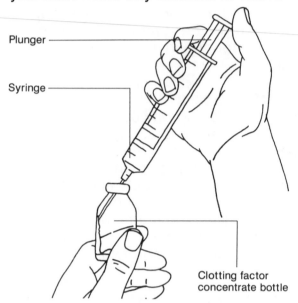

Plunger

Syringe

Clotting factor concentrate bottle

Withdraw air to relieve pressure, and then withdraw the needle. Put a cap on the needle.

If you're using *vacuum bottles,* the idea is the same. Insert the double-ended needle into the water bottle. Then turn the needle and bottle upside down, and insert the other end of the needle into the bottle that contains the concentrate.

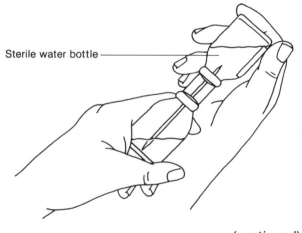

Sterile water bottle

(continued)

Learning self-infusion of clotting factors *(continued)*

Direct the stream of water against the side of the bottle so that you don't make bubbles or foam.

Lift the water bottle off the needle (to release the vacuum). Pull the needle from the concentrate, and rotate or roll the bottle gently in your hands until the powder dissolves completely. Clean the stopper of the concentrate bottle with a new alcohol wipe.

Next, transfer the dissolved concentrate into your syringe that has a needle and a filter. To do this, use the syringe to inject air into the concentrate bottle. Then pull back on the plunger to draw the reconstituted concentrate into the syringe.

5 Wrap the tourniquet around your lower arm about 3 inches above the place where you'll insert the needle into your vein. Clean the area with an alcohol wipe and let it dry.

Then loosen the hub at the end of the butterfly needle tubing to break the vacuum. Uncap the needle and insert it at a 30- to 45-degree angle through your skin into the center of the vein.

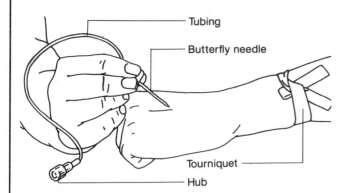

Tubing

Butterfly needle

Tourniquet

Hub

When you see blood return, lower the needle to make it level with your skin. Slide the needle slightly forward so that it won't slip from the vein.

6 Take off the tourniquet and tape the butterfly needle to your skin. Now remove the filter section of your syringe. Attach the syringe part holding the liquid concentrate to the hub of the butterfly needle's tubing. Pull back gently on the plunger of the syringe to fill the tubing with blood. Then infuse the concentrate slowly, as directed by your nurse or doctor.

7 When the infusion is finished, place a gauze pad over the site and remove the needle. *Don't apply pressure to the site as you remove the needle. It can damage the vein.*

8 When you've removed the needle, apply firm pressure to the venipuncture site for 3 to 5 minutes. Make sure bleeding has stopped at the site.

9 To prevent the spread of infection, put used equipment into a special box or plastic container. Return it to the hospital or clinic. Wrap other equipment in plastic and return it also.

Additional instructions

_____

_____

_____

_____

_____

_____

_____

Giving an intramuscular injection

Dear Patient or Caregiver:

Use these instructions to review how to give an intramuscular injection.

Selecting the injection site
First choose the injection site. You can use the thigh, hip, buttock, or upper arm. If you're giving yourself the injection, use the front or side of the thigh. If someone else is giving you the injection, he can use the hip, buttock, or upper arm. If possible, though, he should avoid using the upper arm because the muscle there is small and very close to the brachial nerve.

If a series of injections is necessary, rotate the sites. To reduce pain and improve drug absorption, don't use the same site twice in a row.

Thigh
To find the target, place one hand at your knee and your other hand at your groin. As shown, use the area marked by solid lines for adult injections. Or use the area marked by dotted lines for injections for infants and children.

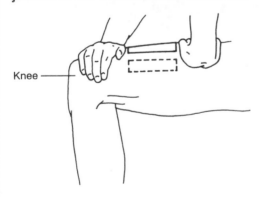

Knee

Hip
To find this site, place your right hand on the patient's left hip (or your left hand on the patient's right hip). Then spread your index and middle fingers to form a V. Your middle finger should be on the highest point of the pelvis, known as the iliac crest. The triangular area shown in the illustration is the injection site.

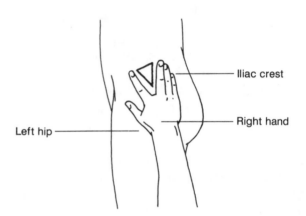

Iliac crest

Right hand

Left hip

Buttock
Imagine lines dividing each buttock into four equal parts. Give the injection in the upper outermost area near the iliac crest, as shown. Don't give it in the sciatic nerve area.

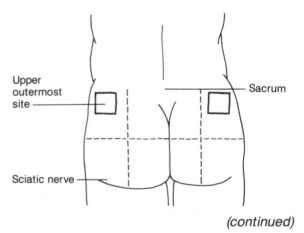

Upper outermost site

Sacrum

Sciatic nerve

(continued)

Giving an intramuscular injection *(continued)*

Upper arm

Locate the injection site by placing one hand at the top of the patient's shoulder and extending your thumb down the patient's upper arm. Place the other hand at armpit level, as shown. The triangular space shown between the hands is the injection area.

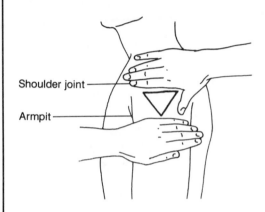

Shoulder joint ——

Armpit ——

Giving the injection

1 Wash your hands and gather the medication, alcohol swabs, syringe, and needle. Make sure you have the right medication. For safety, check the expiration date.

2 Remove the top of the medication bottle, and wipe the rubber stopper with an alcohol swab. Unwrap the syringe, and remove the needle cover.

3 Pull back on the plunger of the syringe until you've drawn air into it in an amount equal to the medication you'll be injecting. Insert the needle into the bottle through the rubber stopper. Then inject the air in the syringe into the bottle without withdrawing the needle. This will prevent formation of a vac-

uum and will make withdrawing the medication easier.

4 Invert the medication bottle. With the needle positioned below the fluid level, draw the medication into the syringe by pulling back on the plunger while you measure the correct amount by checking the markings on the side of the syringe. Then withdraw the needle from the bottle.

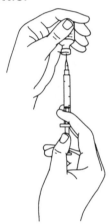

5 Next, check for air bubbles in the syringe. If you see any, hold the syringe with the needle pointing up, and tap the syringe lightly so that the bubbles rise to its top. Then push the plunger to get rid of the air and, if necessary, draw up more medication to obtain the correct amount.

Again hold the syringe with the needle pointing up, and pull back on the plunger just a little bit more. This will cause a tiny air bubble to form inside the syringe; when you inject the medication, this bubble will help clear the needle and keep the medication from seeping out of the injection site. Replace the needle cover.

(continued)

Giving an intramuscular injection *(continued)*

6 Check the injection site for any lumps, depressions, redness, warmth, or bruising on the skin. Then gently tap the site to stimulate nerve endings and reduce the initial pain of injection.

7 Clean the site with an alcohol swab, beginning at the center and wiping outward in a circular pattern to move dirt particles away from the site.

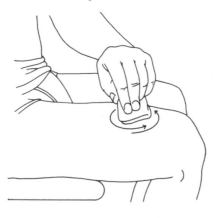

Let the skin dry for 5 to 10 seconds. If it's not dry, the injection might push some of the alcohol into the skin, causing a burning sensation.

8 Remove the needle cover. Now, with one hand, stretch the skin taut

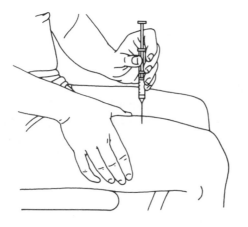

around the injection site. This makes inserting the needle easier and helps disperse the medication after the injection.

With your other hand, hold the syringe and needle at a 90-degree angle to the injection site, as shown in the illustration at the bottom of the left column. Then insert the needle with a quick thrust.

9 Holding the syringe firmly in place, remove the hand stretching your skin and use it to pull back slightly on the plunger. If blood appears in the syringe, you've entered a blood vessel. Take the needle out and press an alcohol swab over the site. Then discard everything and start again. If no blood appears, inject the medication slowly, keeping the syringe and needle at a 90-degree angle. Never push the plunger forcefully.

10 When you've injected all the medication, press an alcohol swab around the needle and injection site, and withdraw the needle at the same angle at which you inserted it.

Using a circular motion (extending from the center outward), massage the site with the alcohol swab to help distribute the medication and promote its absorption.

11 Dispose of the used syringe and needle by returning the cover to the needle. Then, holding the syringe, unscrew or snap off the needle and cover. Put both in a covered container used only for disposal of needles and syringes. Keep the container in a safe place until you can dispose of it; then dispose of it properly.

Caring for a central venous catheter

Dear Patient:

To keep your central venous catheter trouble-free, you must flush the catheter and change the dressing regularly.

How to flush the catheter
Flush the catheter at least once a day to prevent blood clots from forming in it.

1 Gather the following equipment: a bottle of heparin-lock flush solution, a disposable syringe with needle, two alcohol or povidone-iodine swabs, several sterile 4-inch square gauze pads, and tape. Now wash and dry your hands. Open the bottle of heparin-lock flush solution, and wipe the bottle top with an alcohol or povidone-iodine swab. *Don't touch the top after you've cleaned it.*

2 Pick up the syringe, remove the needle cover, and pull back the syringe plunger. Then insert the needle into the heparin solution bottle top, and push down on the plunger. Turn the bottle upside down, as shown, and pull back

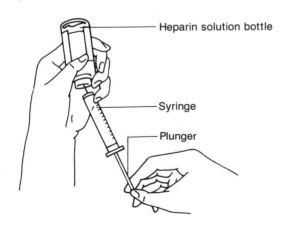

Heparin solution bottle

Syringe

Plunger

on the syringe plunger to fill the syringe with solution. Remove the needle from the bottle, and put the bottle aside. Replace the needle cover.

3 Remove and discard the gauze pad protecting the end of the catheter. Using a clean povidone-iodine or alcohol swab, wipe the end of the catheter. When the end is dry, remove the catheter's clamp. After removing the needle cover, insert the needle into the catheter.

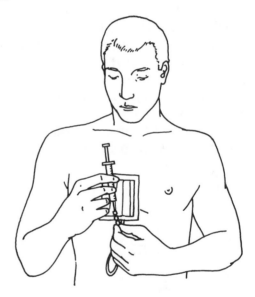

Push down on the syringe plunger to inject the solution into the catheter. Replace the clamp after you withdraw the needle. Wrap the catheter end in a sterile gauze pad, and tape it on top of the dressing.

(continued)

Caring for a central venous catheter *(continued)*

How to change the dressing

Change the dressing over the catheter every other day or whenever it becomes wet or dirty. When you change your dressing, carefully check the skin around the catheter. Call the doctor at once if you see any sign of infection, such as redness, swelling, or pus. Also call him if a fever or pain develops.

1 To change the dressing, obtain a dressing change kit or assemble the supplies recommended by your nurse or doctor. Then wash your hands and remove the soiled dressing. Wash your hands again. (If suggested by your doctor, you may want to put on sterile gloves to avoid possible contamination.)

Clean the skin around the catheter with an alcohol swab, beginning near the catheter and working outward in a circular motion. Repeat the procedure, using a povidone-iodine swab.

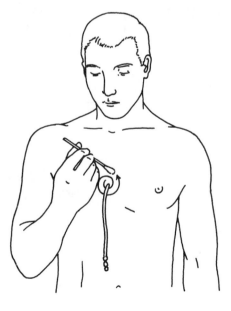

2 Squeeze some povidone-iodine ointment onto a sterile gauze pad. Put the pad over the catheter exit site. Cover it with a dry sterile gauze pad.

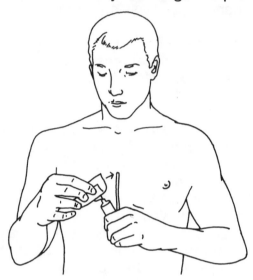

3 Apply adhesive tape over the gauze pads and put an extra layer of tape around the edge (as shown here) to secure the bandage to your skin. Wrap the catheter end in a sterile gauze pad, and tape it on top of the bandage.

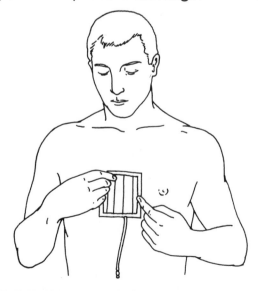

Caring for an implanted port

Dear Patient:

Here are some guidelines for flushing and injecting medication into your implanted port.

Flushing the port

To keep your implanted port trouble-free, flush the port according to your doctor's instructions (usually monthly). Check with your doctor if you develop a fever or if you observe redness, pain, swelling, or pus at the port site.

1 Gather the following equipment: a 10-ml syringe with needle, a bottle of heparin (if you don't have a prefilled syringe), a special needle (called a Huber needle), one or two alcohol swabs, and one or two povidone-iodine swabs. Wash your hands. Open the bottle of heparin, and wipe the top with an alcohol or povidone-iodine swab. *Don't touch the top after you've cleaned it.*

2 Remove the needle cover from the syringe needle, and pull back the syringe plunger, permitting air to enter the syringe. Pull back on the plunger until the amount of air in the syringe equals the amount of solution that you'll withdraw from the heparin bottle.

   Then insert the needle into the heparin bottle top and push down on the plunger. Turn the bottle upside down, and pull back on the syringe plunger to fill the syringe with solution to the correct amount. Now remove the needle from the bottle and put the bottle aside. Be sure to replace the needle cover until you've prepared the injection site.

   Change the needle on the heparin flush syringe to the Huber needle.

3 Locate your port by feeling for the small bump on your skin. (The site is over a bony area, usually on the upper chest.)

4 Clean the injection site with an alcohol swab (allow the site to air dry) and then a povidone-iodine swab. As shown, hold the port between two fingers.

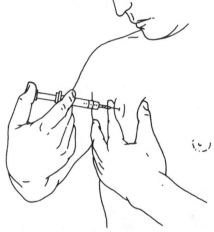

Push the Huber needle firmly through the skin and port septum until it hits the bottom of the port's chamber. Be sure the needle is inserted at a 90-degree angle.

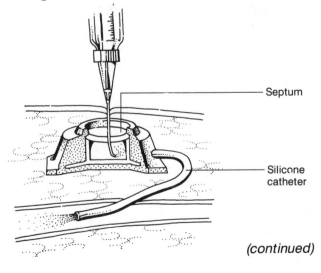

Septum

Silicone catheter

(continued)

Caring for an implanted port *(continued)*

5 Now push down on the syringe plunger, which will inject the heparin solution into the port. You'll normally feel a small amount of resistance. Notify the doctor immediately if the solution will not flow into the port.

6 Remove the needle. To keep the solution from flowing back into the syringe when you remove the needle, continue to push down slowly on the syringe plunger as you withdraw the needle.

Injecting medication into the port

1 Gather the needed equipment: an extension set with a special needle (Huber needle), a clamp, a 10-ml syringe filled with saline solution, a syringe containing the prescribed medication, a sterile needle filled with heparin flush solution, a povidone-iodine swab, and two alcohol swabs.

2 Wash and dry your hands. Attach the 10-ml syringe filled with saline solution to the end of the extension set. Gently push on the plunger of the syringe until the extension tubing and needle are filled with solution and all the air is removed. Make sure all the air is removed by flicking the tubing of the extension set.

3 Locate the port by feeling for the small bump on your skin. Hold the port between two fingers. Clean the site with an alcohol swab and then a povidone-iodine swab.

4 Insert the Huber needle through the skin and port septum until it hits the bottom of the port's chamber. Be sure the needle is inserted at a 90-degree angle.

5 Check for a blood return by pulling back on the syringe that's attached to the extension set.

6 Flush the port with 5 ml of saline solution by pushing down on the plunger of the syringe with the saline solution.

7 Clamp the extension set and remove the saline-filled syringe.

8 Connect the medication-filled syringe to the extension set. Open the clamp and inject the medication, as ordered by your doctor.

9 Check the skin around the needle for swelling and tenderness. If you note these signs, stop the injection and call your doctor.

10 When the injection is complete, clamp the extension set and remove the medication syringe.

11 Attach the saline-filled syringe to the extension set. Then open the clamp and flush the port again with 5 ml of saline solution by pushing down on the plunger of the syringe. Remember to flush the port after each medication injection to minimize medication interactions. Clamp the extension set and remove the syringe. Put a protective cap on the end of the extension set.

12 Tape the needle in place and apply a gauze dressing.

Medications

The teaching aids in this section reflect the most commonly prescribed drugs taken by patients at home. Designed for easy use, these teaching aids explain in simple terms what the patient can expect during drug therapy. For your quick access, they're arranged in alphabetical order.

Each teaching aid follows the same format. An introduction identifies the conditions the medication treats, such as allergy symptoms or high blood pressure. It then lists a few common trade names. When appropriate, the introduction also mentions how the medication works.

Following the introduction, *How to take this drug* specifies the administration directions. This section may also give special instructions on how and when to take the medication, especially if the medication has more than one form.

If your patient sometimes forgets to take his medication, he can refer to *What to do if you miss a dose*. This section lists what steps to take to get back on schedule—such as skipping a dose or adjusting the timing of the next dose—and usually emphasizes not to take double doses.

The following section, *What to do about side effects*, identifies the medication's common and life-threatening reactions—and tells when to call a doctor right away. Next, the section *What you must know about other drugs* will alert your patient to possible drug interactions. He may not think, for instance, that he needs to be concerned about a nonprescription cold medication he's taking. As necessary, the teaching aid will caution him about potentially hazardous nonprescription and prescription drugs.

Special directions covers topics such as other medical conditions the patient should report and tips on how to combat side effects. In the final section, *Important reminders*, pregnant or breast-feeding patients, elderly patients, athletes, and others will find specific information about their use of the medication.

Taking acebutolol

Dear Patient:

Acebutolol will help control your high blood pressure or correct your irregular heartbeat. The label may read Sectral.

How to take acebutolol
Acebutolol comes in long-acting capsules. Carefully read the medication label, and follow the directions exactly. Don't break, chew, or crush the capsule. Swallow it whole.

Always check your pulse rate before taking acebutolol. If it's under 50 beats a minute, call your doctor and don't take the dose.

What to do if you miss a dose
If you forget to take your medication, take it as soon as you remember. But if it's within 4 hours of your next dose, skip the dose you missed and take your next dose at the regular time. Don't take two doses together.

What to do about side effects
Call the doctor *right away* if you have trouble breathing or swallowing. Also call your doctor if you feel very tired or light-headed (a symptom of low blood pressure).

What you must know about other drugs
Tell the doctor what other medications you're taking because they can affect how acebutolol works. For example, taking acebutolol with digoxin (Lanoxin) can slow your heart too much, whereas taking it with indomethacin (Indocin) can reduce acebutolol's effect.

If you take medication for diabetes, check your blood glucose levels carefully. That's because acebutolol can hide signs of low blood glucose levels.

Special directions
• Tell your doctor about medical conditions you have, such as chronic lung disease, diabetes, heart or blood vessel disease, kidney or liver disease, depression, thyroid problems, or an unusually slow heartbeat.
• Tell your doctor and pharmacist if you're allergic to acebutolol or other medications, foods, preservatives, or dyes. Acebutolol may make allergic reactions worse and harder to treat.
• Be sure you know how you react to this medication before driving or performing activities requiring alertness.
• If you feel tired after taking this medication, plan frequent rest periods.
• If you have diabetes, keep a fast-acting carbohydrate, such as a package of raisins, nearby—in case your blood glucose level drops.
• Don't abruptly stop taking acebutolol. Doing so may lead to heart problems.
• Before you have surgery, dental work, or emergency treatment, tell the doctor that you're taking acebutolol.
• Check with your doctor or pharmacist before taking nonprescription drugs.

Important reminders
Notify your doctor if you become pregnant while taking acebutolol.

If you're an athlete, you should know that the National Collegiate Athletic Association and the U.S. Olympic Committee have banned acebutolol's use.

Additional instructions

_____

_____

_____

Taking acetaminophen

Dear Patient:

Known by many names (Anacin-3, Panadol, Tylenol, and others), acetaminophen relieves mild pain and fever.

How to take acetaminophen

Acetaminophen comes in many forms: capsule, oral liquid, tablet, chewable tablet, wafer, and suppository.

Carefully read and follow precautions listed on the package label. If you're an adult, you can take a dose of acetaminophen every 4 hours as needed, but don't exceed eight tablets a day. You may repeat a child's dose every 4 hours (but don't exceed five doses a day).

If you're using a *suppository* that's too soft to insert, run cold water over it or refrigerate it for a few minutes before removing the wrapper and inserting the medication.

What to do if you miss a dose

If you forget to take your medication, take it as soon as you remember. If it's almost time for your next dose, skip the missed dose and resume your regular schedule. Don't take two doses together.

What to do about side effects

Keep in mind that large doses of acetaminophen may cause liver damage. Call the doctor if a rash or hives develop or if your skin turns yellowish.

What you must know about alcohol and other drugs

Don't drink alcoholic beverages when taking acetaminophen because this combination may cause liver damage, especially if you take acetaminophen regularly for a long time.

Check with the doctor or pharmacist before taking any nonprescription drugs. Many contain acetaminophen and count toward your total dosage.

Tell your doctor if you're taking diflunisal (Dolobid), which may increase acetaminophen's effects, or warfarin (Coumadin), which may cause bleeding with long-term acetaminophen use.

Special directions

• Tell the doctor if you have medical problems, particularly if you have diabetes, kidney or liver disease, or blood disorders.
• If acetaminophen doesn't relieve pain after 10 days (adults) or 5 days (children), notify the doctor. If you have new symptoms, if the pain gets worse, or if the pain site appears red and swollen, also contact the doctor.
• If acetaminophen doesn't make a fever go away within 3 days, call the doctor. Also call him if the fever returns or rises or if new symptoms, redness, or swelling occurs.

Important reminders

Give this medication to a child under age 2 only as prescribed by a doctor.

If you have diabetes, check your blood glucose level carefully. Acetaminophen can affect test results, so contact your doctor about unusual changes.

Additional instructions

_____

_____

_____

_____

Taking acetaminophen with butalbital and caffeine

Dear Patient:

This medication is usually prescribed to treat moderately severe tension headaches. The medication label may read Esgic, Fioricet, or Rogesic.

How to take this drug
This drug comes in tablet and capsule forms. Carefully read the medication label and follow the directions exactly. Don't take more than six tablets or capsules in a day. If you don't feel better, call your doctor. Don't increase the dose on your own.

To minimize stomach upset, you may take this drug with milk or meals.

What to do if you miss a dose
If you forget to take your medication, take it as soon as you remember. But if it's almost time for your next dose, skip the missed dose and take the next regular dose. Don't take double doses.

What to do about side effects
If you get allergy symptoms (itching, a rash, difficulty breathing or swallowing), stop taking this drug and notify the doctor *immediately.*

The drug may also cause confusion, dizziness, drowsiness, light-headedness, nausea, stomach pain, and vomiting. If these symptoms persist or increase, contact your doctor.

What you must know about alcohol and other drugs
Don't take this drug with alcoholic beverages, drugs that relax you or make you feel sleepy, antihistamines, or other drugs that may decrease your activity level.

Check with the doctor or pharmacist before taking any nonprescription medications. Many contain acetaminophen and should be counted as part of your total daily dosage. In normal amounts, acetaminophen safely and effectively relieves pain. But in high doses, it can damage the liver.

Tell your doctor if you're taking diflunisal (Dolobid) because it may increase the effects of acetaminophen.

Special directions
• Inform the doctor about your medical history, particularly if you have diabetes, kidney or liver disease, or blood disorders.
• Be aware of your response to this medication before driving or performing other activities requiring alertness.
• Don't stop taking this drug suddenly. Your doctor may recommend reducing the dosage before stopping completely. Don't take more than the prescribed amount, and don't take the medication longer than your doctor directs.

Important reminders
If you're pregnant or breast-feeding, check with your doctor before taking this drug.

If you're an athlete, you should know that the National Collegiate Athletic Association and the U.S. Olympic Committee ban the use of this drug.

Additional instructions

_____

_____

_____

Taking acetaminophen with codeine

Dear Patient:

This medication relieves moderately severe pain. The medication label may read M-Gesic or Tylenol with Codeine.

How to take this drug
You may take this medication as a tablet, capsule, or liquid (usually every 4 to 6 hours). To minimize stomach upset, you may take it with milk or meals.

Carefully read the medication label and follow the directions exactly. If you don't feel better, call the doctor. Don't increase the dose on your own.

What to do if you miss a dose
If you forget to take your medication, take it as soon as you remember. But if it's almost time for your next dose, skip the missed dose and take the next regular dose. Don't take double doses.

What to do about side effects
If you have difficulty breathing or swallowing, a rash, or other signs of an allergic reaction, stop taking this medication and get medical help.

The drug may cause confusion, dizziness, drowsiness, light-headedness, stomach pain, nausea, vomiting, and constipation. If any of these symptoms persist, call the doctor.

What you must know about alcohol and other drugs
Don't take this medication with alcoholic beverages, sedatives, antihistamines, or other drugs that decrease your activity.

Check with the doctor or pharmacist before taking nonprescription medications. Many contain acetaminophen and should be counted toward your daily dosage. In normal amounts, acetaminophen is safe; in high doses, it can damage the liver.

Tell your doctor if you're taking diflunisal (Dolobid) because it may increase acetaminophen's effects.

Special directions
• Tell the doctor about your medical history, particularly head injury, severe headaches, diabetes, kidney or liver disease, or blood disorders.
• Avoid driving and other activities that require mental alertness until you know how this medication affects you.
• To avoid possible constipation, include plenty of fluids and fiber in your diet.
• This medication can be habit-forming. Take just the prescribed amount for only as long as directed.
• Don't take this medication if you're allergic to acetaminophen or to codeine, morphine, or other opiates.

Important reminders
If you're breast-feeding or pregnant, talk to your doctor before taking this medication.

Sharing this medication is against federal law.

If you're an athlete, you should know that the National Collegiate Athletic Association and the U.S. Olympic Committee ban the use of this medication.

Additional instructions

_____

_____

_____

Taking acetaminophen with hydrocodone

Dear Patient:

This medication helps relieve moderately severe pain. The medication label may read Amacodone, Dolacet, or Hydrocet.

How to take this drug
Available in tablets, capsules, and oral liquids, this medication can usually be taken every 4 to 6 hours as needed.

Carefully read the medication label and follow directions exactly. If you don't feel better, call the doctor. Don't increase the dose on your own.

What to do if you miss a dose
If you forget to take your medication, take it as soon as you remember. But if it's almost time for the next dose, skip the missed dose and resume your regular schedule. Don't take double doses.

What to do about side effects
If you have a rash, difficulty breathing, or other signs of an allergic reaction, stop taking the medication and notify the doctor *immediately*.

Other possible side effects include confusion, dizziness, drowsiness, lightheadedness, itching, stomach pain, nausea, vomiting, and constipation. If these symptoms continue or become severe, call the doctor.

What you must know about alcohol and other drugs
Avoid taking this medication with alcoholic beverages, medications that relax or sedate you, antihistamines, and other drugs that decrease your activity level.

Check with the doctor or pharmacist before taking any nonprescription medications. Many contain acetaminophen and should be counted toward your daily dosage. In normal doses, acetaminophen is safe and effective; in high doses, it can damage the liver.

Tell your doctor if you're taking diflunisal (Dolobid) because it may increase acetaminophen's effect.

Special directions
• Inform the doctor about your medical history, especially head injury, severe headaches, diabetes, kidney or liver disease, or blood disorders.
• Avoid driving and other activities that require mental alertness until you know how this medication affects you.
• To combat possible constipation, consume plenty of fluids and fiber.
• This medication may be habit-forming. Take just the amount prescribed only as long as directed.
• Don't take this medication if you're allergic to acetaminophen or to codeine, morphine, or other opiates.

Important reminders
If you're pregnant or breast-feeding, talk to your doctor before taking this medication.

Sharing this medication is against federal law.

If you're an athlete, you should know that the National Collegiate Athletic Association and the U.S. Olympic Committee ban this drug's use.

Additional instructions

_____

_____

_____

Taking acetazolamide

Dear Patient:

This medication helps control glaucoma, certain types of seizures, and heart failure. The medication label may read Ak-Zol, Dazamide, or Diamox.

How to take acetazolamide
This medication comes in tablet, long-acting capsule, and injectable forms.

Carefully check the label, and follow the directions exactly. This medication increases urination, so if you take it once a day, take it in the morning with breakfast. If you take it more than once a day, take the last dose no later than 6 p.m., unless the doctor tells you otherwise.

Take acetazolamide with food or milk to minimize the chance of an upset stomach. If you have difficulty swallowing tablets, you can mix a tablet in 2 teaspoons of hot water and 2 teaspoons of honey or syrup. If you have trouble swallowing capsules, call the doctor.

What to do if you miss a dose
Take it as soon as you remember. But if it's almost time for your next dose, skip the missed dose and take the next dose at the regular time. Don't take double doses.

What to do about side effects
Notify the doctor as soon as possible if you start to bruise or bleed easily or if you develop a fever or sore throat.

Special directions
• Inform your doctor about your medical history, especially if you have Addison's disease, diabetes, gout, or kidney, liver, or lung disease.

• Take only the amount of medication the doctor ordered. If you think you need more, consult your doctor.
• Until you know how this medication affects you, avoid driving or any activity that requires alertness and coordination.
• If this medication causes your body to lose potassium, your doctor may advise consuming potassium-rich foods and fluids, including bananas, potatoes, unsalted peanuts, and orange juice. Or the doctor may order a potassium supplement for you. Don't change your diet, however, without first consulting your doctor.
• If you're taking acetazolamide to control seizures, don't suddenly stop taking it.

Important reminders
If you have diabetes, carefully monitor glucose levels in your blood and urine. This medication may increase glucose levels.

If you become pregnant while taking this medication, notify your doctor.

If you're an athlete, you should know that the National Collegiate Athletic Association and the U.S. Olympic Committee ban acetazolamide's use.

Additional instructions

_____

_____

_____

_____

Taking acetohexamide

Dear Patient:

This medication lowers blood glucose levels. A brand name for acetohexamide is Dymelor.

How to take acetohexamide
This medication comes in tablet form. Carefully read the medication label, and follow the directions exactly. Take it at the same time each day, and don't take more or less than your doctor has ordered.

What to do if you miss a dose
If you forget to take your medication, take it as soon as you remember. If it's almost time for your next dose, skip the missed dose. Take your next dose at the regularly scheduled time. Don't take double doses.

What to do about side effects
This medication may cause low blood glucose levels, especially if you delay or miss a meal or snack, exercise more than usual, or drink a significant amount of alcohol. Symptoms of low blood glucose include cool pale skin, difficulty concentrating, shakiness, headache, cold sweats, and anxiety.

Learn to recognize your reaction to a low blood glucose level so you can take corrective steps quickly.

Check your blood glucose level with a test strip to confirm that it's low. (Be sure to ask your doctor for information if you don't know how to test yourself.) To correct a low blood glucose level, eat or drink something containing sugar, such as glucose tablets or gel, fruit juice, or raisins.

If the symptoms don't subside in 10 or 15 minutes or if you feel worse, eat or drink some more food or liquid that contains a lot of sugar. Also seek medical attention immediately.

Be sure to notify your doctor if your blood glucose levels drop and you have symptoms. That's because the blood glucose–lowering effects of acetohexamide may last for days and your symptoms may recur.

Other possible side effects include nausea, vomiting, mild drowsiness, headache, heartburn, dizziness, diarrhea, constipation, appetite changes, and stomach pain, fullness, or discomfort. These side effects may subside as your body adjusts to the medication. If these effects persist, consult your doctor.

What you must know about alcohol and other drugs
Avoid alcoholic beverages until you have discussed their use with your doctor. Combining acetohexamide and alcohol can make you ill or cause your blood glucose level to drop.

Tell the doctor what other medications you're taking, including nonprescription drugs. Many contain ingredients that interact with acetohexamide to increase or decrease your blood glucose level beyond a safe amount. For example, antidepressants, chloramphenicol (Chloromycetin), sulfa drugs, or oral anticoagulants (blood thinners) may increase your risk of having a low blood glucose level. On the other hand, steroids, glucagon, or thiazide diuretics (water pills) may increase your chances for a high blood glucose level.

(continued)

Taking acetohexamide *(continued)*

Some heart medications (called beta blockers) may make a low blood glucose episode last longer or hide the symptoms of a low glucose level.

What's more, some nonprescription medications (such as aspirin or similar products containing salicylates, appetite control medications, or cold or cough medicines) may affect your glucose level.

Special directions
• Be sure your doctor knows your medical history, especially if you have a heart problem or kidney, liver, or thyroid disease.
• Follow your special meal plan carefully. Diet is the most important part of controlling your diabetes and is necessary for your medication to work.
• Test the amount of glucose in your blood and urine as directed by your doctor. Self-testing helps you keep your diabetes under control and warns you when it's not.
• Don't take any other medication unless it's prescribed or approved by your doctor. This precaution applies especially to nonprescription medications used to treat colds, coughs, asthma, or hay fever. It also applies to appetite control preparations.
• Tell the doctor if you develop an infection because you may need insulin temporarily to control your blood glucose level. Severe infection can cause your glucose level to change rapidly.
• Because this medication may make your skin more sensitive to the sun, wear a sun block (with a skin protection factor [SPF] of at least 15). Also wear protective clothing and sunglasses when you're outside. If you develop a severe reaction from sun exposure,

contact your doctor and stay out of the sun.
• Keep follow-up medical appointments so your doctor can check your progress regularly, especially during the first few weeks that you take acetohexamide.
• Before any kind of surgery, dental work, or emergency treatment, tell the doctor or dentist that you're taking acetohexamide.
• Wear a medical identification tag or bracelet or carry an identification card at all times. Your identification should state that you have diabetes. It should also name your medications.

Important reminders
If you're breast-feeding or you become pregnant, check with your doctor before taking this medication.

If you're an older adult, be aware that you may be more sensitive than younger adults to the effects of acetohexamide.

Additional instructions

_____

_____

_____

_____

_____

_____

_____

_____

Taking acyclovir

Dear Patient:

This medication, which is also called Zovirax, treats infections caused by the herpes virus, such as genital herpes and shingles. It's also given for chicken pox. Although this medication won't cure you, it will make you feel more comfortable and shorten your illness.

How to take acyclovir
Carefully read the label on your medication, which may be in capsule, tablet, liquid (oral suspension), or ointment form. Follow the directions exactly.

Take acyclovir until your prescription is finished, even if your symptoms subside and you begin to feel better. Try not to miss any doses, but don't take the drug more often or longer than directed.

Take the *capsule, tablet,* or *liquid* form of acyclovir with meals to minimize possible stomach upset. If you're taking *liquid* acyclovir, measure each dose accurately by using a measuring spoon. Don't use a household teaspoon.

If you're using *ointment,* wear a disposable glove to apply the medication. Doing this helps prevent spreading the infection to other body areas. Apply enough ointment to cover each herpes blister. A ½-inch strip of ointment will cover about 2 square inches.

What to do if you miss a dose
Take the dose as soon as you remember. But if it's almost time for your next dose, skip the missed one and take the next one at your regularly scheduled time. Don't take two doses together.

What to do about side effects
The drug may cause nausea and vomiting. If these symptoms persist or become worse, contact your doctor.

What you must know about other drugs
Be sure to tell the doctor what other medications you're taking—especially probenecid (Probalan), which may make acyclovir's effects stronger. Also tell the doctor if you're taking zidovudine (also called AZT or Retrovir) because this combination may cause drowsiness.

Special directions
• Avoid sexual activity if either you or your partner has herpes symptoms. Acyclovir will not prevent the spread of herpes between partners. Using a latex condom may help prevent the spread of herpes, but using a spermicidal jelly or a diaphragm probably won't.
• Keep the areas affected by herpes clean and dry. Also, wear loose-fitting clothing to avoid irritating the sores.
• Never apply the ointment form of acyclovir to your eyes.

Important reminder
If you're a woman and have genital herpes, be sure to have a Pap test at least once a year.

Additional instructions

_____

_____

_____

_____

Taking albuterol

Dear Patient:

Albuterol is prescribed for bronchial asthma, chronic bronchitis, emphysema, and other lung disorders. It relieves coughing, wheezing, shortness of breath, and breathing difficulties by improving the flow of air in the lungs. Albuterol is also known as Proventil and Ventolin.

How to take albuterol
You may take albuterol in syrup, tablet, extended-release tablet, or aerosol form. Or you may use an albuterol solution with a nebulizer.

Carefully read the medication label. Follow the directions exactly. Don't increase the amount or frequency of your dose without consulting your doctor.

Don't break or chew an *extended-release tablet;* swallow it whole.

Use your nebulizer or other breathing device exactly as you were taught. Don't take more than two inhalations at a time, unless directed. Wait 1 to 2 minutes after the first inhalation to be sure you need another. If you need another breathing device in less than 2 weeks, you may be taking too much medication. As needed, check with your doctor or pharmacist.

What to do if you miss a dose
Take a missed dose as soon as possible. Take any remaining doses for that day at regularly spaced intervals. Don't take double doses.

What to do about side effects
You may experience tremors, nervousness, dizziness, difficulty sleeping, headaches, or an unusual taste in your mouth. If these symptoms persist, call your doctor.

What you must know about other drugs
Tell your doctor what other medications you're taking because they may affect the way albuterol works. For example, some medications for depression may affect the heart and blood vessels. And some heart medications may keep albuterol from working properly.

Special directions
• If you still have trouble breathing after using albuterol or if your condition is worse, contact your doctor.
• If you're taking two aerosol medications—such as albuterol and an adrenocorticoid drug or ipratropium (Atrovent)—inhale the albuterol first. Wait about 5 minutes and then use the adrenocorticoid or the ipratropium. Taking albuterol first opens your air passages and helps the next medication work better.

Important reminders
If you have diabetes, albuterol may increase your glucose level. Contact your doctor if you notice a change in your blood or urine test results.

Tell your doctor if you're allergic to sulfites. Some albuterol contains sulfites.

Tell your doctor if you become pregnant while taking this medication.

If you're an athlete, you should know that the U.S. Olympic Committee permits the use of inhalation aerosol and inhalation solution forms of albuterol.

Taking allopurinol

Dear Patient:

Allopurinol treats chronic gout (gouty arthritis) by decreasing the amount of uric acid produced by the body. The name on your medication may be Lopurin or Zyloprim.

How to take allopurinol

This medication is available as a tablet. Carefully read your medication label. Follow the directions exactly. To work effectively, allopurinol must be taken regularly as directed by your doctor.

Take allopurinol after a meal if you find that it upsets your stomach. Drink ten to twelve 8-ounce glasses of liquid each day unless your doctor directs otherwise. And continue to take allopurinol even if you take another medication for gout attacks.

What to do if you miss a dose

Take it as soon as you remember. But if it's almost time for your next dose, skip the missed dose and take the next dose at the regular time. Don't take double doses.

What to do about side effects

Contact your doctor *immediately* if you have a rash, skin ulcers, hives, itching, blood in your urine, trouble breathing, chest tightness, or unusual bruising, bleeding, or weakness.

Common side effects include drowsiness, diarrhea, nausea, and vomiting. If any of these symptoms persist or become worse, call your doctor.

What you must know about alcohol and other drugs

Avoid alcoholic beverages or limit the amount you drink. Too much alcohol may increase the uric acid in your blood and decrease the benefit of allopurinol.

Inform your doctor about other medications that you're taking. Combining oral anticoagulants (blood thinners) and allopurinol may increase your risk for abnormal bleeding. Taken with allopurinol, drugs such as azathioprine (Imuran) or mercaptopurine (Purinethol) may increase the chance of serious side effects.

Also consult your doctor before taking nonprescription preparations. Taking too much vitamin C, for instance, may increase your risk for kidney stones.

Special directions

• Until you know how allopurinol affects you, avoid driving and other activities that require alertness.
• Tell the doctor about any other medical problems you may have, particularly diabetes, high blood pressure, or kidney disease, because your dosage of allopurinol may need to be adjusted.
• Have regular checkups so your doctor can monitor your progress and the effects of allopurinol.

Additional instructions

_____

_____

_____

_____

_____

_____

Taking alprazolam

Dear Patient:

This medication is used to relieve anxiety or tension caused by unusual stress. Alprazolam is also known as Xanax.

How to take alprazolam
This medication is available as a tablet. Carefully read your medication label. Follow the directions exactly.

What to do if you miss a dose
If you're using this medication regularly and you miss a dose, take it right away if it's within an hour or so of the scheduled time. Later than that, skip the missed dose and take the next dose at the regular time. Don't take double doses.

What to do about side effects
Alprazolam may make you feel drowsy, dizzy, light-headed, clumsy, unsteady, or less alert than usual. Even if you take this medication at bedtime, you may feel drowsy or sluggish when you wake up. If these feelings persist or become severe, contact your doctor.

What you must know about alcohol and other drugs
Avoid alcoholic beverages and other central nervous system depressants (including hay fever, allergy, or cold remedies), which may cause excessive drowsiness. When taken with alprazolam, cimetidine (Tagamet) may also increase drowsiness.

Tell your doctor about other medications you're taking. Their dosages may need to be adjusted because of combined effects with alprazolam.

Special directions
• See your doctor regularly (at least every 4 months) to evaluate whether you need to continue this medication.
• Let your doctor know that you're taking alprazolam because it may change certain medical test results.
• If you're having dental work that will require an anesthetic, tell your dentist that you're taking alprazolam.
• Don't abruptly stop taking this medication without consulting your doctor. To prevent withdrawal effects, your doctor may reduce your dosage gradually.
• If you think you may have taken an overdose, get emergency help. Overdose signs include continuing slurred speech or confusion, severe drowsiness, and staggering.
• Be sure you know how this medication affects you before you drive or perform other activities requiring alertness.

Important reminders
If you're breast-feeding or pregnant, be sure to tell your doctor before taking this medication.

Children and older adults are more likely to experience side effects with alprazolam.

If you're an athlete, you should know that alprazolam use is banned in most athletic events sponsored by the National Collegiate Athletic Association and the U.S. Olympic Committee.

Additional instructions

_____

_____

_____

Taking aluminum and magnesium hydroxides

Dear Patient:

Called by the brand names Di-Gel, Gelusil, and Maalox, this medication relieves heartburn, acid indigestion, and symptoms of an ulcer. Some of these products contain simethicone, an ingredient that relieves the symptoms of excess gas.

How to take this drug
This medication is available in tablets, capsules, and liquid. Follow the instructions on the package exactly.

If your doctor gave you special instructions on how to use it and how much to take, follow those instructions.

What to do if you miss a dose
If you're taking this medication on a regular schedule, take the missed dose as soon as you remember. However, if it's almost time for your next regular dose, skip the missed dose and resume your regular schedule. Never take two doses together.

What to do about side effects
Constipation or diarrhea may occur. If these problems persist or are bothersome, call your doctor.

What you must know about other drugs
Check with your doctor or pharmacist before taking any other medication because this drug may change the way other medications work or other medications may change the way this drug works.

As a general rule, don't take this drug within 2 hours of taking any other medication by mouth. However, if you're taking tetracycline, ketoconazole (Nizoral), ciprofloxacin (Cipro), or methenamine

(Hiprex), you should wait 3 hours after a dose before taking this drug.

Special directions
• Be sure your doctor knows about your medical history, particularly a bone fracture, appendicitis, colitis, severe constipation, hemorrhoids, an inflamed bowel, intestinal blockage or bleeding, rectal bleeding, a colostomy or an ileostomy, diarrhea, edema, or heart, kidney, or liver disease. This medication may make these conditions worse or cause serious problems.
• If you're using this medication to relieve heartburn or acid indigestion, don't take it for more than 2 weeks unless your doctor tells you to.
• If you're using this medication to relieve symptoms of an ulcer, take it exactly as directed and for the full time of treatment ordered by the doctor. For best results, take it 1 and 3 hours after meals and at bedtime (unless the doctor puts you on a different schedule).
• If your stomach condition doesn't improve or recurs, consult your doctor.
• Have regular checkups so your doctor can check your progress, especially if you're taking this medication for a long time.

Important reminder
If you're an older adult and have bone problems, check with your doctor before taking this medication.

Additional instructions

_____

_____

_____

Taking amantadine

Dear Patient:

Amantadine is used to prevent or treat type A influenza (flu) infections. It's also used to treat Parkinson's disease and stiffness and shaking caused by other medications you may take for some nervous or emotional conditions. Other names for amantadine are Symadine and Symmetrel.

How to take amantadine

Amantadine comes as capsules or a syrup. Carefully read your medication label. Follow the directions exactly.

If you're taking amantadine to prevent or treat influenza, finish all of your medication. If you stop taking it too soon, your symptoms may recur. Take the doses at regular intervals—both day and night. Pour the syrup into a measuring spoon for an accurate dose.

What to do if you miss a dose

Take it as soon as possible. However, if you're within 4 hours of the next dose, skip the missed dose and go back to your regular dosing schedule. Don't take double doses.

What to do about side effects

Contact the doctor *immediately* if you faint, have blurred vision, feel confused, have difficulty urinating, or experience seizures or hallucinations (see, hear, or feel things that others tell you aren't there).

Common side effects include dizziness, distractibility, irritability, difficulty sleeping, and purplish red, lacy spots on your skin. If any of these side effects persist or become severe, contact your doctor.

What you must know about alcohol and other drugs

Avoid alcoholic beverages because they can increase the side effects of amantadine.

Special directions

• Until you know how this medication affects you, avoid driving or other activities that require alertness and clear vision.

• You may feel dizzy, light-headed, or faint if you get up suddenly from a lying or sitting position. Getting up slowly may help.

• Amantadine may cause mouth, nose, and throat dryness. Try using sugarless hard candy or gum, ice chips, or a saliva substitute. If dryness persists after 2 weeks, check with your doctor.

• If you're taking this medication to prevent or treat flu infections and your symptoms continue or worsen within a few days, contact your doctor.

• If you think amantadine is losing its effectiveness for you, call your doctor. Don't adjust your dosage on your own. And don't stop taking your medication suddenly. If you do, your Parkinson's disease or other symptoms may become worse. Your doctor may reduce your dose gradually.

Important reminders

If you're pregnant or breast-feeding, notify your doctor.

Older adults may be especially sensitive to side effects.

Additional instructions

_____

_____

Taking amiloride

Dear Patient:

This medication helps reduce the amount of water in your body without reducing potassium levels. Amiloride may be used to control high blood pressure. A brand name for this medication is Midamor.

How to take amiloride

Amiloride is available in tablet form. Carefully read the medication label. Follow the directions exactly.

Because amiloride increases urination, take it in the morning if you take a single dose daily. If you take more than one dose daily, take the last dose no later than 6 p.m. If this medication upsets your stomach, take it with meals or milk.

What to do if you miss a dose

Take it as soon as possible. But if it's almost time for your next dose, skip the missed dose and go back to your regular schedule. Don't take double doses.

What to do about side effects

This medication may cause headaches, nausea, vomiting, diarrhea, and loss of appetite. If these effects persist or become severe, contact your doctor.

What you must know about other drugs

Tell your doctor if you're taking other medication for high blood pressure, potassium supplements, or another potassium-sparing water pill. If these medications are taken with amiloride, your potassium level could rise dangerously high.

Tell your doctor if you're taking lithium (Lithane) because this combination may increase lithium's side effects.

Check with your doctor before using nonprescription pain relievers because they can interfere with amiloride's effectiveness.

Special directions

• Don't change your diet without checking with your doctor. Increasing your potassium intake by taking a potassium supplement or eating a high-potassium diet is unnecessary and could be dangerous. Symptoms of too much potassium include confusion, nervousness, fatigue, irregular heartbeat, weakness, shortness of breath, and numbness or tingling in your hands, feet, or lips.
• Before surgery (including dental surgery), emergency treatment, or medical tests, tell the doctor or dentist that you're taking amiloride.
• Because amiloride may cause sun sensitivity, avoid direct sunlight when possible, wear protective clothing, and use a sun block (skin protection factor [SPF] 15 or higher). If you develop a severe sun reaction, contact your doctor.

Important reminders

If you become pregnant while taking this medication, notify your doctor.

Symptoms of too much potassium are especially likely in older adults because of possible increased sensitivity to amiloride.

If you're an athlete, you should know that amiloride use is banned by the National Collegiate Athletic Association and the U.S. Olympic Committee.

Additional instructions

_____

_____

_____

Taking amiodarone

Dear Patient:

Your doctor has prescribed amiodarone to correct your irregular heartbeats. The label may read Cordarone.

How to take amiodarone
Amiodarone is available as a tablet. Carefully read the label on your prescription bottle because it tells you how much medication to take. Follow the directions exactly.

What to do if you miss a dose
If you miss a dose of amiodarone, skip the dose completely and go back to your regular dosing schedule. Don't take double doses. If you miss two or more doses in a row, check with your doctor.

What to do about side effects
Check with your doctor *immediately* if you develop a cough, irregular heartbeat, shortness of breath, or painful breathing. Also check with him if you experience malaise, unusual fatigue, nausea, vomiting, increased sensitivity to sunlight, or visual disturbances.

What you must know about other drugs
Tell your doctor if you're taking an anticoagulant (blood thinner), other heart medication, or phenytoin (Dilantin). The effects of these medications may increase if taken with amiodarone.

Special directions
• Visit your doctor regularly to make sure the medication is working properly.
• Carry medical identification that states that you're taking this medication.
• Before surgery (including dental surgery) or emergency treatment, tell the doctor or dentist that you're taking amiodarone.
• Amiodarone increases your skin's sensitivity to sunlight. Avoid direct sunlight, wear protective clothing including a hat and sunglasses, and use a sun block that contains zinc or titanium dioxide. Contact your doctor if you have a severe sun reaction. Keep in mind that your skin may continue to be sensitive to sunlight for several months after you stop taking this medication.
• After you've taken this medication for a long time, your skin may turn blue-gray where it's been exposed to sunlight. This color usually fades (it may take several months) after amiodarone treatment ends.

Important reminders
Tell the doctor if you're breast-feeding or you become pregnant while taking amiodarone.

Older adults may be especially sensitive to side effects and more likely than younger adults to develop thyroid problems when taking amiodarone.

Additional instructions

_____

_____

_____

_____

_____

_____

_____

Taking amitriptyline

Dear Patient:

Your doctor has prescribed amitriptyline to relieve your depression. The label may read Elavil, Endep, or Enovil.

How to take amitriptyline
Amitriptyline comes as a syrup or tablet. Carefully follow the directions on the prescription bottle. They tell you how much and when to take your medication.

Take amitriptyline with food, even for a daily bedtime dose, unless your doctor has told you otherwise.

What to do if you miss a dose
If you miss a dose and you take one dose daily at bedtime, don't take the missed dose in the morning because it may cause disturbing side effects during waking hours. Call your doctor for directions.

If you take more than one dose daily, take the missed dose as soon as possible. But if it's almost time for your next dose, skip the missed dose and go back to your regular schedule. Don't take double doses.

What to do about side effects
Amitriptyline may make you feel drowsy or dizzy. You may experience an irregular or fast pulse, blurred vision, dry mouth, constipation, problems with urinating, or sweating.

You may also feel light-headed or faint if you get up suddenly from a lying or sitting position. Getting up slowly may help. Notify your doctor if any of these effects persist or become severe.

What you must know about alcohol and other drugs
Check with your doctor before combining amitriptyline with alcoholic beverages or nonprescription medications, such as allergy, cold, or other medications that make you sleepy.

Tell your doctor if you're taking other medications. Barbiturates (antianxiety medication) may decrease amitriptyline's effectiveness.

Cimetidine (Tagamet) and methylphenidate (Ritalin) may increase amitriptyline's effect beyond a safe level.

When taken with amitriptyline, epinephrine (Adrenalin) and norepinephrine (Levophed) may increase your blood pressure, and monoamine oxidase (MAO) inhibitors may cause severe excitation, high fever, or seizures.

Special directions
• Be sure to tell your doctor if you have other medical problems. They may affect the use of amitriptyline.
• You may need to take this medication for several weeks before you begin to feel better. See your doctor at regular intervals so he can check your progress and make dosage adjustments.
• Until you know how amitriptyline affects you, don't drive, use machinery, or do anything else that requires alertness. The drowsiness and dizziness usually go away after a few weeks of taking this medication.
• Increase your fluid and fiber intake to help combat constipation. If these steps don't help, your doctor may prescribe a stool softener.

(continued)

Taking amitriptyline *(continued)*

• If this medication causes mouth dryness, use sugarless gum or hard candy, ice chips, or a saliva substitute. However, if your mouth continues to feel dry for more than 2 weeks, check with your doctor or dentist. Continuing mouth dryness may increase the chance of dental disease, including tooth decay, gum disease, and fungus infections.

• Amitriptyline may make your skin more sensitive to sunlight. Sun exposure may cause a rash, itching, redness, other discoloration, or a severe sunburn. Avoid direct sunlight, wear protective clothing including a hat and sunglasses, and use a sun block (skin protection factor [SPF] 15 or higher) on your skin and lips. If you have a severe sun reaction, check with your doctor.

• Amitriptyline may affect some medical test results, so tell your doctor that you're taking this medication.

• Also tell the doctor you're taking this medication before you have surgery, dental work, or emergency treatment.

• Don't stop taking this medication without checking with your doctor. He may reduce the dosage gradually to prevent your condition from becoming worse and to lessen the possibility of withdrawal symptoms, such as headache, nausea, and an overall feeling of discomfort.

• Keep in mind that the effects of this medication may last for 3 to 7 days after you stop taking it.

Important reminders

If you have diabetes and you notice a change in your blood or urine glucose test results, contact your doctor. This medication may affect your glucose levels.

Notify your doctor if you're pregnant or breast-feeding while taking this medication.

Children and older adults may be especially sensitive to amitriptyline's effects.

Additional instructions

_____

_____

_____

_____

_____

_____

_____

_____

_____

_____

_____

_____

_____

_____

Taking amitriptyline with perphenazine

Dear Patient:

Amitriptyline with perphenazine is used to treat certain mental and emotional disorders. The label may read Etrafon or Triavil.

How to take this drug

Take this medication with food or right after meals, unless otherwise directed. Don't increase the dose or take it more often than prescribed.

What to do if you miss a dose

Take it as soon as you remember. However, if you remember within 2 hours of your next dose, skip the missed dose and go back to your regular schedule. Don't take double doses.

What to do about side effects

Call the doctor *immediately* if you develop a fever, bleeding gums, or mouth sores or if you feel extremely tired.

You may also experience dizziness, drowsiness, uncontrolled movements of the arms or legs, light-headedness when changing position, increased pulse rate, constipation, dry mouth, blurred vision, sensitivity to sunlight, and sweating. Contact the doctor if these effects persist or become severe.

What you must know about alcohol and other drugs

Avoid alcoholic beverages or other medications that make you sleepy or relaxed, such as allergy, hay fever, and cold medications; prescription pain and seizure medications; and anesthetics.

Don't take this drug within 2 hours of taking antacids or medication to treat diarrhea. Taking these medications too close together may lessen the effectiveness of amitriptyline with perphenazine.

Special directions

• Be sure to tell your doctor if you have other medical problems. They may affect the use of this medication.
• Tell your doctor about previous allergic or unusual reactions to perphenazine or other antipsychotics or to amitriptyline (Elavil) or other antidepressants.
• Before you have surgery, dental work, or emergency treatment, tell the doctor that you're taking this medication.
• This medication can cause drowsiness, so be sure you know how it affects you before you drive a car or perform other activities that require alertness.
• Get up slowly from a lying or sitting position to prevent dizziness.
• Avoid direct sunlight as much as possible. Wear protective clothing, including sunglasses and a hat, and use a sun block (skin protection factor [SPF] 15 or higher).

Important reminders

If you're breast-feeding or you become pregnant while taking this medication, notify your doctor as soon as possible.

Teenagers and older adults may be especially sensitive to the effects of this medication.

If you're an athlete, you should know that perphenazine use is banned by the National Collegiate Athletic Association and the U.S. Olympic Committee.

Additional instructions

_____

_____

Taking amoxapine

Dear Patient:

Your doctor has prescribed amoxapine to help treat your depression. The label may read Asendin.

How to take amoxapine
Take amoxapine with food, unless the doctor directs you otherwise.

What to do if you miss a dose
If you usually take one dose daily at bedtime, don't take the missed dose in the morning because it may cause disturbing side effects during the day. Call your doctor for instructions.

If you take more than one dose daily, take the missed dose as soon as possible. But if it's almost time for your next dose, skip the missed dose and go back to your regular schedule. Don't take double doses.

What to do about side effects
If you pass small amounts of urine and your hands, ankles, and feet swell, stop taking amoxapine and notify your doctor *immediately.*

Other side effects include drowsiness, dizziness, dry mouth, feeling lightheaded when you stand up, irregular or fast pulse, blurred vision, constipation, and sweating. Notify your doctor if these effects persist or become severe.

What you must know about alcohol and other drugs
Check with your doctor about drinking alcoholic beverages or using nonprescription medications.

Tell your doctor if you're taking other medications. Barbiturates (antianxiety medications) may decrease amoxapine's effectiveness. Cimetidine (Tagamet) and methylphenidate (Ritalin) may increase the effect of amoxapine.

When taken with amoxapine, epinephrine (Adrenalin), a drug used to treat breathing problems, may raise your blood pressure.

Monoamine oxidase (MAO) inhibitors may cause severe excitation, high fever, or seizures when used with amoxapine.

Special directions
• Tell your doctor if you have other medical problems. They may affect the use of amoxapine.
• Don't drive or perform other activities that require alertness until you know how amoxapine affects you.
• Getting up slowly may help prevent dizziness.
• For temporary relief of mouth dryness, use sugarless gum or hard candy, ice chips, or a saliva substitute.
• Avoid direct sunlight if possible. Wear protective clothing and use a sun block (skin protection factor [SPF] 15 or higher). If you have a severe sun reaction, check with your doctor.
• Tell the doctor that you're taking amoxapine before you have medical tests, surgery, dental work, or emergency treatment.

Important reminders
If you have diabetes, contact your doctor if you notice a change in your blood or urine test results. This medication may affect your glucose levels.

If you're breast-feeding or you become pregnant, notify your doctor.

Children and older adults may be especially sensitive to the effects of this medication.

Taking amoxicillin

Dear Patient:

Your doctor has prescribed amoxicillin to treat your bacterial infection. Common brand names are Amoxil, Trimox, and Wymox.

How to take amoxicillin
Finish all your medication even if you feel better. If you stop it too soon, your symptoms may return.

Take amoxicillin on a full or an empty stomach at evenly spaced times during the day and night. This medication works best when you have a constant amount in your blood.

Take the *liquid form* straight or mixed with other liquids. To get the full dose, take it immediately after mixing and drink all the liquid.

Don't break, chew, or crush the *capsule form* of the drug. Swallow it whole. The *chewable tablet form* should be chewed or crushed before swallowing.

What to do if you miss a dose
Take it as soon as possible. If you take two doses daily and it's almost time for your next dose, space the missed dose and your next dose 5 to 6 hours apart. If you're taking three or more doses a day, space the missed dose and the next dose 2 to 4 hours apart. Then go back to your regular schedule.

What to do about side effects
Contact your doctor *immediately* and stop taking this medication if you develop difficulty breathing, a rash, hives, itching, or wheezing. Such symptoms may mean an allergic reaction.

Common side effects include nausea and diarrhea. If they persist or become severe, notify your doctor.

What you must know about other drugs
Tell your doctor about other medications you're taking. Allopurinol (Zyloprim) taken with amoxicillin may make you more likely to develop a rash. Probenecid (Probalan) increases blood levels of amoxicillin—a beneficial side effect.

Special directions
• Inform your doctor if you have kidney, stomach, or intestinal disease or infectious mononucleosis. They may increase the risk of side effects.
• If your symptoms don't improve within a few days or if they become worse, check with your doctor.
• Tell your doctor if you're allergic to other penicillins or cephalosporins, griseofulvin (Fulvicin), or penicillamine (Cuprimine). If you're allergic to amoxicillin, carry medical identification that describes your allergy.
• If you develop severe diarrhea, don't take diarrhea medication without checking with your doctor. It may make your diarrhea worse or last longer.

Important reminders
If you have diabetes, amoxicillin may cause false test results with some urine glucose tests. Call your doctor before changing your diet or the dosage of your diabetes medication.

If you're breast-feeding, discuss with your doctor whether you should continue while taking amoxicillin.

Additional instructions

_____

_____

Taking amoxicillin with clavulanate potassium

Dear Patient:

The combination of amoxicillin with clavulanate potassium helps treat some bacterial infections. The medication label may read Augmentin.

How to take this drug
Take this medication on a full or an empty stomach at evenly spaced times during the day and night. This medication works best when you have a constant amount in your blood. Finish all of the medication prescribed.

If you're taking the *chewable tablets,* crush or chew them well before swallowing.

If you're taking the *oral suspension,* use the dropper that comes with the bottle to measure the correct amount. If your medication doesn't have a dropper, use a specially marked measuring spoon.

What to do if you miss a dose
Take the dose as soon as possible. But if it's almost time for your next dose and you usually take two doses daily, space the missed dose and the next one 5 to 6 hours apart. If you take three or more doses daily, space the missed dose and the next one 2 to 4 hours apart. Then go back to your regular schedule.

What to do about side effects
Contact your doctor *immediately* and stop taking this medication if you experience difficulty breathing, itching, a rash, hives, or wheezing. These effects may indicate that you're allergic to this medication.

You may also have nausea and diarrhea. Contact the doctor if these symptoms persist or become severe.

What you must know about other drugs
Tell your doctor about other medications you're taking. Allopurinol (Zyloprim) taken with this medication may increase your chances of developing a rash. Probenecid (Probalan) increases blood levels of amoxicillin—a beneficial side effect.

Special directions
• Inform your doctor if you have kidney, stomach, or intestinal disease or infectious mononucleosis. They may increase the risk of side effects.
• Tell your doctor if you're allergic to other penicillins or cephalosporins, griseofulvin (Fulvicin), or penicillamine (Cuprimine). If you're allergic to this medication, carry medical identification that describes your allergy.
• If you develop severe diarrhea, don't take diarrhea medication without checking with your doctor. Diarrhea medications may make your diarrhea worse or last longer.

Important reminders
If you have diabetes, this medication may cause false test results with some urine glucose tests. Call your doctor before changing your diet or the dosage of your diabetes medication.

If you're breast-feeding, discuss with your doctor whether you should continue taking this medication.

Additional instructions

_____

_____

_____

Taking ampicillin

Dear Patient:

Ampicillin is used to treat bacterial infections. The label may read Omnipen, Polycillin, or Totacillin.

How to take ampicillin

Take all the prescribed medication, even if you feel better. If you stop it too soon, your symptoms may return. Take it at evenly spaced times day and night. Try not to miss a dose because ampicillin works best when you have a constant amount in your blood.

Take ampicillin with a full glass (8 ounces) of water on an empty stomach either 1 hour before or 2 hours after a meal unless otherwise directed.

If you're taking the *liquid form,* use a specially marked measuring spoon to measure the correct dose.

If you're taking the *capsule form,* don't break, chew, or crush the capsules. Swallow them whole.

Don't use ampicillin after the expiration date on the label. It may not work properly after that date.

What to do if you miss a dose

Take it as soon as possible. But if it's almost time for your next dose and you normally take two doses daily, space the missed dose and the next dose 5 to 6 hours apart. If you take three or more doses a day, space the missed dose and the next dose 2 to 4 hours apart. Then go back to your regular schedule.

What to do about side effects

Contact your doctor *immediately* and stop taking this medication if you have difficulty breathing, a rash, hives, itching, or wheezing. These effects may mean that you're allergic to ampicillin.

You may also have nausea and diarrhea. If these symptoms persist or become severe, notify your doctor.

What you must know about other drugs

Tell your doctor about other medications you're taking. Allopurinol (Zyloprim) taken with this medication may increase your chances of developing a rash. Probenecid (Probalan) increases blood levels of ampicillin—a beneficial side effect.

Special directions

• If your symptoms don't improve within a few days or if they become worse, check with your doctor.

• Tell your doctor if you're allergic to other penicillins or cephalosporins, griseofulvin (Fulvicin), or penicillamine (Cuprimine). If you're allergic to this medication, carry medical identification that describes your allergy.

• Ampicillin may interfere with the effectiveness of oral contraceptives (birth control pills) containing estrogen. Use a different or additional birth control while you're taking ampicillin.

• If you develop severe diarrhea, don't take any diarrhea medication without checking with your doctor. Diarrhea medications may make your diarrhea worse or last longer.

Important reminders

If you have diabetes, ampicillin may cause false test results with some urine glucose tests. Check with your doctor before changing your diet or the dosage of your diabetes medication.

If you're breast-feeding, tell your doctor before taking this medication.

Taking aspirin

Dear Patient:

Aspirin is used to relieve pain and reduce fever. It may also be used to relieve some symptoms caused by arthritis (rheumatism).

Aspirin may be used to lessen the chance of heart attack, stroke, or other problems that may occur when blood clots block a blood vessel. However, don't take aspirin for these purposes unless ordered by your doctor because doing so may increase your chance of serious bleeding.

Aspirin has many brand names, including Aspergum, Empirin, and Ecotrin.

How to take aspirin

Aspirin is available in capsules, tablets, chewable tablets, chewing gum tablets, delayed-release (enteric-coated) tablets, extended-release tablets, and suppositories.

Take aspirin after meals or with food (except for enteric-coated tablets and suppositories) to lessen stomach irritation. Take the *tablets* and *capsules* with a full glass (8 ounces) of water. Don't lie down for 15 to 30 minutes after taking the medication to prevent irritation that may lead to trouble swallowing.

Chewable tablets may be chewed, dissolved in liquid, crushed, or swallowed whole. *Enteric-coated tablets* must be swallowed whole. Check with your pharmacist about how *extended-release tablets* should be taken. Some may be broken into pieces (not crushed) before swallowing—others must be swallowed whole.

If you're using a *suppository* and it's too soft to insert, chill it in the refrigerator for 30 minutes or run cold water over it before you remove the foil wrapper. To insert it, first wash your hands; then remove the foil wrapper. Lie on your side and draw your knees up toward your chest. With your index finger, push the suppository—rounded end first—into your rectum as far as you can.

What to do if you miss a dose

If you're taking this medication regularly and you miss a dose, take it as soon as you remember. However, if it's almost time for your next dose, skip the missed dose and go back to your regular schedule. Don't take double doses.

What to do about side effects

Call your doctor *immediately* and stop taking this medication if you experience difficulty breathing; wheezing; flushing, redness, or other changes in skin color; hives; itching; or swelling of eyelids, face, or lips. These effects may mean that you're allergic to aspirin.

Also, call your doctor *immediately* and stop taking this medication if you have ringing in your ears or hearing loss because you may have too much aspirin in your system (aspirin toxicity).

You may also experience nausea, stomach problems, or easy bruising. If these symptoms persist or become severe, notify your doctor.

What you must know about alcohol and other drugs

Check with your doctor about drinking alcoholic beverages while taking aspirin because this combination may cause stomach problems.

(continued)

Taking aspirin *(continued)*

If you're taking other medications, check with your doctor before taking aspirin. Ammonium chloride increases blood levels of aspirin products, which may lead to aspirin toxicity. Antacids in high doses make aspirin less effective. Corticosteroids (for example, prednisone) cause aspirin to be eliminated from the body more rapidly, making aspirin less effective.

Anticoagulants (blood thinners) shouldn't be used with aspirin because they may increase your risk of bleeding. Aspirin may increase the effect of oral antidiabetic medication, causing low blood glucose reactions.

Special directions
• Tell your doctor if you have other medical problems. They may affect the use of aspirin. Don't give aspirin to children or teenagers who have fever or other symptoms of a viral infection because of the risk of developing Reye's syndrome. Check with the doctor.
• Don't use aspirin if it has a strong, vinegar-like odor. This odor means the medication is breaking down and is no longer effective.
• Don't use the chewable forms of aspirin for 7 days after having your tonsils removed, a tooth pulled, or other dental or mouth surgery.
• Don't place aspirin directly on a tooth or gum surface because it may cause a burn and erode the tooth enamel.
• Check the labels of all nonprescription and prescription medications and skin products, such as shampoo, for aspirin, other salicylates, or salicylic acid.

Count these products as part of your total aspirin dosage for the day. Pepto-Bismol (bismuth subsalicylate) is an example of a commonly used nonpre-scription medication that contains salicylates. Using salicylate-containing products while taking aspirin may lead to an overdose.
• See your doctor at regular intervals if you're taking aspirin for more than 10 days (5 days for children) or if you're taking large amounts.
• *If you're taking aspirin to relieve pain* and the pain lasts for more than 10 days (5 days for children) or gets worse, new symptoms occur, or redness or swelling occurs, call your doctor.
• *If you're taking aspirin to reduce a fever* and the fever lasts for more than 3 days, returns, or gets worse; new symptoms occur; or redness or swelling occurs, call your doctor.
• *If you're taking aspirin for a sore throat* and your throat is very painful or the pain lasts for more than 2 days or occurs with or is followed by fever, headache, rash, nausea, or vomiting, call your doctor.
• *If you're taking aspirin to lessen the chance of heart attack, stroke, or other problems caused by blood clots,* take only the amount ordered by your doctor. Talk to your doctor if you need medication to relieve pain, fever, or the symptoms of arthritis because he may not want you to take extra aspirin.
• Don't take aspirin for 5 days before surgery (including dental surgery) unless otherwise directed by your doctor or dentist. Taking aspirin during this time may cause bleeding problems.
• If you have rectal irritation from using suppositories, contact your doctor.

Taking aspirin with butalbital and caffeine

Dear Patient:

This combination medication helps to relieve pain and to slow down the nervous system. It's known by several brand names, including Fiorinal.

How to take this drug

This medication is available as tablets and capsules. Take it exactly as ordered. Don't increase your dose or take more of it, and don't take it longer than ordered by the doctor. If you take too much of this medication, it may cause stomach problems, become habit-forming, or lead to medical problems due to an overdose.

To reduce stomach irritation, take this medication with meals or an 8-ounce glass of milk or water.

What to do if you miss a dose

If you take this medication regularly and you miss a dose, take it as soon as you remember. However, if it's almost time for your next dose, skip the missed dose and resume your regular schedule. Never take double doses.

What to do about side effects

If you have difficulty breathing, itching, a rash, or other signs of an allergic reaction, stop taking this medication and notify the doctor *immediately.*

Side effects may include stomach and intestinal symptoms, such as abdominal pain caused by gas, heartburn, indigestion, and nausea. If these side effects persist or become severe, contact the doctor.

What you must know about alcohol and other drugs

Don't drink alcoholic beverages while taking this medication because the mixture may irritate your stomach. Also, the mixture of alcohol and butalbital increases nervous system effects.

Check with the doctor before taking other medications that slow the nervous system—medications for colds or hay fever and other allergies; prescription pain and seizure medications; muscle relaxants; and other medications that make you feel relaxed or sleepy. These medications can increase the effect of butalbital.

Special directions

• Other medical problems may affect the use of this medication. Tell your doctor if you have anemia, gout, peptic ulcer or other stomach problems, or heart, kidney, or liver disease because using this medication may make these conditions worse. Also tell him if you have vitamin K deficiency.
• Don't take this medication if it has a strong, vinegar-like odor. This odor means the medication is breaking down and is no longer effective.
• Before surgery (including dental surgery) or emergency treatment, tell your doctor or dentist that you're taking this medication. Your doctor may tell you to stop taking it for 5 days before surgery to prevent bleeding problems.
• Because this medication may make you dizzy, drowsy, or light-headed, don't drive, operate machinery, or perform other activities that require alertness until you know how this medication affects you.

(continued)

Taking aspirin with butalbital and caffeine *(continued)*

• If you think you or anyone else may have taken an overdose, get emergency help immediately. Symptoms of overdose include hearing loss, confusion, ringing or buzzing in your ears, severe excitement or dizziness, seizures, and difficulty breathing.

• If you're taking this medication regularly or in large amounts, don't stop taking it without checking with your doctor. Abruptly stopping this medication may cause withdrawal symptoms.

Important reminders

If you have diabetes and take this medication regularly, it may cause false urine glucose test results. Check with your doctor if you notice any unusual changes in the test results.

If you become pregnant or you're breast-feeding while taking this medication, notify your doctor.

Never give a child or a teenager with a fever or other signs of a viral infection, such as flu or chicken pox, medication containing aspirin. Contact the doctor as soon as possible. Aspirin may cause a serious illness called Reye's syndrome.

Children are especially sensitive to the effects of this medication, especially if they have a fever or have lost large amounts of body fluids from vomiting, diarrhea, or sweating.

Older adults are also especially sensitive to the effects of this medication and may develop more side effects than younger adults. They may show signs of confusion, depression, or overexcitement.

If you're an athlete, you should know that the National Collegiate Athletic Association and the U.S. Olympic Committee limit the amount of caffeine that can be present in the urine of athletes.

Additional instructions

_____

_____

_____

_____

_____

_____

_____

_____

_____

_____

_____

_____

_____

_____

_____

_____

Taking aspirin with codeine

Dear Patient:

This medication is used to treat moderate to severe pain. Brand names include Emcodeine and Empirin with Codeine.

How to take aspirin with codeine
To reduce stomach irritation, take this medication with food or an 8-ounce glass of milk or water.

What to do if you miss a dose
If you take this medication regularly and you miss a dose, take it as soon as you remember. However, if it's almost time for your next dose, skip the missed dose and go back to your regular schedule. Don't take double doses.

What to do about side effects
If you have trouble breathing, itching, a rash, or other signs of an allergic reaction, stop taking this medication and notify the doctor *immediately.*

Side effects may include intestinal symptoms, including abdominal pain caused by gas, heartburn, indigestion, and nausea. If these symptoms persist or become severe, contact your doctor.

What you must know about alcohol and other drugs
Don't take this medication with alcoholic beverages because the codeine in it can slow down your nervous system, which could make you extremely drowsy. Also, the mixture of alcohol and aspirin may irritate your stomach.

Tell your doctor about other medications you're taking because some may interact with aspirin with codeine. Medications that make your urine less acidic, such as antacids, also increase urination, which leaves aspirin with codeine less time to work.

Check with your doctor before taking other medications that slow the nervous system, such as medications for colds or hay fever and other allergies, prescription pain and seizure medications, muscle relaxants, and other medications that make you feel relaxed or sleepy.

Taking this medication with anticoagulants (blood thinners) may increase your risk of bleeding.

If you have diabetes, keep in mind that aspirin taken regularly may increase the effects of oral antidiabetic medications. Check with your doctor to see whether your antidiabetic medication dosage needs adjustment.

Taking this medication with acetaminophen (Tylenol) may put you at risk for unwanted side effects.

Special directions
• Tell your doctor if you've ever had an unusual or allergic reaction to aspirin or codeine.
• Inform the doctor if you have other medical problems. For instance, if you have gout, aspirin products can worsen this disorder and reduce the effects of other medications used to treat gout. If you have gallbladder disease, the codeine in this medication may cause serious side effects.
• Check the labels of all nonprescription and prescription medications for aspirin, other salicylates, or salicylic acid. Pepto-Bismol (bismuth subsalicylate) is an example of a commonly used nonprescription medication that contains salicylates. Contact your doctor if

(continued)

Taking aspirin with codeine *(continued)*

you're taking a product that contains a narcotic, aspirin, or other salicylates because combining these medications can lead to overdose.
• Don't take this medication if it smells like vinegar. This odor means that the aspirin is breaking down and losing its effectiveness.
• Some people become drowsy when taking this medication. Be sure you know how you respond to this medication before you perform activities that require alertness, such as driving or operating machinery.
• This medication may cause dizziness and light-headedness. Move slowly when you change from a lying or sitting position.
• Tell your doctor or dentist that you're taking this medication before surgery (including dental surgery) or emergency treatment. Because this medication may cause bleeding problems, your doctor may instruct you to stop taking it 5 days before surgery.
• Don't suddenly stop taking this medication if you've been taking it regularly. Your doctor may want to reduce your dosage gradually to avoid withdrawal effects.

Important reminders
If you become pregnant while taking this medication, notify the doctor as soon as possible. Don't take aspirin in the last 3 months of your pregnancy unless directed by your doctor.

If you're breast-feeding, tell the doctor before you take this medication.

Never give a child or teenager with a fever or other signs of a viral infection, such as chicken pox or flu, medication containing aspirin. Contact the doctor

as soon as possible. Aspirin may cause a serious illness called Reye's syndrome.

Keep in mind that children are especially sensitive to the effects of this medication, especially if they have a fever or have lost large amounts of body fluids from vomiting, diarrhea, or sweating. Also, the codeine in this medication may make children unusually excited or restless.

Older adults are especially susceptible to the side effects of this medication, particularly breathing problems.

If you're an athlete, you should know that the National Collegiate Athletic Association and the U.S. Olympic Committee ban the use of codeine.

Additional instructions

_____

_____

_____

_____

_____

_____

_____

_____

_____

_____

_____

Taking astemizole

Dear Patient:

Astemizole is used to relieve or prevent the symptoms of hay fever and other allergies. The brand name for this medication is Hismanal.

How to take astemizole
This medication is available as a tablet. Take it on an empty stomach 1 hour before or 2 hours after meals.

What to do if you miss a dose
If you take this medication regularly and you miss a dose, take it as soon as possible. However, if it's almost time for your next dose, skip the missed dose and go back to your regular schedule. Don't take double doses.

What to do about side effects
You may experience headaches, drowsiness, nervousness, dry mouth, dizziness, nausea, or diarrhea. Contact your doctor if these symptoms persist or become severe.

What you must know about alcohol and other drugs
Check with your doctor before drinking alcoholic beverages because the combined effects of alcohol and this medication may increase the risk of drowsiness.

If you're taking this medication regularly, be sure to tell your doctor if you're taking large amounts of aspirin at the same time (for example, for arthritis). This medication may mask warning signs—such as ringing in the ears—that you're taking too much aspirin.

Special directions
• Tell your doctor if you have other medical problems, especially asthma, an enlarged prostate, urinary tract blockage or difficulty urinating, or glaucoma. They may affect the use of astemizole.
• Make sure you know how you react to this medication before you drive, use machinery, or perform other activities that require alertness.
• Inform the doctor that you're taking this medication before you have skin tests for allergies because this medication may affect the test results.

Important reminders
Tell your doctor if you're breast-feeding or you become pregnant while taking this medication.

Be aware that children and older adults are especially sensitive to the effects of astemizole.

Additional instructions

_____

_____

_____

_____

_____

_____

_____

_____

_____

Taking atenolol

Dear Patient:

Atenolol is used to treat high blood pressure, relieve chest pain caused by angina, and prevent another heart attack in recent heart attack victims. The brand name is Tenormin.

How to take atenolol
Swallow the tablet whole—don't crush, break, or chew it.

Your doctor may tell you to check your pulse rate before and after taking atenolol. If it's much slower than usual, call him before the next dose.

Try not to miss doses. Some conditions become worse when this medication isn't taken regularly.

What to do if you miss a dose
Take it as soon as possible. However, if it's within 8 hours of your next dose, skip the missed dose and resume your regular schedule. Don't take double doses.

What to do about side effects
Contact the doctor *immediately* if you have trouble breathing, swollen ankles, or a sudden weight gain of 3 pounds or more (signs that you're retaining water) or if your blood pressure rises.

You may feel light-headed and extremely tired and have a slow pulse rate. If these symptoms persist or become severe, contact your doctor.

What you must know about other drugs
Tell your doctor if you're taking other medications. If you're taking other medications to lower your blood pressure, atenolol may lower your blood pressure too much. If you're taking digoxin (Lanoxin), your pulse rate may become dan-

gerously slow. Indomethacin (Indocin) may make atenolol less effective.

If you're taking an antidiabetic medication or insulin, check your blood glucose level carefully because atenolol can hide low blood glucose levels.

Special directions
• Tell your doctor if you have other medical problems, especially breathing problems, diabetes, kidney or liver disease, depression, or thyroid problems.
• If you have allergies to medications, foods, preservatives, or dyes, this medication may worsen allergic reactions and make them harder to treat.
• Because atenolol may make you drowsy, avoid driving, using machinery, or performing other activities that require alertness.
• You may be especially sensitive to cold while taking atenolol, especially if you have blood circulation problems.
• Don't suddenly stop taking this medication because your condition may worsen. Your doctor may reduce the amount you're taking gradually.
• Before surgery (including dental surgery), emergency treatment, or medical tests, tell the doctor or dentist that you're taking atenolol.
• Check with your doctor before taking nonprescription medications.

Important reminders
Contact your doctor if you become pregnant while taking this medication.

Older adults are especially sensitive to this medication and likely to experience side effects.

If you're an athlete, you should know that atenolol use is banned by the National Collegiate Athletic Association and the U.S. Olympic Committee.

Taking atropine

Dear Patient:

Your doctor has prescribed atropine to relieve your stomach and intestinal cramps or spasms. It's also used with antacids or other medications to treat peptic ulcer.

The ophthalmic (eye) form of atropine is used to dilate (enlarge) the pupil and to treat certain eye inflammations. Your container may be labeled Atropisol or Ocu-Tropine.

How to take atropine
Atropine is available in tablet form and also as an ophthalmic solution and an ophthalmic ointment. Carefully check your prescription label. Follow the directions exactly.

Take *tablets* 30 minutes to 1 hour before meals, unless your doctor instructs otherwise.

If you're using *eyedrops,* wash your hands first. With your middle finger, apply pressure to the inner corner of the eye (continue applying pressure with this finger for 2 to 3 minutes after using the medication). Tilt your head back and, with the index finger of the same hand, pull the lower eyelid away from the eye to form a pouch. Squeeze the drops into the pouch and gently close the eye. Don't blink. Keep the eye closed for 1 to 2 minutes so the medication will be absorbed.

If you're applying *eye ointment,* wash your hands, then pull the lower eyelid away from the eye to form a pouch. Squeeze a thin strip of ointment into the pouch. Gently close your eyes, and keep them closed for 1 to 2 minutes to allow the medication to be absorbed.

Wash your hands immediately after using eyedrops or ointment. And if you gave this medication to an infant or a child, also wash his hands and any other place the medication may have touched. Don't let any of the medication enter his mouth.

To keep the medication germfree, don't let the applicator tip touch any surface. Also keep the container tightly closed.

What to do if you miss a dose
If you forget to take your tablet or to use your ophthalmic atropine, do so as soon as you remember. But if it's almost time for your next dose, skip the missed dose and resume your normal schedule. Don't take or apply double doses.

What to do about side effects
If you're taking the *tablet* form, make sure family members know to contact the doctor *immediately* if you become so sleepy that you can't be roused.

More common side effects (with the tablet form) include difficulty sleeping, dizziness, rapid pulse rate, palpitations, chest pain, dry mouth, constipation, and blurred vision. If these symptoms persist or worsen, call the doctor.

Common side effects associated with the *ophthalmic* form include blurred vision and sensitivity to light. If these symptoms persist or worsen, contact your doctor.

What you must know about other drugs
Tell the doctor about other medications you're taking. Atropine taken with methotrimeprazine (Levoprome) can cause involuntary body movements, such as

(continued)

Taking atropine *(continued)*

twitching, changes in muscle tone, and abnormal posture.

Don't take oral atropine within 2 to 3 hours of taking antacids or diarrhea medications. Taking these medications too close together may prevent atropine from working properly.

Special directions
For oral atropine
• If you think you may have taken an overdose, get emergency help at once.
• Make sure you know how you react to this medication before driving or performing activities that require alertness.
• Because you may sweat less while taking oral atropine, your body temperature may increase. Take extra care not to become overheated during exercise or in hot weather because it may result in heatstroke. Also, hot baths or saunas may make you feel dizzy or faint while you're taking atropine.
• If you feel dizzy, light-headed, or faint when getting up from a bed or chair, rising slowly may lessen this problem.
• To relieve mouth dryness, use sugarless hard candy or gum, ice chips, or a saliva substitute. If dryness persists for more than 2 weeks, check with your doctor or dentist. Continuing mouth dryness increases the risk of dental disorders.
• Check with your doctor before you begin using new medications (prescription or nonprescription) or if you develop new medical problems while taking atropine.
• Check with your doctor before you stop using atropine. The doctor may want you to reduce your dosage gradually. Stopping atropine abruptly may cause unpleasant withdrawal effects,

such as vomiting, sweating, and dizziness.

For ophthalmic atropine
• Make sure you know how you react to this medication before driving or performing other activities requiring alertness and clear vision.
• Protect light-sensitive eyes by wearing sunglasses and avoiding bright lights.
• Blurred vision and light sensitivity may last for several days after you stop using this medication. If these effects persist longer, notify your doctor.

Important reminders
If you're breast-feeding, be aware that oral atropine may reduce milk flow and that ophthalmic atropine can cause such side effects as rapid pulse rate, fever, or dry skin in breast-feeding infants. Discuss these possibilities with your doctor.

Children (especially those with blond hair and blue eyes) and older adults are especially sensitive to ophthalmic atropine and its side effects.

Additional instructions

_____

_____

_____

_____

_____

_____

_____

Taking azathioprine

Dear Patient:

Also called Imuran, azathioprine decreases the body's natural immunity. This helps to prevent a rejection reaction after organ transplantation. It's also used to treat rheumatoid arthritis.

How to take azathioprine
Check the label on your prescription bottle; follow the directions exactly.

What to do if you miss a dose
If your dosing schedule is once a day, don't take the dose you missed and don't double the next dose. Instead, resume your normal dosing schedule and check with your doctor.

If you're taking more than one dose a day, take the missed dose as soon as you remember it. If it's time for your next dose, take both doses together, then resume your usual schedule. If you miss more than one dose, notify your doctor.

If you vomit after taking a dose, notify your doctor, who will instruct you either to take the dose again or to wait until the next scheduled dose.

What to do about side effects
Notify your doctor *immediately* if you have a fever, chills, wet cough, or other symptoms of infection; black stools; bloody urine; unusual bruising or bleeding; or increased tiredness or weakness.

What you must know about other drugs
Tell your doctor about other medications you're taking. If you're taking allopurinol (Zyloprim), you'll need a lower azathioprine dose.

Special directions
• Tell your doctor if you have other medical problems. They may affect the use of azathioprine.
• Schedule regular checkups so that your doctor can monitor azathioprine therapy and check for side effects.
• Don't stop taking azathioprine without first consulting your doctor.
• During and after azathioprine therapy, don't receive any vaccinations unless your doctor approves. Azathioprine increases your risk of getting the infection that the vaccine prevents.
• Caution close associates who receive the oral polio vaccine that they could pass the polio virus to you. If you can't avoid people who have received this vaccine, wear a protective mask over your nose and mouth.
• Because azathioprine increases your risks of infection and bleeding, take precautions:
—Avoid people with known infections.
—Call your doctor immediately if you think you're getting sick.
—Be careful not to cut yourself using a toothbrush, dental floss, or a razor.
—Avoid touching your eyes or nose.
—Avoid contact sports or other activities in which bruising or injury can occur.

Important reminders
If you become pregnant, stop taking azathioprine and notify your doctor. Also, don't breast-feed while taking this medication.

Additional instructions

Injecting aztreonam

Dear Patient:

Aztreonam is used to treat bacterial infections. This medication is available in a vial and must be given by an intramuscular injection. The medication label may read Azactam.

How to inject aztreonam
Carefully check the label on your prescription vial. This label tells you how much aztreonam to inject and when to inject it. Follow the directions exactly. If you don't know how to give yourself an intramuscular injection, have someone who is skilled in giving an injection give you your medication.

Inject the drug deeply into a large muscle mass, such as the upper outer quadrant of your buttock or the outer side portion of your thigh.

To help clear up your infection completely, you must complete the full course of prescribed aztreonam therapy, even if you begin to feel better after a few days.

For this medication to be most effective, it must be administered at evenly spaced times as directed.

What to do if you miss a dose
If you miss a dose of your medication, contact your doctor for instructions.

What to do about side effects
Tell the doctor *immediately* if you develop pain, swelling, or redness at the injection site.

Also stop using this medication and tell the doctor *immediately* if you experience difficulty breathing, wheezing, a tight feeling in your chest, difficulty swallowing, hives, a rash, or itching. These symptoms indicate that you may be having an allergic reaction to aztreonam.

Some common side effects of aztreonam include abdominal or stomach cramps, nausea, vomiting, and diarrhea. If these symptoms persist or become severe, notify your doctor.

What you must know about other drugs
Tell your doctor about other medications you're taking. Furosemide (Lasix) or probenecid (Benemid, Benn, Probalan, or Robenecid) may raise the amount of aztreonam in your blood.

Special directions
• Tell your doctor if you have other medical problems, especially liver or kidney disease. These and other medical problems may affect your use of aztreonam.
• Check with your doctor before you begin taking any new medication—either a prescription or a nonprescription preparation.
• Contact your doctor if you develop new medical problems while using aztreonam.

Additional instructions

_____

_____

_____

_____

_____

_____

_____

Taking baclofen

Dear Patient:

Baclofen is used to relax certain muscles and relieve the spasms, cramping, and tightness caused by disorders such as multiple sclerosis or some spinal injuries. A brand name for baclofen is Lioresal.

How to take baclofen

Baclofen comes in tablet form. Read your medication label carefully. Follow the directions exactly. To prevent possible stomach upset, take baclofen with milk or meals.

What to do if you miss a dose

Take it as soon as you remember, as long as it's within about an hour of the scheduled dose. If you don't remember until later, skip the dose you missed and resume your normal dosing schedule. Don't take double doses.

What to do about side effects

Common side effects include drowsiness, dizziness, weakness, fatigue, seizures, and nausea. Contact your doctor if seizures develop or if other side effects persist or worsen.

What you must know about alcohol and other drugs

Tell your doctor if you drink alcoholic beverages and take other medications that depress the central nervous system (antidepressants, antihistamines, and barbiturates, for example). These increase baclofen's side effects.

Special directions

• Tell your doctor if you have other medical problems, particularly diabetes, seizure disorder, kidney disease, mental or emotional problems, stroke, and brain disorders.
• Make sure you know how you react to this medication before you drive, operate machinery, or do anything else that could be hazardous if you aren't alert, well coordinated, and able to see well.
• Don't abruptly stop taking this medication; unwanted side effects may occur. Ask your doctor how to gradually reduce your dosage before stopping completely.

Important reminders

If you have diabetes, baclofen may raise your blood glucose level. Check your blood glucose level carefully; if you notice a change, tell your doctor.

If you're breast-feeding or you become pregnant while taking this medication, contact your doctor.

Older adults are especially sensitive to baclofen and may experience more side effects.

If you're an athlete, you should know that baclofen is banned by the National Collegiate Athletic Association and the U.S. Olympic Committee. Its use may disqualify you from certain amateur athletic events.

Additional instructions

_____

_____

_____

_____

_____

Taking beclomethasone

Dear Patient:

Beclomethasone comes in an aerosol form for oral inhalation (Beclovent, Vanceril) and in aerosol or spray form for nasal use (Beconase, Vancenase).

The oral inhalant helps to prevent asthma attacks. Keep in mind that it can't relieve an asthma attack that has already started.

The nasal form helps to relieve the stuffy nose and irritation related to hay fever, other allergies, and other nasal problems. It also helps to prevent nasal polyps from growing back after they've been surgically removed.

How to take beclomethasone

Before using your medication, carefully read the directions that come with the container. Follow them exactly. If you don't understand the directions or aren't sure how to use the medication, check with your doctor or pharmacist.

For this medication to work, you must take it every day at regular intervals as your doctor prescribes. Keep in mind that up to 4 weeks may pass before you feel the medication's full effects.

What to do if you miss a dose

Take it as soon as you remember. But if it's almost time for your next dose, skip the missed dose and resume your normal dosing schedule. Don't take double doses.

What to do about side effects

Nasal beclomethasone may cause mild, transient nasal burning and stinging. If this persists or becomes severe, contact your doctor.

Special directions

• Tell your doctor if you have other medical problems, particularly lung disease or infections of the mouth, nose, sinuses, throat, or lungs.

For the oral inhalant

• Notify your doctor if you experience unusual stress; if you have an asthma attack that doesn't improve after you take a bronchodilator; if signs of mouth, throat, or lung infection occur; if your symptoms don't improve; or if your condition worsens.
• Carry a medical identification card stating that you're taking beclomethasone and may need additional medication in an emergency situation, during a severe asthma attack or other illness, or when you're under unusual stress.
• Before surgery (including dental surgery) or emergency treatment, tell the doctor or dentist that you're taking beclomethasone.
• If you're also using a bronchodilator inhalation aerosol, use it first and then wait about 5 minutes before taking beclomethasone, unless directed otherwise by your doctor.

For the nasal form

• If you're taking this medication for more than a few weeks, see your doctor regularly.
• Check with your doctor if you develop signs of a nasal, sinus, or throat infection; if your symptoms don't improve within 3 weeks; or if your condition worsens.

Additional instructions

_____

_____

Taking belladonna with phenobarbital

Dear Patient:

The combination of belladonna alkaloids and phenobarbital (also called Chardonna-2) relieves cramping from stomach and intestinal spasms and also decreases stomach acid.

How to take this drug
This medication comes in tablet form. Carefully read the label on your prescription bottle. Follow the directions exactly. Unless your doctor gives you other instructions, take the medication 30 to 60 minutes before meals.

What to do if you miss a dose
Take it as soon as you remember. But if it's almost time for your next dose, skip the missed dose and resume your normal dosing schedule. Never take double doses.

What to do about side effects
If you experience itching or a rash, unusual bleeding or bruising, a sore throat and fever, eye pain, or yellowish eyes or skin, stop taking the medication and call your doctor *immediately.*

Other side effects include constipation; mouth, nose, throat, or skin dryness; decreased sweating; dizziness; and drowsiness. Call your doctor if these symptoms persist or become worse.

What you must know about alcohol and other drugs
Don't take this medication with alcoholic beverages or medications that can cause drowsiness (for example, medications for hay fever and other allergies or colds), seizure medication, sleeping medication, or muscle relaxants.

Avoid taking this medication within 1 hour of taking an antacid or diarrhea medication. Taking these medications too close together decreases the effectiveness of belladonna with phenobarbital.

Special directions
• Tell your doctor if you have other medical problems. They may affect the use of this medication.
• Check with your doctor before taking any new medications, either prescription or nonprescription, while taking belladonna with phenobarbital.
• Make sure you know how you respond to this medication before you drive or perform other activities requiring alertness.
• If you experience increased sensitivity to light, wear sunglasses and avoid bright lights.
• Avoid becoming overheated because the belladonna alkaloids in this medication may cause you to sweat less and thus increase your body temperature.

Important reminders
If you're pregnant or breast-feeding, check with your doctor before taking this medication.

Children and older adults are especially sensitive to the effects of this medication.

Additional instructions

_____

_____

_____

_____

Taking benztropine

Dear Patient:

Benztropine relieves symptoms of Parkinson's disease and controls reactions to medications that cause Parkinson-like symptoms. The brand name is Cogentin.

How to take benztropine
Follow the directions on your prescription exactly. To lessen stomach upset, take benztropine with meals, unless your doctor directs otherwise.

What to do if you miss a dose
Take it as soon as you remember. But if you remember within 2 hours of your next scheduled dose, skip the missed dose and resume your normal dosing schedule. Don't take double doses.

What to do about side effects
Common side effects include constipation and dry mouth. If these effects persist or worsen, contact your doctor.

What you must know about alcohol and other drugs
Check with your doctor before drinking alcoholic beverages or taking nonprescription medications. Also tell your doctor about other medications you're taking. Amantadine (Symadine, Symmetrel); phenothiazines, such as chlorpromazine (Thorazine); and tricyclic antidepressants, such as imipramine (Tofranil), may increase your risk of benztropine side effects.

Don't take benztropine within 1 hour of antacids or medication for diarrhea. Doing so may reduce benztropine's effectiveness.

Special directions
• Be sure to tell your doctor if you have other medical problems. They may affect the use of benztropine.
• If you think you've taken an overdose of benztropine, get help *at once.*
• If your eyes are sensitive to light, wear sunglasses and avoid bright lights.
• Make sure you know how you react to benztropine before performing activities that require clear vision and alertness.
• If you feel dizzy or light-headed when arising, get up slowly.
• Avoid becoming overheated because benztropine may make you sweat less and thus increase your body temperature.
• To relieve dry mouth, use sugarless hard candy or gum, ice chips, or a saliva substitute. Consult your dentist if dryness persists because it increases the risk of tooth decay and other disorders.
• Have regular checkups, especially during the first few months you're taking benztropine, so that your doctor can adjust the dosage to meet your needs.
• Don't stop taking benztropine abruptly. Check with your doctor, who may direct you to gradually reduce the dosage.

Important reminders
If you're breast-feeding, check with your doctor before taking benztropine.

Children and older adults may be especially sensitive to benztropine and more likely to experience side effects.

Additional instructions

_____

_____

_____

Taking bethanechol

Dear Patient:

Bethanechol is used to treat certain bladder or urinary tract disorders. It stimulates urination and complete bladder emptying. The label may read Duvoid, Urabeth, or Urecholine.

How to take bethanechol
Bethanechol comes in tablet form. Carefully follow the directions for how much medication to take and when to take it.

Unless your doctor directs otherwise, take bethanechol on an empty stomach (either 1 hour before or 2 hours after meals) to minimize possible nausea and vomiting.

What to do if you miss a dose
If you forget to take your medication and you remember within an hour or so of the scheduled dosing time, take it right away. But if you don't remember until 2 or more hours after your scheduled dosing time, skip the dose you missed and resume your normal dosing schedule. Don't take double doses.

What to do about side effects
Common side effects include abdominal cramps and diarrhea. If these symptoms persist or become severe, contact your doctor.

Less common side effects include tearing, headache, flushing, sweating and, rarely, shortness of breath or wheezing. If you experience a breathing problem, contact your doctor right away.

What you must know about other drugs
Tell your doctor about other medications you're taking. For example, anti-cholinergic agents—such as atropine or propantheline (Pro-Banthine), procainamide (Pronestyl), and quinidine (CinQuin)—may decrease bethanechol's effectiveness.

Special directions
• Inform your doctor if you have other medical problems because bethanechol may aggravate some disorders.
• You may feel dizzy, light-headed, or faint, especially when arising from a lying or sitting position. To minimize this problem, try getting up slowly.

Important reminder
Contact your doctor if you become pregnant while taking bethanechol.

Additional instructions

_____

_____

_____

_____

_____

_____

_____

_____

_____

_____

Taking bisacodyl

Dear Patient:

Bisacodyl is used to relieve constipation. Brand names include Dacodyl, Deficol, Dulcolax, Fleet Bisacodyl, and Theralax.

How to take bisacodyl

Bisacodyl is available in tablet, enema, powder for rectal solution, and suppository forms.

Follow your doctor's instructions. Also follow the manufacturer's package directions exactly if you're using the Fleet enema, powder for rectal solution, or suppository form.

Whichever bisacodyl form you use, drink six to eight 8-ounce glasses of liquid daily to help soften your stools.

Take the *tablet* on an empty stomach for rapid effect. Because the tablets are specially coated to prevent stomach irritation, don't chew, crush, or take them within an hour of drinking milk or taking antacids. You may want to take tablets at bedtime to produce results the next morning.

If you're using a *suppository* and it's too soft to insert, chill it for 30 minutes or run cold water over it before removing the foil wrapper. To insert it, first wash your hands, then remove the wrapper and moisten the suppository with cold water. Lie on your side and use your finger to gently push the suppository into your rectum.

To use the *enema,* first lubricate your anus with petroleum jelly (Vaseline). Then lie on your side and gently insert the rectal tip of the enema applicator. Squeeze all the solution from the enema bottle.

What to do about side effects

Common side effects include nausea, vomiting, abdominal cramps and, with the suppository, a burning sensation in the rectum. If these symptoms persist or worsen, contact your doctor. Also notify the doctor if you notice rectal bleeding, blistering, pain, burning, itching, or other irritation you didn't have before using this medication.

Special directions

• If you have other medical problems, check with your doctor before using bisacodyl.
• Don't use bisacodyl or other laxatives if you have stomach or lower abdominal pain, cramping, bloating, soreness, nausea, or vomiting. Instead, notify your doctor as soon as possible.
• Don't use bisacodyl within 2 hours of taking other medications; doing so can reduce other medications' effects.
• Never use bisacodyl for more than 1 week unless your doctor prescribes it.
• If a change in bowel function persists longer than 2 weeks or keeps returning, check with your doctor before using bisacodyl.
• Don't use bisacodyl unless you need it. Overusing laxatives may damage bowel structures, foster dependence, and cause weakness, poor coordination, dizziness, and light-headedness.

Important reminder

Don't use bisacodyl in children under age 6 unless prescribed by a doctor.

Additional instructions

_____

_____

Taking bromocriptine

Dear Patient:

By regulating certain hormones, bromocriptine treats menstrual problems, enhances fertility in some women, and stops breast milk production. It's also used for Parkinson's disease, acromegaly (overproduction of growth hormone), and pituitary disorders. The label may read Parlodel.

How to take bromocriptine
This medication comes in capsules and tablets. Carefully read the medication label, and follow the directions exactly. If bromocriptine upsets your stomach, try taking it with meals or milk.

What to do if you miss a dose
Take it as soon as you remember (within 4 hours of the scheduled dosing time). After a longer time, skip the missed dose and resume your normal schedule. Don't take double doses.

What to do about side effects
Contact your doctor if you suddenly become short of breath or have chest pain, blurred vision, headache, or severe nausea and vomiting.

Common effects include dizziness, headache, abdominal cramps, and light-headedness. If these symptoms persist or become severe, call the doctor.

What you must know about alcohol and other drugs
Avoid alcoholic beverages when taking bromocriptine. The combination may cause unwanted side effects. Also tell your doctor about other prescription and nonprescription medications you're taking. Other drugs may intensify or decrease bromocriptine's effect or require dosage changes.

Special directions
• Tell your doctor if you have other medical problems, particularly uncontrolled high blood pressure, liver disease, or emotional illness. They may affect the use of bromocriptine.
• Have regular checkups so your doctor can monitor your condition and bromocriptine's effects.
• Make sure you know how you react to this medication before you perform activities requiring alertness.
• If you feel dizzy or faint when arising from bed or a chair, get up slowly.
• To relieve dry mouth, use sugarless hard candy or gum, ice chips, or a saliva substitute. Persistent dryness increases the risk of tooth decay and other mouth disorders.
• Bromocriptine may take several weeks to become effective. Don't stop the drug or reduce your dosage without consulting your doctor.
• When treating infertility, your doctor may advise birth control measures (other than oral contraceptives) at first. Later, you can determine when to stop using birth control.

Important reminders
If you're pregnant or breast-feeding, consult your doctor before taking bromocriptine.

Older adults may be more sensitive to this drug and its side effects.

Additional instructions

_____

_____

Taking brompheniramine with phenylpropanolamine

Dear Patient:

This medication relieves a stuffy or runny nose and sneezing from colds and allergies. Brand names include Bromatap, Bromatapp, and Dimetapp.

How to take this drug
This medication comes in tablet, extended-release tablet, and elixir forms. Carefully read the medication label, and follow the directions exactly. Take the medication with food, milk, or water to reduce stomach upset.

Swallow an extended-release tablet whole; don't break, crush, or chew it. If you can't swallow it, consult the doctor, nurse, or pharmacist.

What to do if you miss a dose
Take it as soon as you remember. If it's almost time for your next dose, skip the dose you missed and resume your normal dosing schedule. Never take double doses.

What to do about side effects
Call the doctor *immediately* if you have a rapid or irregular heartbeat, a tight chest, sore throat, fever, unusual tiredness or weakness, or unusual bleeding or bruising.

Common side effects include a dry mouth, thick phlegm, drowsiness and, possibly, nervousness, restlessness, and insomnia. If these effects persist, call your doctor.

What you must know about alcohol and other drugs
Tell your doctor about other medications you're taking. Taking this drug with alcoholic beverages and other medications that depress the central nervous system (such as antihistamines and pain and seizure medications) increases the side effects of all. And taking this drug with appetite suppressants increases the risk of overdose. Signs of overdose include difficulty breathing, severe drowsiness, persistent headache, and seizures.

Special directions
• Inform the doctor if you have asthma, heart or blood vessel disease, high blood pressure, glaucoma, diabetes, an overactive thyroid, or urinary problems. Also report any allergic or unusual reactions to antihistamines.
• Know how you respond to this medication before you drive or perform other activities requiring alertness.
• If you have trouble sleeping, take the day's last dose a few hours before bedtime.
• Relieve dry mouth with ice chips or sugarless gum or hard candy.

Important reminders
If you're pregnant or breast-feeding, consult your doctor about using this medication.

Use this medication cautiously in young children and older adults.

If you're an athlete, you should know that the National Collegiate Athletic Association and the U.S. Olympic Committee disqualify athletes from competitions if urine samples contain excess phenylpropanolamine.

Additional instructions

_____

_____

Taking bumetanide

Dear Patient:

Bumetanide stimulates urination and reduces water in your body. The label may read Bumex.

How to take bumetanide
Carefully check your medication label. Follow the directions exactly. So that urination doesn't interrupt your sleep, take your single daily dose in the morning after breakfast. If you're taking more than one dose a day, take the last dose before 6 p.m. unless directed otherwise by your doctor.

What to do if you miss a dose
Take it as soon as you remember unless it's almost time for your next dose. Then you should skip the dose you missed and resume your normal dosing schedule. Don't take double doses.

What to do about side effects
Common side effects include fatigue, dizziness, light-headedness, and fainting. If these symptoms persist or become severe, contact your doctor.

What you must know about other drugs
Tell your doctor about other medications you're taking. Taking some antibiotics with bumetanide increases your risk of hearing problems. Probenecid (Probalan), indomethacin (Indocin), and some analgesics may decrease bumetanide's effects.

Special directions
• Before taking bumetanide, inform your doctor if you have other medical problems.
• Because this medication may reduce electrolytes needed by your body (such as potassium, chloride, sodium, calcium, and magnesium), have your blood tested regularly.
• To replace lost potassium, eat foods and drink beverages containing potassium (for example, citrus fruits and orange juice). Or take a potassium supplement or other medication prescribed by your doctor to minimize potassium loss.
• To prevent excessive water and potassium loss, call your doctor if you experience persistent vomiting or diarrhea.
• To help relieve dizziness or light-headedness, get up slowly from bed or a chair, limit the amount of alcoholic beverages you drink, and take care not to get overheated. If the problem persists or worsens, tell your doctor.
• Before surgery (including dental surgery) or emergency treatment, inform the doctor or dentist that you're taking bumetanide.

Important reminders
If you have diabetes, check your blood glucose levels carefully and notify your doctor if you note any changes.

If you become pregnant while taking bumetanide, tell your doctor promptly.

Older adults are especially sensitive to this medication and its side effects.

If you're an athlete, be aware that the National Collegiate Athletic Association and the U.S. Olympic Committee ban the use of bumetanide.

Additional instructions

_____

_____

_____

Taking buspirone

Dear Patient:

This medication (also called BuSpar) is used to treat certain anxiety disorders and to relieve anxiety symptoms.

How to take buspirone
Carefully check your medication label. Follow the directions exactly. Be aware that you may not feel buspirone's full effects until 1 to 2 weeks after you begin taking it.

What to do if you miss a dose
If you forget to take your medication, take it as soon as you remember. But if it's almost time for your next dose, skip the dose you missed and resume your regular dosing schedule. Never take double doses.

What to do about side effects
Common side effects include drowsiness and dizziness. If these symptoms persist or worsen, notify your doctor.

What you must know about alcohol and other drugs
Tell your doctor about other medications you're taking. Buspirone taken with alcoholic beverages and other central nervous system depressants, such as sleeping pills, some cold or allergy medications, and tranquilizers, can cause drowsiness. When taken with monoamine oxidase (MAO) inhibitors, such as isocarboxazid (Marplan), buspirone may raise your blood pressure.

Special directions
• Inform your doctor about your medical history, especially drug abuse or dependency or kidney or liver disease. These and other medical problems may affect the use of buspirone.
• If you're taking this medication regularly for a long time, schedule regular checkups so your doctor can monitor your progress and buspirone's effects.
• Make sure you know how you react to this medication before you drive, operate machinery, or perform other activities requiring physical coordination and alertness.
• If you think you may have taken an overdose of this medication, get emergency help at once.

Important reminder
If you're an athlete, be aware that the National Collegiate Athletic Association and the U.S. Olympic Committee ban the use of buspirone in certain competitions.

Additional instructions

_____

_____

_____

_____

_____

_____

_____

_____

_____

_____

Taking captopril

Dear Patient:

Captopril helps control high blood pressure and congestive heart failure. The label may read Capoten.

How to take captopril

Carefully read the medication label. Follow the directions exactly. Take captopril 1 hour before meals unless your doctor directs otherwise.

What to do if you miss a dose

Take it as soon as you remember. But if it's almost time for your next scheduled dose, skip the dose you missed and take your next dose at the scheduled time. Don't take double doses.

What to do about side effects

Contact your doctor *immediately* and stop taking this medication if you have a fever, chills, hoarseness, sudden trouble swallowing or breathing, or a swollen face, mouth, hands, or feet. These symptoms may indicate an allergic reaction.

A common side effect is a dry, continuing cough. If it persists or worsens, notify your doctor.

What you must know about other drugs

Tell the doctor about other medications you're taking. Some antacids and analgesics may decrease captopril's effectiveness. Captopril taken with digoxin (Lanoxin) can increase the risk of toxic effects. And taking potassium supplements with captopril increases your risk for having too much potassium.

Special directions

• See your doctor regularly to monitor captopril's effectiveness and to check for side effects.

• Don't stop taking this medication on your own even if you feel better. Although high blood pressure may not produce symptoms, you may still need ongoing treatment.

• Remember to follow any prescribed special diet that will help this medication lower your blood pressure.

• Don't take new medications (prescription or nonprescription) without first consulting your doctor.

• Dizziness, light-headedness, or even fainting may follow the first dose of this medication, especially if you have been taking a diuretic (water pill). These side effects may also follow heavy sweating, which depletes body water and lowers blood pressure. Avoid becoming overheated.

• Notify your doctor promptly if you become sick while taking this medication, especially if you have severe or continuing vomiting or diarrhea, which can cause rapid body water loss and low blood pressure.

• Before medical tests, surgery (including dental surgery), or emergency treatment, tell the doctor or dentist that you're taking captopril.

Important reminders

If you become pregnant while taking captopril, tell your doctor, who may change your prescription to another blood pressure medication. If you're breast-feeding, discuss the use of captopril with your doctor.

Additional instructions

_____

_____

Taking carbamazepine

Dear Patient:

This medication controls some types of seizures. It's also used to treat trigeminal neuralgia pain. The label may read Epitol or Tegretol.

How to take carbamazepine
Carbamazepine comes in oral suspension, tablet, and chewable tablet forms. Carefully read your medication label. Follow the directions exactly. Take carbamazepine with meals.

What to do if you miss a dose
Take it as soon as you remember. If it's almost time for your next dose, skip the dose you missed and take the next dose at the scheduled time. Never take double doses. If you miss more than one dose a day, check with your doctor.

What to do about side effects
Consult the doctor *at once* if you have abnormal blood test results or signs of infection (fever, chills, cough) or unusual bleeding (bruises or bloody urine or stools).

Common side effects include dizziness, drowsiness, clumsiness, nausea, vertigo (sensation that objects are spinning), mouth sores, and rashes. If these symptoms persist or worsen, notify your doctor.

What you must know about alcohol and other drugs
Be sure to tell your doctor about other medications you're taking. Alcoholic beverages and central nervous system depressants (such as sleeping pills and cold remedies) may reduce alertness and coordination. Some drugs may decrease or increase carbamazepine's effects and the effects of other drugs you take.

Special directions
• As a pain reliever, carbamazepine works only for certain kinds of pain. Don't take it for other discomfort.
• If you're taking carbamazepine for seizures, don't stop using it without consulting your doctor, who may reduce the dosage gradually.
• Have regular checkups to monitor your progress and make dosage changes.
• Know how you react to carbamazepine before driving or performing other activities requiring alertness.
• Your sensitivity to sunlight may increase, especially at first. Protect yourself from the sun. If you have a severe reaction, notify your doctor.
• Before medical tests, surgery, dental work, or emergency treatment, tell the doctor that you're taking carbamazepine.
• Carry an identification card or bracelet that states you're taking carbamazepine.

Important reminders
If you have diabetes, carbamazepine may affect your urine glucose levels.

If you're pregnant or breast-feeding, consult the doctor before taking carbamazepine.

Children and older adults may be especially sensitive to this medication.

If you're an athlete, you should know that carbamazepine is banned by the National Collegiate Athletic Association and the U.S. Olympic Committee.

Additional instructions

_____

_____

Taking carisoprodol

Dear Patient:

This medication relaxes your muscles and relieves the pain and discomfort of strains, sprains, and other muscle injuries. The label may read Rela, Sodol, or Soridol.

How to take carisoprodol
Carisoprodol comes in tablet form. Carefully read your medication label. Follow the directions exactly.

What to do if you miss a dose
If you forget to take your medication and remember within an hour or so of the scheduled dosing time, take the dose you missed right away. But if you don't remember until later, skip the missed dose and resume your normal dosing schedule. Don't take double doses.

What to do about side effects
Common side effects include drowsiness, dizziness, and skin changes. If these symptoms persist or worsen, call your doctor.

What you must know about alcohol and other drugs
Tell your doctor if you're taking other medications. Avoid taking carisoprodol with alcoholic beverages or other drugs that depress the central nervous system (such as sleeping pills and cold remedies). Doing so can cause increased drowsiness and dizziness.

Special directions
• Before you start to take carisoprodol, tell your doctor if you have other medical problems. They may affect the use of this medication.

• If you're taking this medication for more than a few weeks, see your doctor regularly to check your progress.
• Make sure you know how you react to carisoprodol before you drive, operate machinery, or perform other activities requiring alertness and coordination.

Important reminders
If you become pregnant while taking carisoprodol, tell your doctor.

If you're breast-feeding, be aware that carisoprodol passes into breast milk and can cause drowsiness and stomach upset in breast-feeding infants; discuss its use with your doctor.

If you're an athlete, be aware that carisoprodol is banned by the National Collegiate Athletic Association and the U.S. Olympic Committee. Its use could result in your disqualification from amateur athletic competitions.

Additional instructions

_____

_____

_____

_____

_____

_____

_____

Taking cefaclor

Dear Patient:

Cefaclor is used to treat infections caused by bacteria. The label may read Ceclor.

How to take cefaclor
Carefully check the label on your pre-scription bottle, which contains either capsules or a liquid.

Follow the directions exactly. Take your daily doses at evenly spaced times over 24 hours, as your doctor pre-scribes. If this medication upsets your stomach, you may take it with food. If you're taking the liquid, shake the bottle well. Then use a medicine dropper or a measuring spoon to pour each dose ac-curately.

What to do if you miss a dose
If you forget to take your medication and your dosing schedule is one dose a day, space the missed dose and the next scheduled dose 10 to 12 hours apart. If you're taking two doses a day, space the missed dose and the next dose 5 to 6 hours apart. If you're taking three or more doses a day, space the missed dose and the next dose 2 to 4 hours apart. After taking the dose you missed, resume your normal dosing schedule.

What to do about side effects
Common side effects include diarrhea, nausea, and a rash. If these persist or worsen, contact your doctor.

What you must know about other drugs
Tell your doctor if you're taking other medications. Probenecid (Probalan) may increase cefaclor's effects.

Special directions
• Before starting to take cefaclor, inform your doctor if you have other medical problems. They may affect the use of this medication.
• To help clear up your infection com-pletely, take the medication for the full course of treatment, even if you begin to feel better after a few days. If you stop taking it too soon, your infection may recur.
• If your symptoms don't improve within a few days or if you feel worse, notify your doctor.
• If you have mild diarrhea, you may take a diarrhea medication containing kaolin or attapulgite (Kaopectate or Dia-sorb)—but no other type. Another type may increase or prolong diarrhea. Se-vere diarrhea is a serious side effect; if it occurs, check with your doctor before taking any more diarrhea medication.

Important reminders
If you have diabetes, be aware that cefa-clor may cause false results with some urine glucose tests. Check with your doctor before changing your diet or the dosage of your diabetes medication.

If you're breast-feeding, consult your doctor before using cefaclor.

Additional instructions

_____

_____

_____

_____

_____

Taking cefuroxime axetil

Dear Patient:

This medication is an antibiotic used to treat various infections, but not colds or flu. The label may read Ceftin.

How to take cefuroxime axetil
This medication comes in tablet form. Carefully check your medication label, and follow the directions exactly. Take the medication on a full stomach. If you can't swallow the tablet, you may crush it and mix it with a small amount of food.

What to do if you miss a dose
If you forget to take your medication, take it as soon as you remember. If it's almost time for your next dose and your dosing schedule is two times a day, space the dose you missed and the next scheduled dose 5 to 6 hours apart. Then resume your normal dosing schedule.

What to do about side effects
Occasionally, this medication produces serious side effects, including allergic reaction, anemia, and colitis. If you have a fever, rash, itchy skin, restlessness, or difficulty breathing, stop taking the medication and *immediately* seek emergency medical care.

If you experience fatigue, weakness, pale skin, nausea, vomiting, appetite loss, and diarrhea, report these effects to your doctor promptly.

What you must know about other drugs
Tell your doctor about other medications you're taking. Probenecid (Probalan) may increase the amount of cefuroxime in your blood.

Special directions
• Tell your doctor if you're allergic to this medication or other medications, especially other antibiotics.
• Inform your doctor if you have other medical problems, particularly kidney disease.
• Avoid taking diarrhea medication without first consulting your doctor. Many diarrhea medications can increase or prolong diarrhea.
• Check with your doctor before taking new medications (prescription or non-prescription) or if you develop new medical problems.
• To be sure that the infection clears up completely, take this medication for the entire time your doctor prescribes, even if your symptoms subside.
• If your symptoms don't subside within a few days or if you feel worse, call your doctor.

Important reminder
If you're pregnant or breast-feeding, consult your doctor before taking this medication.

Additional instructions

_____

_____

_____

_____

_____

_____

Taking cephalexin

Dear Patient:

This antibiotic is used to treat various infections, but not colds or flu. Brand names include Keflet, Keflex, and Keftab.

How to take cephalexin

Cephalexin comes in tablets, capsules, and an oral suspension. Carefully check your medication label. This tells you how much to take at each dose and when to take it. Follow the directions exactly.

Take tablets or capsules with food or milk to decrease possible stomach upset.

Store the suspension in the refrigerator. Keep the bottle closed tightly and shake it well before using. Discard unused suspension after 14 days.

What to do if you miss a dose

Take it as soon as you remember. But if it's almost time for your next dose and your dosing schedule is three or more times a day, space the dose you missed and the next scheduled dose 2 to 4 hours apart. Then resume your normal dosing schedule.

What to do about side effects

Occasionally, this medication produces serious side effects, including allergic reaction, anemia, and colitis. If you experience a fever, rash, itching, restlessness, or difficulty breathing, stop taking the medication and seek emergency medical care *immediately.*

If you experience fatigue, weakness, pale skin, nausea, vomiting, loss of appetite, or diarrhea, report these effects to your doctor promptly.

What you must know about other drugs

To ensure that you benefit from treatment, tell your doctor about other medications you're taking. Probenecid (Probalan) may increase the effects of cephalexin.

Special directions

• Tell your doctor if you're allergic to this medication or other medications, especially other antibiotics.
• Inform your doctor if you have other medical problems, particularly kidney disease.
• Check with your doctor before taking new medications (prescription or nonprescription) or if new medical problems develop.
• Avoid taking diarrhea medication without consulting your doctor. Many diarrhea medications can increase or prolong diarrhea.
• To be sure that your infection clears up completely, take your medication for the entire time your doctor prescribes, even if your symptoms subside.
• If symptoms don't subside in a few days or if they worsen, call your doctor.

Important reminder

If you're pregnant or breast-feeding, check with your doctor before taking this medication.

Additional instructions

_____

_____

_____

_____

Taking chloral hydrate

Dear Patient:

Chloral hydrate is used to help calm you and help you sleep. Brand names include Aquachloral Supprettes and Noctec.

How to take chloral hydrate

Chloral hydrate comes in capsule, syrup, and suppository forms. Follow directions on the label exactly. To aid sleep, take chloral hydrate 15 to 30 minutes before bedtime. Take the *capsule* form after meals. Swallow it whole, and drink a full glass (8 ounces) of liquid to minimize possible stomach upset. For the same reason, mix a *syrup* dose in half a glass of liquid before taking.

If you're using a *suppository* and it's too soft to insert, chill it briefly or run cold water over it before removing the foil wrapper. To insert it, first wash your hands, then remove the wrapper and moisten the suppository with cold water. Lie on your side and use your finger to gently push the suppository into your rectum.

What to do if you miss a dose

If you forget to take your medication, skip the missed dose. Take the next scheduled dose. Don't take double doses.

What to do about side effects

Common side effects include drowsiness, dizziness, a hangover-like feeling, and nausea. If these effects persist or worsen, tell your doctor. If you experience serious side effects, such as extreme drowsiness, swallowing or breathing difficulties, or seizures, stop taking the medication and get emergency medical care *immediately.*

What you must know about alcohol and other drugs

Avoid drinking alcoholic beverages while taking chloral hydrate. It can lead to an overdose. Tell your doctor about other medications you're taking. Certain drugs that cause drowsiness (for example, allergy and cold medications, pain relievers, muscle relaxants, and anesthetics) can increase chloral hydrate's effects. And chloral hydrate will increase the effects of anticoagulants (blood thinners).

Special directions

• Tell your doctor if you have other medical problems, including drug dependency or heart, liver, stomach, intestinal, kidney, blood, and emotional disorders. They may affect the use of this medication.
• Also, let your doctor know if you've ever had allergic reactions to drugs or foods.
• Check with your doctor before taking new medications or if you develop new medical problems.
• Make sure that you know how you react to this medication before you drive or perform other activities that require alertness.
• Take this medication only as directed. Overuse can lead to dependency. Also, don't stop taking this medication without consulting your doctor, who may adjust the dosage to prevent withdrawal effects.

Important reminder

If you're pregnant or breast-feeding, check with your doctor before taking this medication.

Taking chloramphenicol

Dear Patient:

Chloramphenicol treats specific severe infections. Because it may cause serious side effects, the doctor prescribes it only when other antibiotics are ineffective. It is never used for minor infections or to prevent infection.

Common brand names include Ak-Chlor Ophthalmic, Chloromycetin, Chloromycetin Ophthalmic, Chloromycetin Otic, Chloroptic S.O.P., and Ophthoclor Ophthalmic.

How to take chloramphenicol
Chloramphenicol comes in capsules, liquids, eardrops, eyedrops or eye ointment, and skin creams. Carefully read your medication label, and follow the directions exactly.

Take *capsules* with a full glass of water on an empty stomach, either 1 hour before or 2 hours after a meal. Don't open the capsule because chloramphenicol has an unpleasant taste.

To take the *liquid form,* use a special measuring spoon to make sure you pour an accurate dose.

Wash your hands before and after applying medication to your eyes, ears, or skin. Keep eye, ear, and skin medications as germfree as possible. Don't touch a dropper tip or let it touch anything, including your eye or ear. After using ointment, wipe the tip of the tube with a clean tissue. Keep all containers tightly closed.

To use *eardrops,* lie down or tilt your head so the infected ear is up. Gently pull your earlobe up and back (down and forward for children) to straighten the ear canal; then squeeze the drops into the ear canal. Keep your head tilted for 1 to 2 minutes. Then put a sterile cotton ball into your ear opening to hold the medication in.

To use *eyedrops or eye ointment,* gently clean any crusted matter from your eyes. Sit down, and if you're using eyedrops, tilt your head back. Gently pull down your lower lid to create a pocket. Carefully squeeze eyedrops or a thin strip of ointment into the pocket, then close your eyes gently. Don't blink. Keep your eyes closed for 1 to 2 minutes. After applying ointment, your vision may be blurred for a few minutes.

Before applying *skin cream,* wash the site with soap and water and dry it thoroughly.

What to do if you miss a dose
If you forget to take your *capsule* or *liquid,* take it as soon as you remember. But if it's almost time for your next dose and your dosing schedule is two doses a day, space the missed dose and the next dose 5 to 6 hours apart. If you take three or more doses a day, space the missed dose and the next dose 2 to 4 hours apart. Then resume your normal dosing schedule.

If you miss a dose of *ear, eye,* or *skin medication,* take it as soon as you remember. But if it's almost time for your next dose, skip the dose you missed and take your next dose at the scheduled time.

What to do about side effects
Serious blood problems (such as severe anemia, infections, and abnormal bleeding) may occur, particularly with long-term use of the *capsule, liquid, or*

(continued)

Taking chloramphenicol *(continued)*

cream forms. Promptly report fever, weakness, confusion, bleeding, sore throat, or mouth sores to your doctor.

If you develop signs and symptoms of an allergic reaction—fever, rash, itching, restlessness, difficulty swallowing or breathing—stop taking the medication and seek emergency medical care *immediately.*

Also stop using the medication and seek emergency medical care *immediately* if you're giving this medication to an infant who develops a swollen abdomen, breathing difficulties, extreme sleepiness, or grayish skin.

When using *eye medication,* be alert for itching, swelling, or persistent burning. With *ear medication,* be alert for ear pain or fever. With *skin cream,* watch for a rash, itching, or burning. If these effects occur, stop taking the medication and call your doctor.

What you must know about other drugs
Discuss other medications you're taking with your doctor. Acetaminophen (Tylenol), for example, affects the amount of chloramphenicol circulating in the blood, which may increase the drug's effects.

Special directions
• Inform the doctor if you have other medical problems, especially kidney or liver disease, bleeding problems, porphyria, or glucose-6-phosphate dehydrogenase (G6PD) deficiency. Before using chloramphenicol eardrops, tell the doctor if you've ever had a punctured or ruptured eardrum. Also report any allergic reactions to chloramphenicol or other medications or food.
• To ensure that your infection clears up completely, take this medication for the entire time prescribed, even when your symptoms subside.
• Have regular checkups and blood tests (especially if you're taking capsules or liquid chloramphenicol) so your doctor can monitor the medication's effectiveness and check for complications.
• If you don't notice improvement in a few days or if your symptoms worsen, notify your doctor.
• Check with your doctor before taking new medications (prescription or nonprescription) or if you develop new medical problems.
• Because of possible bleeding problems, be careful when brushing and flossing your teeth. If possible, delay dental procedures until you stop taking this medication.
• Don't share this medication—including the eye, ear, or skin forms—with anyone. Also, use separate washcloths and towels to prevent spreading the infection.

Important reminder
If you're pregnant or breast-feeding, tell your doctor before taking chloramphenicol.

Additional instructions

_____

_____

_____

_____

_____

_____

Taking chlordiazepoxide

Dear Patient:

Chlordiazepoxide is used to relieve mild to moderate anxiety and tension. Brand names may include Libritabs and Librium.

How to take chlordiazepoxide
This medication comes in tablets and capsules. Carefully read the medication label, and follow the directions exactly. Take this medication only as your doctor prescribes. Taking too much may lead to dependency.

What to do if you miss a dose
Take it as soon as you remember. But if it's almost time for the next dose, skip the dose you missed and take your next dose at the regular time. Don't take double doses.

What to do about side effects
You may feel drowsy or have a hang-over-like feeling. If these symptoms persist or worsen, tell your doctor.

What you must know about alcohol and other drugs
Remember to tell your doctor about other medications you're taking. And avoid using alcoholic beverages with this drug. Chlordiazepoxide increases the effects of alcohol and other drugs that depress the nervous system, including some allergy and cold remedies, seizure medications, and pain relievers.

Special directions
• Before starting chlordiazepoxide, inform the doctor if you're allergic to other medications (such as other benzodiazepines).

• Also inform the doctor about your medical history because certain disorders may affect chlordiazepoxide therapy. For example, a brain disease increases the risk for side effects, and sleep apnea may worsen with this medication.
• Make sure that you know how you respond to this medication before driving or performing other activities requiring alertness.
• If you think that this drug isn't helping you after a few weeks, consult your doctor. Don't increase the dosage on your own.
• If you're taking this medication for a long time, don't suddenly stop taking it; unpleasant withdrawal symptoms may occur. Consult your doctor to help you gradually reduce the dosage before completely stopping chlordiazepoxide.

Important reminders
If you're pregnant or breast-feeding, tell your doctor before taking chlordiazepoxide.

Children and older adults who take chlordiazepoxide may experience more side effects.

If you're an athlete, you should know that the National Collegiate Athletic Association and the U.S. Olympic Committee ban the use of chlordiazepoxide. Taking it may disqualify you from amateur athletic competitions.

Additional instructions

_____

_____

_____

Taking chlorothiazide

Dear Patient:

Chlorothiazide helps control high blood pressure. Also, by increasing urination, this drug relieves the body of excess water. The label may read Diuril.

How to take chlorothiazide

Read your medication label, and follow the directions exactly. Take a single daily dose in the morning after breakfast. If you're taking more than one dose a day, schedule the last dose by 6 p.m., unless your doctor directs otherwise.

If you're taking the liquid form, remember to shake the bottle well before pouring a dose.

What to do if you miss a dose

If you forget to take your medication, take it as soon as you remember. If it's almost time for your next dose, skip the dose you missed, and take your next dose at the regular time. Don't take double doses.

What to do about side effects

If you develop a persistent fever, sore throat, joint pain, unusual bruising or bleeding, or extreme listlessness or fatigue, stop taking chlorothiazide and call the doctor *immediately.*

More common side effects include jitteriness, muscle cramps, numbness and tingling, weakness, fatigue, increased urination and thirst, and sensitivity to sunlight. If these symptoms persist or worsen, call your doctor.

What you must know about other drugs

Tell your doctor about other medications (prescription and nonprescription) you're taking because some may reduce chlorothiazide's effectiveness.

Special directions

• Tell the doctor if you have other medical problems, particularly diabetes, gout, lupus, pancreatitis, and kidney or liver disease. Also report any allergies you have.
• If the doctor prescribes a special low-sodium diet (to help reduce your blood pressure), follow it closely.
• When you take this medication, your body will lose water and potassium. To prevent complications, your doctor may recommend potassium-rich foods (such as citrus fruits and bananas), a potassium supplement, or another medication.
• Notify your doctor if you have severe or continuing vomiting or diarrhea. These conditions can lead to increased potassium and water loss.
• If you're sensitive to light, protect yourself from direct sunlight.

Important reminders

Don't take this medication if you're pregnant or breast-feeding.

If you have diabetes, monitor your blood glucose levels carefully.

Older adults are especially sensitive to the effects of this medication.

If you're an athlete, you should know that the National Collegiate Athletic Association and the U.S. Olympic Committee ban the use of chlorothiazide.

Additional instructions

_____

_____

_____

_____

Taking chlorpheniramine

Dear Patient:

This medication can relieve or prevent hay fever and other allergy symptoms. Common brand names include Aller-Chlor, Chlorate, and Chlor-Trimeton.

How to take chlorpheniramine
This medication comes in tablet, chewable tablet, timed-release tablet or capsule, and syrup forms. Carefully read the medication label. Follow the directions exactly. To reduce possible stomach upset, you can take this medication with food or a full glass of milk or water.

If you're taking the timed-release tablets or capsules, swallow them whole — don't break, chew, or crush them. If you have trouble swallowing, consult your doctor, nurse, or pharmacist.

What to do if you miss a dose
If you forget to take your medication, take it as soon as you remember. If it's almost time for the next dose, skip the dose you missed, and take your next dose at the regular time. Don't take double doses.

What to do about side effects
You may feel jittery or drowsy, and your mouth may be dry. If these symptoms persist or worsen, tell your doctor.

What you must know about alcohol and other drugs
Tell your doctor about other medications you're taking. Avoid taking chlorpheniramine with alcoholic beverages, medications that depress the nervous system (some allergy and cold remedies, seizure medications, and pain relievers), and monoamine oxidase (MAO)

inhibitors, such as isocarboxazid (Marplan). Doing so increases unwanted side effects. Keep in mind, too, that chlorpheniramine may hide unwanted side effects of high-dose aspirin therapy (for arthritis, for example), such as ringing in the ears.

Special directions
• Before you undergo allergy tests, tell the doctor that you're taking this medication. Chlorpheniramine may affect test results.
• Relieve a dry mouth with ice chips or sugarless gum or hard candy.
• Make sure you know how you respond to this medication before you drive or perform other activities requiring alertness.

Important reminders
If you're breast-feeding, tell your doctor before taking this medication.

Children and older adults are especially sensitive to this medication's side effects.

Additional instructions

_____

_____

_____

_____

_____

_____

_____

_____

Taking chlorpromazine

Dear Patient:

Chlorpromazine is used to treat persistent hiccups, mild withdrawal from alcohol, tetanus, and certain mental and emotional disorders. The label may read Thorazine.

How to take chlorpromazine

Chlorpromazine comes in tablet, sustained-release capsule, concentrate, syrup, and suppository forms. Carefully read the medication label. Follow the directions exactly. You may take oral forms of this medication with food, milk, or water to minimize stomach upset.

Swallow a sustained-release capsule whole. Don't crush, chew, or break it.

Mix the concentrated form in 2 to 4 ounces of water, soda, juice, milk, pudding, or applesauce.

What to do if you miss a dose

If you forget to take your medication and you're taking one dose a day, take it as soon as you remember that day. If you don't remember it until the next day, skip the dose you missed and take your next regular dose.

If you're taking more than one dose a day and you remember it within an hour or so of the scheduled time, take it right away. If you don't remember it until later, skip the missed dose and take your next dose at the regular time.

What to do about side effects

If you have a persistent fever, sore throat, joint pain, or unusual bruising or bleeding, stop taking this medication and call the doctor *at once.*

Other possible side effects include unusual movements, such as lip smacking or jumpy arms and legs, blurred vision, dry mouth, constipation, inability to urinate, and sensitivity to sunlight. If any of these symptoms persist or worsen, call your doctor.

What you must know about alcohol and other drugs

Avoid alcoholic beverages or other drugs that depress the central nervous system because chlorpromazine intensifies their effect.

Tell the doctor about other medications you're taking because chlorpromazine may change the effects of other drugs. For example, it decreases the effects of drugs that lower blood pressure and prevent blood clots.

Special directions

• Check with your doctor before taking new medications (prescription or nonprescription).
• Before surgery, dental work, or emergency treatment, tell the doctor or dentist that you're taking this drug.
• Be sure of your response to this medication before performing activities requiring alertness and clear vision.
• If you become extra sensitive to light, protect yourself from direct sunlight.
• To relieve dry mouth, use ice chips or sugarless gum or hard candy.

Important reminders

If you're pregnant or breast-feeding, tell your doctor before using chlorpromazine.

Children and older adults are especially sensitive to side effects from chlorpromazine.

Taking chlorpropamide

Dear Patient:

Because you have diabetes, your doctor has prescribed chlorpropamide to lower your blood glucose level. Brand names for this drug include Diabinese and Glucamide.

How to take chlorpropamide
Chlorpropamide comes in tablets. Take it exactly as ordered. Don't take more or less of it. And take it at the same time each day.

What to do if you miss a dose
Take it as soon as possible. But if it's almost time for your next dose, skip the missed dose and take the next one on schedule. Don't take two doses together.

What to do about side effects
Low blood glucose may occur while you use this medication. Watch for symptoms, such as cool pale skin, difficulty concentrating, shakiness, headache, cold sweats, or feelings of anxiety.

If your blood glucose level drops too low, eat or drink something sugary, such as glucose tablets or fruit juice. If you don't feel better within 15 minutes, eat or drink some more sugary food and call your doctor *right away*.

Tell your doctor if you experience nausea, vomiting, or heartburn. Also tell him if you develop a rash or other allergic reactions.

What you must know about alcohol and other drugs
Avoid drinking alcohol, except in amounts your doctor permits, because combined use of chlorpropamide and alcohol may make you ill or cause your blood glucose level to drop.

Talk to your doctor before taking any other prescription or nonprescription medications. Many medications can react with chlorpropamide to make your blood glucose too high or too low. In general, you need to avoid certain antidepressants; sulfonamides (sulfa medications); chloramphenicol (Chloromycetin), an antibiotic; blood thinners; steroids; glucagon (a hormone); and water pills.

Also, taking chlorpropamide with certain medications for high blood pressure may cover up symptoms of low blood glucose or make a bout of low blood glucose last longer. In addition, aspirin-containing products, appetite-control medications, and cough or cold medications may alter your blood glucose control.

Special directions
• Tell your doctor if you have other medical problems, especially if you're taking insulin. Let him know if you have a heart, liver, or kidney condition.
• Carefully follow your special meal plan because this is the most important part of controlling your diabetes. It's also necessary for chlorpropamide to work well.
• Test for glucose in your blood or urine as your doctor directs. Regular testing lets you know your diabetes is under control—and warns you when it's not.
• This medication may increase your sensitivity to sunlight, so limit your exposure to the sun.

Important reminders
If you're pregnant, check with your doctor before taking this medication. Don't use chlorpropamide if you're breast-feeding. If you're an older adult, you may be especially prone to chlorpropamide's side effects.

Taking cholestyramine

Dear Patient:

Your doctor has prescribed cholestyramine to lower your blood cholesterol level and to remove substances called bile acids from your body. Other names for this medication include Cholybar, Questran, and Questran Light.

How to take cholestyramine

Cholestyramine comes as a chewable bar and a powder.

If you're taking the *powder* form of this medication, follow these steps:
• First, mix the medication with liquid. Never take it in its dry form because you might choke.
• Place the prescribed dose in 2 ounces of any beverage and stir thoroughly.
• Add an additional 2 to 4 ounces of beverage and again mix thoroughly (it won't dissolve). Drink the liquid.
• After drinking all the liquid, rinse the glass with a little more liquid and drink that also.

You may also mix the powder with milk in hot or regular breakfast cereals or in thin soups. Or add it to pulpy fruits, such as crushed pineapple or fruit cocktail.

If you're taking the *chewable bar* form of this medication, chew each bite well before swallowing.

Don't stop taking cholestyramine without first checking with your doctor.

What to do if you miss a dose

Take it as soon as possible. But if it's almost time for your next dose, skip the missed dose and take the next dose on schedule. Don't double dose.

What to do about side effects

You may experience constipation, nausea, or rashes. Check with your doctor if these symptoms persist or become bothersome.

What you must know about other drugs

Tell your doctor about other medications you're taking. Many medications may not be absorbed well if taken at the same time as cholestyramine. Examples include acetaminophen (Tylenol), certain blood thinners, beta blockers, corticosteroids, digoxin (Lanoxin), fat-soluble vitamins (A, D, E, and K), iron preparations, some water pills, and thyroid hormone. If possible, take cholestyramine 2 hours before or after taking other medication to prevent this problem.

Special directions

• Because cholestyramine can make certain medical problems worse, tell your doctor if you have gallbladder disease or a history of constipation or digestive problems.
• Also let your doctor know if you're allergic to tartrazine (a yellow food dye) because the powder form of this medication contains tartrazine.
• This medication may not work well if you're very overweight, so you may be advised to go on a reducing diet. However, check with your doctor before starting any diet.

Important reminders

If you're pregnant or breast-feeding, check with your doctor before taking this medication. If you're an older adult, you may be especially prone to side effects.

Taking cimetidine

Dear Patient:

This medication treats ulcers and may prevent their return. It may also be used to treat Zollinger-Ellison disease, an illness in which the stomach makes too much acid. The medication label may read Tagamet.

How to take cimetidine
Cimetidine is available as an oral solution or tablets.

Carefully check the prescription label, and follow the directions as ordered. If you're taking this medication once a day, take it at bedtime, unless otherwise directed. If you're taking two doses a day, take one in the morning and one at bedtime. If you're taking more than two doses a day, take them with meals and at bedtime for best results.

What to do if you miss a dose
Take it as soon as possible. But if it's almost time for your next dose, skip the missed dose and take your next dose as scheduled. Don't double dose.

What to do about side effects
Contact your doctor *immediately* if you've been told that your complete blood count is abnormal or you develop signs and symptoms of infection or bleeding. A common side effect is mild, temporary diarrhea. If this symptom doesn't go away or becomes severe, call your doctor.

What you must know about other drugs
Tell your doctor about other medications you're taking. Antacids may interfere with the absorption of cimetidine.

Also, cimetidine can interfere with the breakdown of other medications in your body, including warfarin (Coumadin), a blood thinner; phenytoin (Dilantin), a seizure medication; some sedatives; theophylline (Theo-Dur), an asthma medication; and propranolol (Inderal), a heart and high blood pressure medication.

Special directions
• Tell your doctor if you have other medical problems, especially kidney and liver disease.
• Realize that several days may pass before cimetidine begins to relieve your stomach pain. In the meantime, you may take antacids, unless your doctor has told you not to use them. Wait 30 minutes to 1 hour between taking the antacid and cimetidine.
• Tell the doctor that you're taking this medication before you have skin tests for allergies or tests to determine how much acid your stomach produces.
• Avoid cigarette smoking because it reduces the effectiveness of cimetidine.
• Contact your doctor if your ulcer pain continues or gets worse while taking cimetidine.

Important reminders
If you're pregnant or breast-feeding, talk to your doctor before you use this medication. If you're an older adult, you may be especially prone to cimetidine's side effects.

Additional instructions

_____

_____

Taking cinoxacin

Dear Patient:

This medication helps treat and prevent infections of the urinary tract. The medication label may read Cinobac.

How to take cinoxacin
Available in capsule form, cinoxacin is typically taken in two to four doses daily. Follow your doctor's directions exactly. Take this medication with meals or snacks, unless otherwise directed by your doctor.

Take your doses at evenly spaced times, day and night, to keep a constant amount of cinoxacin in your body.

Continue taking this medication for the full time of treatment, even if you start to feel better. If you stop taking it too soon, your infection might return.

What to do if you miss a dose
Take it as soon as possible. But if it's almost time for your next dose, adjust your dosing schedule as follows.

If you're taking two doses a day, space the missed dose and the next dose 5 to 6 hours apart.

If you're taking three or more doses a day, space the missed dose and the next dose 2 to 4 hours apart. Then resume your regular dosing schedule.

What to do about side effects
This medication may make you dizzy or cause headache, nausea, vomiting, or abdominal pain. Check with your doctor if you have these side effects, especially if they persist or become severe.

What you must know about other drugs
Tell your doctor about other medications you're taking. If you take probenecid (Probalan), a gout medication, you may be at special risk for cinoxacin's side effects.

Special directions
• Because certain medical problems may interfere with the use of cinoxacin, tell your doctor if you have other medical problems, especially kidney disease. Let him know if you've ever had an allergic reaction to this medication.
• If your symptoms don't improve within a few days or if they get worse, check with your doctor.
• This medication makes some people dizzy. Be sure you know how you react to cinoxacin before you drive, use machines, or perform other hazardous activities that require alertness.

Important reminders
If you're pregnant or breast-feeding, don't take this medication without checking first with your doctor.

Don't give cinoxacin to children under age 12 unless otherwise directed by your doctor because it may interfere with bone development.

Additional instructions

_____

_____

_____

_____

_____

_____

Taking ciprofloxacin

Dear Patient:

Your doctor has ordered ciprofloxacin to treat a bacterial infection in your body. The label may read Cipro.

How to take ciprofloxacin
This medication is available in tablets.

Carefully check the label on your prescription, and follow the directions exactly. Take your dose with a full glass of water. You may take it with meals or on an empty stomach. Take this medication at evenly spaced times, day and night, to keep a constant amount in your body.

Keep taking ciprofloxacin for the full time of treatment, even if you begin to feel better after a few days. If you stop taking it too soon, your symptoms may return.

What to do if you miss a dose
Take it as soon as possible. But if it's almost time for your next dose, skip the missed dose and take your next dose on schedule. Don't double dose.

What to do about side effects
Call your doctor *right away* if you experience a seizure while taking this medication. Check with your doctor if you have nausea, diarrhea, or a skin rash.

What you must know about other drugs
Tell your doctor about other medications you're taking. Antacids containing magnesium hydroxide or aluminum hydroxide may decrease the absorption of ciprofloxacin. Therefore, if you take these antacids, take them 2 hours before or after taking ciprofloxacin. Probenecid (Probalan), a gout medication, may increase the risk of side effects from ciprofloxacin. Ciprofloxacin may increase the blood levels of theophylline (Theo-Dur), an asthma medication, which could lead to side effects.

Special directions
• Before taking ciprofloxacin, tell your doctor if you have other medical problems, especially conditions that cause seizures. Also reveal if you've ever had an allergic reaction to ciprofloxacin or another medication.
• Drink several extra glasses of water every day while taking this medication, unless your doctor gives you other directions. Drinking extra water will help to prevent side effects.
• If your symptoms don't improve within a few days or if they become worse, check with your doctor.
• Ciprofloxacin may make you more sensitive than usual to sunlight, so limit your exposure to direct sun.
• This medication may make you dizzy or drowsy. Make sure you know how you react to it before you drive, use machines, or perform other activities that require full alertness.

Important reminders
Don't take this medication if you're pregnant or breast-feeding unless instructed by your doctor. Also, don't give it to infants, children, or adolescents unless instructed by your doctor.

Additional instructions

_____

_____

Taking clemastine

Dear Patient:

Your doctor has prescribed clemastine to relieve your hay fever or other allergy. If you're taking the *syrup* form, the label may read Tavist. If you're taking the *tablets,* the label may read Tavist-1.

How to take clemastine
Carefully check the prescription label, and take the medication exactly as ordered. Take it with food, water, or milk to lessen stomach irritation.

What to do if you miss a dose
If you take this medication regularly and you miss a dose, take it as soon as possible. But if it's almost time for your next dose, skip the missed dose and take your next dose on schedule. Don't double dose.

What to do about side effects
Call your doctor *immediately* if you've been told your complete blood count is abnormal or if you develop a fever, shortness of breath, or bleeding. This medication may also make you feel drowsy or cause dryness of your mouth. Call your doctor if these symptoms persist or become severe.

What you must know about alcohol and other drugs
Don't drink alcoholic beverages while taking this medication. Doing so could cause you to become oversedated.

Tell your doctor about other medications you're taking. Depressants (medications that slow down your central nervous system) may increase the sedative effect of clemastine. Don't use clemastine if you take monoamine oxidase (MAO) inhibitors.

Also let your doctor know if you take large amounts of aspirin, such as for arthritis pain. Clemastine may cover up warning signs of aspirin overdose.

Special directions
• Because this medication can aggravate certain conditions, tell your doctor if you have other medical problems, especially asthma, glaucoma, an enlarged prostate, bladder problems, or difficulty urinating. Also reveal if you have heart disease, an overactive thyroid, diabetes, or stomach ulcers.
• Inform the doctor that you're taking this medication before you have skin tests for allergies because clemastine may alter the test results.
• Make sure you know how you react to clemastine before you drive, use machines, or perform other activities that require alertness.
• If you experience dry mouth with this medication, try using sugarless hard candy or gum, ice chips, or a saliva substitute. If your dry mouth lasts for more than 2 weeks, check with your doctor or dentist.

Important reminders
If you're pregnant or breast-feeding, don't use clemastine unless your doctor instructs you otherwise.

Be aware that children and older adults are especially sensitive to the effects of clemastine and therefore more likely to develop side effects.

Additional instructions

_____

_____

Taking clindamycin

Dear Patient:

Your doctor has prescribed clindamycin to treat your bacterial infection. If you're taking the *oral* form of this medication, such as a capsule or liquid, the label may read Cleocin. If you're applying *topical* clindamycin to your skin, the label may read Cleocin T Gel, Cleocin T Lotion, or Cleocin T Topical Solution.

How to take clindamycin
If you're taking *capsules,* take them with a full glass (8 ounces) of water or with meals. If you're using the *oral solution,* measure your dose with a specially marked measuring spoon, not a household teaspoon.

Before you apply topical clindamycin, wash the affected skin and pat dry. If you're using the *gel* or *lotion,* apply a thin film of medication.

If you're using the *topical solution,* wait 30 minutes after washing or shaving before applying this medication because the alcohol it contains may sting.

Avoid getting this medication in your eyes, nose, or mouth.

Keep taking your medication for the full time of treatment, even if you start to feel better. Stopping too soon might allow your infection to return.

What to do if you miss a dose
If you miss an *oral* dose, take it as soon as possible. But if it's almost time for your next dose (and you take three or more doses a day), space the missed dose and the next dose 2 to 4 hours apart. Then go back to your regular dosing schedule.

If you miss a *topical* dose, apply it as soon as possible. But if it's almost time for your next dose, skip the missed dose and apply your next dose on schedule.

What to do about side effects
Call your doctor *right away* if you have:
• severe, bloody diarrhea
• abdominal pain, with vomiting
• black, tarry, or bloody stools
• signs of an allergic reaction: chest tightness, wheezing, hives, itching, or a rash.

Check with your doctor if you have nausea, mild diarrhea, or difficulty swallowing.

What you must know about other drugs
Tell your doctor about other medications you're taking. Erythromycin (another antibiotic) may prevent clindamycin from working properly. Also avoid the use of kaolin (an ingredient in some diarrhea medications) because it decreases the absorption of clindamycin.

Special directions
• Tell your doctor if you have other medical problems, especially diseases of the liver, kidney, stomach, or intestines. Also reveal if you have asthma or allergies.
• Before having surgery (including dental surgery) with a general anesthetic, tell the doctor or dentist in charge that you're taking clindamycin.

Important reminder
If you're pregnant or breast-feeding, check with your doctor before using this medication.

Additional instructions

_____

_____

Taking clofibrate

Dear Patient:

Your doctor has prescribed clofibrate to lower the cholesterol and triglyceride (fatlike substances) levels in your blood. Brand names include Abitrate and Atromid-S.

How to take clofibrate
This medication comes in capsules. Take clofibrate exactly as your doctor orders. Don't break, chew, or crush the capsules—swallow them whole. Take clofibrate with food or right after meals to lessen possible stomach upset.

Don't stop taking clofibrate abruptly without first checking with your doctor.

What to do if you miss a dose
Take it as soon as possible. But if it's almost time for your next dose, skip the missed dose and take your next dose on schedule. Don't double dose.

What to do about side effects
Call your doctor *immediately* if you develop flulike symptoms, such as fever or aches and pains.

Check with your doctor if you gain weight or experience diarrhea, heartburn, increased appetite, nausea, or vomiting.

What you must know about other drugs
Tell your doctor about other medications you're taking. Clofibrate can increase the effects of certain medications, including water pills, blood thinners, and diabetes medication. Clofibrate also shouldn't be used with certain cholesterol-lowering drugs, such as lovastatin (Mevacor).

Clofibrate may not work properly if you take birth control pills or rifampin (Rifadin), a tuberculosis medication. Also, taking clofibrate with probenicid (Probalan), a gout medication, may cause serious side effects.

Special directions
• Tell your doctor if you have other medical problems, especially kidney or liver disease or peptic ulcers.
• When you stop using clofibrate, your blood fat levels may rise again. To prevent this, your doctor may want you to follow a special diet.
• Keep all appointments for follow-up visits so your doctor can check to make sure your medication is working well. Also have your blood cholesterol and triglyceride levels measured regularly.

Important reminders
If you're pregnant or think you may be, check with your doctor before taking this medication. Also, don't use clofibrate if you're breast-feeding because it can cause unwanted side effects in the breast-feeding infant.

Don't give this medication to children under age 2 because cholesterol is needed for normal development.

Additional instructions

_____

_____

_____

_____

_____

Taking clonazepam

Dear Patient:

Your doctor has prescribed this medication to help your condition. Clonazepam acts on the nervous system to prevent seizures. A common brand name for clonazepam is Klonopin.

How to take clonazepam
Clonazepam is available in tablet form. Carefully check the prescription label, and follow the directions exactly. Don't take more than the prescribed amount.

Take this medication faithfully every day in regularly spaced doses.

What to do if you miss a dose
If you're taking this medication regularly and you miss a dose, take it as soon as possible. However, if it's almost time for your next dose, skip the missed dose and take your next dose on schedule. Don't double dose.

What to do about side effects
Get emergency help *at once* if you have the following signs of overdose: slurred speech, confusion, severe drowsiness, and staggering.

Also call your doctor *at once* if this medication starts to slow your breathing or makes breathing difficult. Check with your doctor if you become drowsy, your mouth starts to water, or you notice odd changes in your behavior.

What you must know about alcohol and other drugs
Tell your doctor about other medications you're taking. Don't drink alcoholic beverages while taking clonazepam because the combination may cause oversedation. For the same reason, avoid other central nervous system depressants (that slow down your nervous system) while using clonazepam. Examples of depressants include sleeping pills, tranquilizers, narcotic painkillers, and many cold and flu medications.

Special directions
• Tell your doctor about your medical history, especially if you have liver or lung disease, kidney problems, or glaucoma.
• See your doctor regularly to determine if you need to continue taking this medication because it may become habit-forming.
• Your doctor may want you to carry medical identification stating that you're taking this medication.
• Before any medical tests, tell the doctor that you're taking clonazepam because it may alter the test results.
• Because this medication can make you drowsy, make sure you know how you react to it before you drive, use machines, or perform other hazardous activities that require alertness.

Important reminders
If you're pregnant or breast-feeding, check with your doctor before taking this medication.

If you're an athlete, you should know that use of clonazepam is banned by the National Collegiate Athletic Association and the U.S. Olympic Committee.

Additional instructions

_____

_____

Taking clonidine

Dear Patient:

Your doctor has prescribed clonidine to treat your high blood pressure. If you're taking the *tablet* form of this medication, the label may read Catapres. If you're using the *skin patch,* the label may read Catapres-TTS.

How to take clonidine
If you're taking the *tablets,* take them at the same times each day. Even if you feel well, continue to take clonidine exactly as directed.

If you're using the *skin patch,* apply it to a clean, dry, hairless area on your upper arm or chest. Change the patch every 7 days or as often as your doctor orders. Place the patch at a different site every week to prevent skin irritation. Be sure to read the instructions that come with the patches.

What to do if you miss a dose
Take it as soon as you remember. Then go back to your regular dosing schedule.

If you miss two or more tablet doses in a row or if you miss changing the skin patch for 3 or more days, check with your doctor right away. If you go too long without clonidine, your blood pressure may rise, possibly causing unpleasant effects.

What to do about side effects
Call your doctor *at once* if you experience a severe headache, visual changes, or extreme dizziness. Also check with your doctor if you become drowsy or constipated or your mouth feels dry.

If you're using the skin patch, you may experience itching or a rash. If these symptoms persist or become severe, call your doctor.

What you must know about alcohol and other drugs
Don't drink alcoholic beverages, except in amounts permitted by your doctor, while taking clonidine because the combination may cause oversedation. Similarly, central nervous system depressants, such as sleeping pills and tranquilizers, may cause oversedation when used with clonidine.

If you're taking clonidine with propranolol (Inderal) or other beta blockers, these medications may raise your blood pressure when taken together. Also, clonidine may not work properly when taken with certain antidepressants.

Special directions
• Tell your doctor if you have other medical problems, especially heart or kidney disease, diabetes, or depression.
• Keep all appointments for follow-up visits, so your doctor can check your progress.
• If you're using the skin patch, keep it on while showering, bathing, or swimming. If it loosens, cover it with the extra adhesive provided.
• Because clonidine may make you drowsy, make sure you know how you react to it before you drive, use machines, or perform other hazardous activities that require alertness.

Important reminders
If you're pregnant or breast-feeding, check with your doctor before taking this medication. If you're an older adult, realize that this medication may make you dizzy or faint. Take care to prevent falls.

Taking clorazepate

Dear Patient:

Your doctor has prescribed clorazepate to help your condition. This medication is used to prevent seizures in people with seizure disorders and to relieve extreme feelings of nervousness or tension. Brand names include Gen-XENE, Tranxene-SD, and Tranxene T-Tab.

How to take clorazepate
This medication comes in tablet or capsule form.

Follow your doctor's instructions exactly. Don't take more, and don't take it more often or longer than the label directs because this medication can be habit-forming.

If you're taking clorazepate for a seizure disorder, take it every day in regularly spaced doses, as ordered.

What to do if you miss a dose
Take it as soon as possible. But if it's almost time for your next dose, skip the missed dose and take your next dose on schedule. Don't double dose.

What to do about side effects
Get emergency help *at once* if you have these symptoms of an overdose: slurred speech, confusion, severe drowsiness, and staggering. Check with your doctor if this medication makes you feel drowsy, lethargic, or like you have a hangover.

What you must know about alcohol and other drugs
Tell your doctor about other medications you're taking. Avoid alcoholic beverages and other central nervous system depressants (medications that slow down your nervous system) while taking clorazepate because this combination may cause oversedation. Cimetidine (Tagamet), an ulcer medication, may also cause increased drowsiness when used with clorazepate.

Special directions
• Tell your doctor if you have other medical problems, especially glaucoma, myasthenia gravis, Parkinson's disease, or kidney or liver disease. Also reveal if you have a history of mental illness or drug abuse.
• If you're taking this medication for a long time, don't stop taking it without first checking with your doctor.
• If you're taking clorazepate for a seizure disorder, your doctor may want you to carry medical identification stating that you're taking it.
• Before you have medical tests, tell the doctor that you're taking clorazepate because this drug may alter the test results.
• Because this medication can make you drowsy, make sure you know how you react to it before you drive, use machines, or perform other hazardous activities that require alertness.

Important reminders
If you're pregnant or breast-feeding, check with your doctor before taking this medication. If you're an older adult, be aware that you may be especially prone to side effects.

If you're an athlete, you should know that clorazepate use is banned by the National Collegiate Athletic Association and the U.S. Olympic Committee.

Taking clotrimazole

Dear Patient:

Your doctor has prescribed clotrimazole to treat your fungal infection. If you're taking clotrimazole *lozenges,* the label may read Mycelex Troches. If you're using a *topical lotion, cream,* or *solution* on your skin, the medication may be called Lotrimin or Mycelex. If you're taking this medication for a *vaginal* infection, the label may read Gyne-Lotrimin.

How to take clotrimazole

If you're taking the *lozenge* form, hold the lozenge in your mouth and allow it to dissolve slowly and completely. This may take 15 to 30 minutes. Try not to swallow your saliva during this time. Don't chew the lozenges or swallow them whole.

If you're applying *topical* clotrimazole to your skin, apply enough to cover the area, and rub it in gently. Avoid getting it in your eyes. Don't put a bandage over the treated area unless instructed by your doctor.

If you're using the *vaginal* form, fill the applicator with cream to the level indicated or unwrap a tablet, wet it with lukewarm water, and place it on the applicator.

Continue to take your medication, even if your symptoms clear up in a few days. Otherwise, your infection may return. Because fungal infections may be slow to clear up, you may need to take your medication every day for several weeks or more.

What to do if you miss a dose

Take it as soon as possible. However, if it's almost time for your next dose, skip the missed dose and take your next dose on schedule.

What to do about side effects

If you're using the *lozenges,* check with your doctor if you experience nausea and vomiting.

If you're applying the *topical* form of this medication, call your doctor if redness, blistering, or swelling occurs. Also call if the treated area burns or stings.

If you're using the *vaginal* form, check with your doctor if you feel burning or irritation in your vagina.

Special directions

• Tell your doctor if you have other medical problems, especially liver disease. Also mention if you're allergic to this medication.
• If you're using the lozenges and your symptoms don't go away within 1 week or they become worse, check with your doctor. If you're using clotrimazole for a skin infection, check with your doctor if your symptoms haven't gone away within 4 weeks.
• If you're using the lozenges, tell the doctor before you have liver tests; this medication may alter the test results.

Important reminders

Don't give clotrimazole lozenges to children under age 5. They may be too young to use them safely.

If you're pregnant, don't use the vaginal form of this medication without first checking with your doctor.

Additional instructions

Taking cloxacillin

Dear Patient:

Your doctor has prescribed cloxacillin (a form of penicillin) to treat your bacterial infection. Brand names include Cloxapen and Tegopen.

How to take cloxacillin
This medication comes in capsules and an oral solution. If you're taking the *capsules,* don't break, chew, or crush them—swallow them whole. If you're taking the *oral* solution, use a dropper or specially marked measuring spoon to measure each dose accurately.

Take your dose with a full glass (8 ounces) of water on an empty stomach, either 1 hour before or 2 hours after meals, unless your doctor tells you otherwise. Don't take your dose with fruit juice or carbonated drinks; doing so may prevent cloxacillin from working.

Keep taking your medication, even after you start to feel better. Stopping too soon may allow your infection to return.

What to do if you miss a dose
Take it as soon as possible. But if it's almost time for your next dose, adjust your dosing schedule as follows.

If you take two doses a day, space the missed dose and the next dose 5 to 6 hours apart.

If you take three or more doses a day, space the missed dose and the next dose 2 to 4 hours apart.

Then resume your regular dosing schedule.

What to do about side effects
Call your doctor *at once* if you develop any symptoms of an allergic reaction to this medication, such as difficulty breathing, skin rash, hives, itching, or wheezing.

If you develop nausea, heartburn, or diarrhea, check with your doctor, especially if these symptoms persist or become severe.

What you must know about other drugs
Tell the doctor about other medications you're taking. If you're taking probenecid (Probalan), a gout medication, your blood levels of cloxacillin may increase. This may or may not be a beneficial effect; check with your doctor.

If you develop severe diarrhea, don't take any diarrhea medications without first checking with your doctor. Some of these medications may make your diarrhea worse.

Special directions
• Tell your doctor about your medical history, especially if you're allergic to other antibiotics, including penicillins, cephalosporins, and griseofulvin. Also reveal if you have kidney disease.
• If you become allergic to cloxacillin, you should carry medical identification stating this.
• Before you have medical tests, tell the doctor that you're taking cloxacillin because this medication may interfere with some test results.

Important reminder
If you're pregnant or breast-feeding, check with your doctor before using this medication.

Additional instructions

_____

_____

Taking colestipol

Dear Patient:

Your doctor has prescribed colestipol to lower your blood cholesterol level. The label may read Colestid.

How to take colestipol

This medication comes in powder form.

Never take colestipol in its dry form because it might cause choking. Instead, follow these steps:

• Add the proper amount of colestipol to at least 3 ounces of your favorite drink. However, if you use a carbonated drink, slowly mix the powder in a large glass to prevent excess foaming.

• Stir until the medication is completely mixed (it won't dissolve). Then drink.

• After drinking all the liquid, rinse the glass with a little more liquid and drink that also, to make sure you get all the medication.

You may also mix colestipol with thin soups, milk in hot or cold cereals, or pulpy fruits, such as crushed pineapple, pears, or fruit cocktail.

What to do if you miss a dose

Take it as soon as possible. But if it's almost time for your next dose, skip the missed dose and go back to your regular dosing schedule. Don't double dose.

What to do about side effects

Constipation is the most common side effect of this medication. If it persists or becomes severe, check with your doctor about decreasing your dosage of colestipol.

What you must know about other drugs

Tell your doctor about other medications you're taking. Colestipol may decrease the absorption of any medication that you take by mouth. Therefore, if you take another oral medication, take it least 1 hour before or 4 hours after you take colestipol. Also, certain drugs for diabetes may prevent colestipol from working properly.

Special directions

• Tell your doctor about your medical history, especially if you have problems with your liver, gallbladder, or digestive tract.

• Carefully follow the special diet your doctor has given you, which is necessary for colestipol to work properly.

• See your doctor regularly so that he can check your cholesterol level and decide if you should continue to take this medication.

• If constipation develops, eat more fiber-rich foods, such as fruits, vegetables, and whole-grain cereals. Also, check with your doctor about using a stool softener.

• Don't stop taking colestipol without first checking with your doctor. When you stop taking it, your blood cholesterol level may rise again. Your doctor may want you to follow a special diet to help prevent this from happening.

Important reminders

If you're pregnant, check with the doctor before taking this medication. If you're an older adult, be aware that you may be especially sensitive to side effects from colestipol.

Additional instructions

_____

_____

Taking co-trimoxazole

Dear Patient:

Your doctor has precribed this antibiotic medication to treat your bacterial infection. Brand names include Bactrim, Cotrim, Septra, and Sulfamethoprim.

How to take co-trimoxazole

Co-trimoxazole is available in tablets and an oral suspension. Take the tablets or oral suspension with a full glass (8 ounces) of water.

If you have trouble swallowing the *tablet* form, you may crush it and take it with water. If you're taking the *oral suspension,* shake the bottle well before using. Use a specially marked spoon or dropper, not a household teaspoon, to measure the correct dose.

Keep taking co-trimoxazole, even after you begin to feel better. If you stop too soon, the infection may return.

What to do if you miss a dose

Take it as soon as possible. However, if it's almost time for your next dose, adjust your schedule as follows.

If you're taking two doses a day, space the skipped dose and the next dose 6 hours apart.

If you're taking three or more doses each day, space the skipped dose and the next dose 2 to 4 hours apart.

Then resume your regular schedule.

What to do about side effects

Get emergency help *at once* if you have symptoms of an allergic reaction, such as difficulty breathing, wheezing, or hives.

Stop taking this medication and call your doctor *right away* if you have a persistent fever, a sore throat, or joint pain; feel extremely tired; start to bleed; or start to bruise easily. Check with your doctor if you experience skin problems, nausea, vomiting, or diarrhea.

What you must know about other drugs

You shouldn't take this medication with vitamin C because it may make co-trimoxazole ineffective. Taking co-trimoxazole can increase the effects of certain medications, especially blood thinners and certain drugs for diabetes. Co-trimoxazole may also prevent birth control pills from working well. Use another form of birth control.

Special directions

• Tell your doctor about your medical history, especially if you have kidney or liver problems, porphyria, severe allergies, asthma, or acquired immunodeficiency syndrome (AIDS). Also reveal if you're allergic to this medication or other sulfa drugs.
• Drink extra water—up to 3 to 4 quarts daily—to prevent side effects, such as kidney stones, from this medication.
• Co-trimoxazole may make you more sensitive to sunlight, so try to avoid exposure to direct sunlight.

Important reminders

If you're pregnant or breast-feeding, talk to your doctor before using this medication.

If you have diabetes and take co-trimoxazole, be aware that you may need to test your urine glucose with a glucose enzymatic test, such as Clinistix or Tes-Tape, because copper sulfate tests may give false-positive results.

Taking cromolyn

Dear Patient:

Cromolyn is used to prevent asthma attacks, to relieve allergies, and to treat a rare condition called mastocytosis. Cromolyn comes in several forms: oral capsules (called Gastrocrom), nasal solution or powder (Nasalcrom), inhalation (Intal), or eyedrops (Opticrom).

How to take cromolyn
If you're taking the *oral capsules,* dissolve the capsule contents in 4 ounces of hot water. Stir until the powder completely dissolves and the solution is clear. Add an equal amount of cold water to the solution. Don't mix your dose with fruit juice, milk, or foods. Doing so may prevent your medication from working well.

If you're using the *inhalation aerosol,* read the directions before using. Keep the spray away from your eyes.

If you're using *capsules for inhalation,* never swallow them. Read the directions before using the special inhaler.

If you're using the *solution for inhalation,* use this medication only in a power-operated nebulizer with an adequate flow rate and a face mask or mouthpiece. Make sure you understand exactly how to use it. Hand-operated nebulizers aren't used with this medication.

If you're using the *nasal* forms, first clear your nasal passages by blowing your nose. To use the nasal forms, you need special spray devices. Read the package instructions.

To use the *eyedrops,* wash your hands, then tilt your head back and pull the lower eyelid away from the eye to form a pouch. Squeeze the drops into the pouch and close the eye. Don't blink. Keep the treated eye closed for 1 to 2 minutes. Don't touch the applicator tip to any surface.

Don't use cromolyn more often than your doctor ordered. It may take at least 1 week before you feel better if you have hay fever. If you have chronic allergic rhinitis, it may take up to 1 month.

What to do if you miss a dose
Take it as soon as possible. Then take any remaining doses for that day at regularly spaced intervals. Don't double dose.

What to do about side effects
If you're using the powder form for nasal inhalation, *call for emergency help* if you start to wheeze and have difficulty breathing after using this medication.

Any form may make you cough or cause soreness or dryness of the mouth and throat. If these symptoms persist, call your doctor.

What you must know about other drugs
If you have asthma, you may be taking cromolyn along with an adrenocorticoid (such as cortisone [Cortone Acetate] or prednisone [Deltasone]). If so, don't stop taking the adrenocorticoid, even if your asthma seems better, unless your doctor tells you to do so.

Special directions
• Tell your doctor if you have other medical problems, especially asthma or diseases of the heart, kidney, or liver.
• If your mouth or throat feels dry or irritated after using cromolyn, gargle after each dose.

Important reminder
If you're pregnant or breast-feeding, check with your doctor before taking this medication.

Taking cyclobenzaprine

Dear Patient:

This medication is a muscle relaxant. It's given to relieve muscle pain, stiffness, and discomfort caused by strains, sprains, or injuries. The label may read Flexeril.

How to take cyclobenzaprine
Cyclobenzaprine comes in tablet form. Carefully check the label on your prescription bottle, which tells you how much medication to take. Follow the directions exactly as ordered.

What to do if you miss a dose
If you remember within an hour or so of the missed dose, take it right away. Then go back to your regular dosing schedule. But if you don't remember until later, skip the missed dose and take your next dose on schedule. Don't take two doses together.

What to do about side effects
Drowsiness is the most common side effect of cyclobenzaprine. If it persists or becomes severe, call your doctor. Also check with your doctor if you develop constipation, heartburn, or abdominal pain, or if your mouth feels dry.

What you must know about alcohol and other drugs
Avoid drinking alcohol while you're taking cyclobenzaprine because the combination may cause oversedation. For the same reason, avoid using other central nervous system depressants (medications that slow down your nervous system), such as tranquilizers, sedatives, sleeping aids, and many medications for hay fever, colds, and flu.

Check with your doctor before you take other prescription or nonprescription medications.

Special directions
• Tell your doctor if you have other medical problems, especially heart, kidney, or liver disease; an overactive thyroid gland; glaucoma; or difficulty urinating.
• Because cyclobenzaprine can cause drowsiness, make sure you know how you react to it before you drive, use machines, or perform other activities that require alertness.
• If this medication makes your mouth feel dry, you may use sugarless hard candy or gum, ice chips, or a saliva substitute. However, if your dry mouth lasts for more than 2 weeks, check with your doctor or dentist. Continuing dryness of the mouth may increase the chance of tooth decay, gum disease, and fungal infections.
• If you're constipated from using cyclobenzaprine, try drinking several extra glasses of water daily. If that doesn't help, check with your doctor about using a stool softener.

Important reminder
If you're an athlete, be aware that use of this medication is banned in biathlon and modern pentathlon events by the U.S. Olympic Committee.

Additional instructions

_____

_____

_____

Taking cyclosporine

Dear Patient:

To keep your transplant functioning normally, your doctor has prescribed cyclosporine. This medication is also known as Sandimmune.

How to take cyclosporine

Cyclosporine comes in liquid or capsules. If you take the *liquid* form, measure your dose precisely. Each milliliter of liquid contains 100 milligrams of cyclosporine. Store the liquid at room temperature to prevent it from becoming too thick.

If you wish, mix your dose in a glass container with fruit juice (preferably at room temperature) or milk to make it taste better. Stir it well and drink it immediately. Then rinse the glass with a little more liquid and drink that also to make sure you take all the medication.

If you take the *capsules,* you should know that they come in two strengths: 25 milligrams and 100 milligrams. You may be taking some of both strengths to obtain an exact dose. Swallow the capsules whole. Don't chew or open them.

Take your dose at the same time each day, preferably in the morning. Take it with meals if it causes nausea.

What to do if you miss a dose

If you forget to take a dose or if you vomit soon after taking it, call your doctor *right away*. Follow his instructions for getting back on schedule. Never skip a dose or take two doses together.

What to do about side effects

Call your doctor *right away* if you:
• have chills or a fever

• need to urinate frequently
• notice your heart beating irregularly
• feel unusually weak or tired or if your legs feel unusually heavy or weak
• see blood in your urine
• have a seizure
• experience breathing problems.
   Also check with your doctor if you have:
• diarrhea or stomach pain with nausea and vomiting
• swollen, tender, or bleeding gums
• headaches or dizziness (indicating a rise in blood pressure)
• shaky or trembling hands
• a change in hair texture.

What you must know about other drugs

Check with your doctor before you take other medications, including nonprescription preparations. Also tell your doctor before you have any immunizations (vaccinations) while you're being treated with cyclosporine and after you stop taking it.

Special directions

• Tell your doctor if you have other medical problems, especially high blood pressure or liver or kidney disease.
• If cyclosporine causes unwanted hair growth, remove it with a depilatory.
• Keep all appointments for follow-up tests so your doctor can detect side effects early.
• See your dentist regularly, and inform him that you're taking cyclosporine.

Important reminder

If you're pregnant or breast-feeding, check with your doctor before taking cyclosporine.

Taking danazol

Dear Patient:

Your doctor has prescribed this medication to treat your condition. Danazol helps treat many medical problems, including endometriosis, breast cysts, and a rare condition called hereditary angioedema. The label may read Danocrine.

How to take danazol
Carefully check the prescription label and follow the directions exactly. For danazol to help you, you must take it regularly for the full time of treatment ordered by your doctor.

What to do if you miss a dose
Take it as soon as possible. However, if it's almost time for your next dose, skip the missed dose and take your next dose on schedule. Don't double dose.

What to do about side effects
If you're female, tell your doctor *right away* if you develop any masculinizing side effects while taking danazol. These effects include weight gain, increased hair growth on your body, a decrease in breast size, voice deepening, and oiliness of your skin or hair.

Special directions
• Tell your doctor if you have other medical problems, especially kidney, heart, or liver disease. If you're female, also reveal if you have a history of abnormal vaginal bleeding.
• See your doctor for regular checkups to make sure that danazol doesn't cause unwanted effects.
• If you're taking this medication for endometriosis or breast cysts, your menstrual period may be irregular, or you may not have a menstrual period while you're taking danazol. This is to be expected. However, if regular menstruation doesn't begin within 60 to 90 days after you stop taking this medication, check with your doctor.
• If you're female, don't use birth control pills while taking danazol. Select a birth control method that doesn't contain hormones, such as a diaphragm.
• If you're taking danazol for breast cysts, examine your breasts regularly. Check with your doctor right away if you detect unusual changes in how your breasts feel.
• Danazol may increase your sensitivity to sunlight, so limit your exposure to the sun.

Important reminders
If you're pregnant or think you may be, don't take danazol. Continued use of danazol during pregnancy may cause malelike changes in female babies. For the same reason, check with your doctor before you use this medication if you're breast-feeding.

If you have diabetes, be aware that danazol may affect your glucose levels. If you notice a change in the results of your blood or urine glucose test, call your doctor.

If you're an older man, you should know that taking danazol may increase your risk of developing prostate enlargement or cancer.

If you're an athlete, you should know that the use of danazol is banned by the U.S. Olympic Committee.

Additional instructions

_____

_____

Taking dantrolene

Dear Patient:

Your doctor has prescribed a muscle relaxant called dantrolene to help your condition. Dantrolene relieves muscle spasms, cramping, and tightness caused by multiple sclerosis, cerebral palsy, stroke, and other conditions. The label may read Dantrium.

How to take dantrolene
If you're taking the *capsule* form, take your dose with milk or meals to help prevent digestive upset.

If you have trouble swallowing the capsules, follow these steps:
• Empty the number of capsules needed for one dose into a small amount of fruit juice or other liquid.
• Stir gently to mix the powder with the liquid. Then drink right away.
• Rinse the glass with a little more liquid and drink that also to make sure you've taken the entire dose.

What to do if you miss a dose
If you remember within an hour or so of the missed dose, take it right away. Then go back to your regular dosing schedule. But if you don't remember until later, skip the missed dose and take your next dose on schedule. Don't double dose.

What to do about side effects
Call your doctor *at once* if your skin or eyes start to turn yellow, if you develop a fever, or if your skin feels itchy. These symptoms could be signs of hepatitis, a liver disorder. Check with your doctor if you feel dizzy or drowsy or have muscle weakness. Also call if you have diarrhea or constipation.

What you must know about alcohol and other drugs
Don't drink alcohol while taking dantrolene because the combination may lead to oversedation. For the same reason, avoid other central nervous system depressants (medications that slow your nervous system), such as sleeping pills, tranquilizers, muscle relaxants, narcotic pain relievers, and many cold, flu, and allergy remedies.

Special directions
• Tell your doctor if you have other medical problems, especially lung, heart, or liver disease.
• See your doctor for regular checkups, especially if you're taking dantrolene for a long time. You may need to have certain blood tests to check for unwanted side effects.
• Because dantrolene can make you drowsy or dizzy, make sure you know how you react to it before you drive, use machines, or perform other activities that could be dangerous if you're not alert.

Important reminders
If you're pregnant or breast-feeding, check with your doctor before using dantrolene.

If you're an athlete, you should know that dantrolene is banned by the National Collegiate Athletic Association and the U.S. Olympic Committee.

Additional instructions

_____

_____

Taking desipramine

Dear Patient:

Your doctor has prescribed desipramine to help relieve your depression. Brand names include Norpramin and Pertofrane.

How to take desipramine
Desipramine comes in capsules and tablets. Follow your doctor's instructions exactly. Don't take more of it or take it more often or longer than directed. Take your dose with food, even for a bedtime dose, unless your doctor has told you to take it on an empty stomach.

Don't stop taking this medication suddenly; check with your doctor first.

What to do if you miss a dose
If you miss a dose, adjust your dosing schedule as follows.

If you take one dose a day at bedtime, don't take the missed dose in the morning. It may cause disturbing side effects during waking hours. Instead, check with your doctor.

If you take more than one dose a day, take the missed dose as soon as possible. However, if it's almost time for your next dose, skip the missed dose and take your next dose on schedule. Don't double dose.

What to do about side effects
Check with your doctor if this medication makes you feel drowsy, dizzy, or light-headed, especially when you get up suddenly from a lying or sitting position. Also call if you experience an irregular or fast heartbeat, blurred vision, dry mouth, constipation, difficulty urinating, or unusual sweating.

What you must know about alcohol and other drugs
Check with your doctor about drinking alcoholic beverages while taking desipramine. Also tell your doctor if you're taking other medication. Desipramine may not work well if taken with barbiturates (sedatives). Taking the ulcer drug cimetidine (Tagamet) may increase the risk of side effects from desipramine.

Other drugs that you may need to avoid while taking this medication are methylphenidate (Ritalin), epinephrine (Adrenalin), and certain drugs used to treat depression and other psychiatric disorders.

Special directions
• Tell your doctor if you have other medical problems, especially heart, liver, or kidney disease; breathing problems; an overactive thyroid; diabetes; or an enlarged prostate.
• Don't drive, use machines, or perform other activities that require alertness until you know how desipramine affects you.
• If desipramine makes you feel faint when you get up from a sitting or lying position, get up slowly.
• Before you have any medical tests, tell the doctor in charge that you're taking desipramine because the drug may affect some test results.

Important reminders
If you're pregnant or breast-feeding, check with your doctor before you take desipramine. If you have diabetes, this medication may affect your glucose levels. If you notice a change in the results of your blood or urine glucose test, call your doctor.

Taking desmopressin

Dear Patient:

Your doctor has prescribed a hormone called desmopressin to help your condition. Desmopressin is used to prevent or control symptoms associated with diabetes insipidus, such as frequent urination, increased thirst, and water loss. Brand names include DDAVP and Stimate.

How to take desmopressin

If you're using the *nasal solution* form, first read the patient directions in the package. Before you administer your dose, gently blow your nose to clear your nasal passages.

If you're using the *injection* form, follow your doctor's instructions.

What to do if you miss a dose

If you miss a dose, adjust your dosing schedule as follows.

If you take one dose a day, take the missed dose as soon as possible. Then go back to your regular dosing schedule. But if you don't remember the missed dose until the next day, skip the missed dose and go back to your regular dosing schedule.

If you take more than one dose a day, take the missed dose as soon as possible. Then go back to your regular dosing schedule. However, if it's almost time for your next dose, skip the missed dose and take your next dose on schedule. Don't double dose.

What to do about side effects

Generally, desmopressin causes few side effects. But check with your doctor if you experience any unwanted effects,

such as headache, runny nose, nausea, or skin flushing, especially if these symptoms persist or seem severe.

Special directions

• Tell your doctor if you have other medical problems, especially heart or blood vessel disease, high blood pressure, or a stuffy nose caused by a cold or an allergy.
• If you're using the *nasal solution* form, check with your doctor if you develop a runny nose from a cold or an allergy. Nasal congestion can interfere with the absorption of this medication.
• If you experience a mild headache from taking this medication, you may take aspirin or acetaminophen (Tylenol), unless your doctor gives you other instructions.
• Your doctor may ask you to check your weight daily to determine if your body is holding enough water.

Important reminders

If you're pregnant or breast-feeding, check with your doctor before taking this medication. If you're an older adult, you may be especially prone to desmopressin's side effects.

Additional instructions

_____

_____

_____

_____

_____

Using ophthalmic dexamethasone

Dear Patient:

Your doctor has prescribed dexamethasone to treat your eye problem. If you're using dexamethasone *eyedrops,* the medication label may read Maxidex Ophthalmic Suspension. If you're using the *eye cream* or *ointment,* the label may read Decadron Phosphate Ophthalmic or Maxidex Ophthalmic.

How to use dexamethasone

If you're using *eyedrops,* follow these steps.
• First, wash your hands. Shake your bottle of eyedrops.
• Tilt your head back, and pull the lower eyelid away from the eye to form a pouch.
• Squeeze the correct number of drops into the pouch and gently close your eye. Don't blink.
• Repeat on the other eye, if directed.
• Keep your eyes closed for 1 to 2 minutes to allow the medication to be absorbed. If you think you didn't get a drop into your eye, use another drop.

If you're using *eye cream* or *ointment,* follow the steps above given for eyedrops, but don't tilt your head back to use the cream or ointment.

Try to keep your medication as germ-free as possible. Don't touch the applicator tip to any surface, including your eye. Keep the container tightly closed between uses.

What to do if you miss a dose

Administer the medication as soon as possible. Then use any remaining medication for that day at regularly spaced intervals. But if it's almost time for your next dose, skip the missed one and go back to your regular schedule.

What to do about side effects

Stop using the medication and call your doctor *right away* if you notice any changes in vision. Tell your doctor if you develop further problems with your eyes, such as blurred vision, burning, stinging, redness, or wateriness.

Special instructions

• Tell your doctor if you have other medical problems with your eyes, such as a corneal abrasion or glaucoma. Also tell him if you're allergic to this or other medications.
• Once your eye infection is cured, don't save your medication and use it for a new eye infection. Always check with your doctor first.
• Don't share this medication with family members, even if they have symptoms that resemble yours. If a family member has the same symptoms, call the doctor.
• Don't rub or scratch around your eye area while taking this medication. You might accidently hurt your eye.
• Keep all appointments for follow-up visits with your doctor.

Additional instructions

_____

_____

_____

_____

_____

_____

_____

Taking oral dexamethasone

Dear Patient:

Your doctor has prescribed oral dexamethasone to treat your condition. The label may read Decadron, Deronil, or Dexone.

How to take dexamethasone
Dexamethasone comes in tablet, oral solution, and elixir forms. Carefully check the label on your prescription bottle, and follow the directions exactly. Don't take dexamethasone more often than ordered.

Take your medication with food to prevent stomach irritation. If you're taking only one dose daily, take it in the morning for best results.

Don't stop taking dexamethasone suddenly. Check with your doctor first.

What to do if you miss a dose
Take it as soon as possible. Then take any remaining doses for that day at regularly spaced intervals. But if it's almost time for your next dose, skip the missed one and take the next one on schedule. Don't double dose.

What to do about side effects
Call your doctor *at once* if you have trouble breathing or start to retain water because the medication may be causing a serious heart problem.

Check with your doctor if you experience mood changes or difficulty sleeping. Also call if you feel weak, are unusually thirsty, urinate frequently, or lose weight despite eating regularly.

What you must know about other drugs
Tell your doctor about other medications you're taking, including nonprescription drugs. Your doctor may want you to avoid certain pain relievers, such as aspirin, because they can increase the risk of stomach problems.

Your doctor also may need to adjust your dose of dexamethasone if you take barbiturates (found in some sleeping pills and medications for seizure disorders) or certain other drugs. Also, check with your doctor before you have any vaccinations.

Special directions
• Tell your doctor if you have other medical problems, especially a fungal infection, ulcers, high blood pressure, diabetes, or diseases of the kidney, liver, blood, bones, or other organs.
• Keep all appointments for follow-up visits.
• Your doctor may want you to carry a medical identification card stating that you're using this medication and that you may need additional medication during an emergency, a severe asthma attack or other illness, or unusual stress.

Important reminder
If you're pregnant or breast-feeding, check with your doctor before using dexamethasone.

Additional instructions

_____

_____

_____

_____

_____

Applying topical dexamethasone

Dear Patient:

Your doctor has prescribed dexamethasone to treat your skin or scalp problem. The brand names for this medication include Decaderm, Decaspray, and Decadron.

How to apply dexamethasone

Topical dexamethasone is available in spray, gel, and cream forms. First, read the patient instructions provided in your medication package. Follow the directions exactly as ordered. Before applying your medication, wash the affected skin gently.

If you're using the *gel* or *cream,* apply a thin coat of medication. Rub in the gel or cream gently to avoid injuring your skin. If you're treating a hairy area, part the hair and apply the medication directly to the affected area. Keep the medication away from your eyes, mouth, nose, and other mucous membranes.

If you're using the *spray,* shake the can well. Then spray while moving the nozzle over the affected area. Take care not to get the spray in your eyes or inhale it.

If you've used your fingers to apply your medication, be sure to wash your hands when you're finished.

Don't wrap the treated skin with a bandage or other tight dressing, unless your doctor has told you to do so.

What to do if you miss an application

Apply the medication as soon as possible. But if it's almost time for your next application, skip the missed one and apply the next one on schedule.

What to do about side effects

Check with your doctor if you experience skin reactions to this medication, including a rash, itching, burning, redness, or dryness. Also report signs of skin infection, such as redness, pain, and oozing.

Special directions

• Tell your doctor if you have other medical problems, especially poor circulation.
• Keep all appointments for follow-up visits, so your doctor can check your progress and detect unwanted side effects early.
• If you're using this medication to treat diaper rash in a young child, don't cover the child's bottom with a tight-fitting diaper or plastic pants.

Important reminder

Check with your doctor before applying this medication on children.

Additional instructions

_____

_____

_____

_____

_____

_____

_____

Taking diazepam

Dear Patient:

Your doctor has prescribed diazepam to help your condition. Because diazepam causes relaxation, it's helpful for treating severe tension or anxiety as well as muscle spasms. It's also used to prevent seizures. The label may read Valium, Valrelease, or Zetran.

How to take diazepam

Diazepam comes in extended-release capsules, an oral solution, and tablets. Carefully check the prescription label, and follow the directions exactly as ordered. Don't increase your dose. If you're taking the *extended-release capsules,* don't crush, break, or chew them—swallow them whole.

If you're taking diazepam regularly, don't suddenly stop taking your medication without first checking with your doctor.

What to do if you miss a dose

Take it right away if you remember within an hour or so of the missed dose. However, if you don't remember until later, skip the missed dose and take your next dose on schedule. Don't double dose.

What to do about side effects

Get emergency help *at once* if you suddenly start to feel very unwell and experience difficulty breathing, faintness, or a dramatic change in your heart or pulse rate.

Check with your doctor if this medication makes you feel drowsy, lethargic, or like you have a hangover. Also call if you start to stagger when you walk.

What you must know about alcohol and other drugs

Don't drink alcoholic beverages while taking diazepam because the combination may cause oversedation. For the same reason, avoid other central nervous system depressants (medications that slow down your nervous system), such as sleeping pills, tranquilizers, and many cold and flu medications. Taking diazepam with the ulcer drug cimetidine (Tagamet) may also lead to increased drowsiness.

Special directions

• Tell your doctor if you have other medical problems, such as glaucoma, myasthenia gravis, Parkinson's disease, and liver or kidney problems. Also mention if you have a history of drug addiction or psychological problems.
• See your doctor regularly to determine if you need to continue taking this medication because if too much is taken, it may become habit-forming.
• Before you have medical tests, tell the doctor that you're taking diazepam because it may alter the test results.
• Make sure you know how you react to diazepam before you drive, use machines, or perform other activities that could be dangerous if you're not fully alert.

Important reminders

If you're pregnant or breast-feeding, check with your doctor before taking this medication. If you're an older adult, realize that you may be especially prone to diazepam's side effects.

If you're an athlete, you should know that diazepam is banned by the National Collegiate Athletic Association and the U.S. Olympic Committee.

Taking diclofenac

Dear Patient:

Your doctor has prescribed diclofenac to relieve joint pain, swelling, and stiffness caused by arthritis. The label may read Voltaren.

How to take diclofenac
Take this medication with milk, meals, or a full glass (8 ounces) of water. Also, avoid lying down for about 15 to 30 minutes after taking this medication. This helps prevent irritation of your esophagus (food tube). Swallow the tablets whole—don't chew or break them.

What to do if you miss a dose
Take it as soon as possible. However, if it's almost time for your next dose, skip the missed dose and take your next dose on schedule. Don't double dose.

What to do about side effects
Get emergency help *at once* if you have symptoms of an allergic reaction, such as wheezing, difficulty breathing, hives, itching, or a rash. Also call your doctor *right away* if you hear ringing or buzzing in your ears.

Be aware that diclofenac can cause serious bleeding from the digestive tract, including ulcers. Stop taking this medication and check with your doctor *at once* if you have any of these warning signs: severe abdominal or stomach pain; black, tarry stools; severe, continuing nausea or heartburn; or vomiting of blood or material that looks like coffee grounds.

Check with your doctor if you feel drowsy or have a headache, abdominal discomfort, or diarrhea.

What you must know about alcohol and other drugs
Avoid alcoholic beverages while taking diclofenac because stomach problems are more likely to occur.

Tell your doctor about other medications you're taking. If you take blood thinners, taking diclofenac may increase your risk of bleeding. Also, don't take aspirin or acetaminophen (Tylenol) for more than a few days while taking this medication, unless your doctor tells you otherwise.

Diclofenac may increase the toxicity of certain drugs, including cyclosporine (Sandimmune), an antibiotic; digoxin (Lanoxin), a heart medication; lithium (Lithane), a drug for manic-depressive disorder; and methotrexate (Mexate), a cancer drug.

Diclofenac may also interfere with the effects of water pills. If you have diabetes, your doctor may need to adjust your medications for this disease.

Special directions
• Tell your doctor if you have other medical problems, especially ulcers, porphyria, or liver or kidney disease. Also tell him if you're allergic to diclofenac, aspirin, or other medications.
• Know how you react to diclofenac before you drive, use machines, or perform other activities that could be dangerous if you're not fully alert.

Important reminders
If you're pregnant or breast-feeding, don't take this medication without your doctor's consent.

If you're an older adult, realize that you may be especially prone to side effects from diclofenac.

Taking dicloxacillin

Dear Patient: /

Your doctor has prescribed dicloxacillin to treat your bacterial infection. The label may read Dycill, Dynapen, or Pathocil.

How to take dicloxacillin

This antibiotic medication comes in capsule and oral suspension forms.

If you're taking the *capsule* form, don't break, chew, or crush the capsule—swallow it whole.

If you're taking the *oral suspension,* use a dropper or specially marked measuring spoon to measure each dose accurately.

Take your medication with a full glass (8 ounces) of water on an empty stomach, either 1 hour before or 2 hours after meals, unless otherwise directed by your doctor.

Continue to take your medication, even after you start to feel better. Stopping too soon may allow your infection to return.

What to do if you miss a dose

Take it as soon as possible. But if it's almost time for your next dose, adjust your dosage schedule as follows.

If you take two doses a day, space the missed dose and the next dose 5 to 6 hours apart.

If you take three or more doses a day, space the missed dose and the next dose 2 to 4 hours apart. Then resume your regular dosing schedule.

What to do about side effects

Call your doctor *at once* if you develop any of the following signs of an allergic reaction: difficulty breathing, a rash, hives, itching, or wheezing.

Check with your doctor if you experience nausea, heartburn, or diarrhea, especially if these symptoms persist or become severe.

What you must know about other drugs

Tell the doctor about other medications you're taking. Probenecid (Probalan), a gout medication, may increase the effects of dicloxacillin. This effect may or may not be beneficial; check with your doctor.

Special directions

• Tell your doctor if you have a history of kidney problems or if you're allergic to this medication or other antibiotics.
• If you become allergic to this medication, you should carry a medical identification card or wear a medical identification bracelet stating this.
• If you develop severe diarrhea, don't take any diarrhea medication without first checking with your doctor. Diarrhea medications may make your diarrhea worse or last longer. For mild diarrhea, you may take a diarrhea medication containing kaolin or attapulgite.
• Tell the doctor that you're taking dicloxacillin before you have medical tests because this medication may alter test results.

Important reminder

If you're pregnant or breast-feeding, check with your doctor before taking this medication.

Additional instructions

_____

_____

Taking dicyclomine

Dear Patient:

Your doctor has prescribed dicyclomine to relieve your digestive cramps or spasms. This medication is often part of the treatment for stomach ulcers. The label may read Antispas, Bentyl, or Dibent.

How to take dicyclomine
Dicyclomine comes in capsule, syrup, and tablet forms. Carefully read the instructions on the prescription label and follow them exactly. Take this medication 30 minutes to 1 hour before meals, unless your doctor directs otherwise.

If you're taking dicyclomine in the *capsule* form, don't break, chew, or crush it—swallow it whole.

Check with your doctor before you stop using this medication. Your doctor may want to reduce your dosage gradually to prevent unwanted effects.

What to do if you miss a dose
Take it as soon as possible. But if it's almost time for your next dose, skip the missed dose and take your next dose on schedule. Don't double dose.

What to do about side effects
Check with your doctor if you have any of the following side effects: headache, dizziness, palpitations, constipation, difficulty urinating, or impotence.

What you must know about other drugs
Don't take dicyclomine within 2 to 3 hours of taking antacids or medication for diarrhea because these medications may make dicyclomine ineffective.

Special directions
• Tell your doctor if you have other medical problems, especially GI, heart, liver, or kidney disease; glaucoma; or an overactive thyroid. Also mention if you have a history of urinary problems.
• Because you may not sweat as much while taking dicyclomine, your body temperature may increase. Therefore, take care not to become too hot during exercise or hot weather because overheating could cause heatstroke. For the same reason, hot baths or saunas may make you dizzy or faint while you're taking dicyclomine.
• Make sure you know how you react to dicyclomine before you drive, use machines, or perform other activities that could be dangerous if you're not fully alert.
• If this medication makes your mouth feel dry, use sugarless hard candy or gum, ice chips, or a saliva substitute. If your mouth dryness lasts for more than 2 weeks, check with your doctor or dentist.

Important reminders
If you're pregnant or breast-feeding, check with your doctor before taking this medication.

If you're an older adult, realize that you may be especially prone to side effects from dicyclomine.

Additional instructions

_____

_____

_____

_____

Taking diethylpropion

Dear Patient:

Your doctor has prescribed short-term use of this medication to treat your obesity. The label may read M-Orexic, Tenuate, or Tepanil.

How to take diethylpropion
Diethylpropion comes in the form of tablets and extended-release tablets. Carefully check the label on your prescription bottle and follow the directions exactly as ordered. Take the last dose for each day about 4 to 6 hours before bedtime to help prevent insomnia. Don't break, crush, or chew tablets—swallow them whole.

Don't stop taking this medication suddenly without first checking with your doctor. Your doctor may want to decrease your dose gradually to prevent withdrawal symptoms.

What to do if you miss a dose
Before you start taking diethylpropion, ask your doctor for instructions on what to do if you miss a dose.

What to do about side effects
Check with your doctor if you become nervous or experience a rapid heartbeat or palpitations while taking this medication, especially if your symptoms persist or become severe.

What you must know about other drugs
Tell your doctor if you're taking other medications. Certain medications to treat depression (known as monoamine oxidase [MAO] inhibitors) may increase your blood pressure to a dangerous level when used with diethylpropion.

Special directions
• Before you begin using diethylpropion, tell your doctor if you have other medical problems.
• See your doctor at regular intervals to make sure this medication doesn't cause unwanted effects.
• Because this medication may make you dizzy or drowsy, make sure you know how you react to it before you drive or use machines that could be dangerous if you're not fully alert.
• Before having any kind of surgery, dental treatment, or emergency treatment, tell the doctor or dentist that you're taking diethylpropion.
• If you're taking diethylpropion for a long time and think you may be dependent on it, check with your doctor. Some signs of dependence are a strong desire or need to continue taking this medication, a need to increase the dose to receive its effects, or withdrawal side effects when you stop taking it.

Important reminders
If you're pregnant or breast-feeding, don't take this medication without your doctor's approval.

If you have diabetes, be aware that diethylpropion may affect your glucose levels. If you notice a change in the results of your urine or blood glucose test, call your doctor.

If you're an athlete, you should know that this medication is banned by the National Collegiate Athletic Association and the U.S. Olympic Committee.

Additional instructions

_____

_____

Taking diflunisal

Dear Patient:

Your doctor has prescribed diflunisal to relieve your pain. This medication, which is similar to aspirin, is often used to treat osteoarthritis symptoms, such as joint swelling, stiffness, and pain. The label may read Dolobid.

How to take diflunisal

Diflunisal comes in tablet form. Take diflunisal with food or an antacid and a full glass (8 ounces) of water. Don't crush or break the tablet—swallow it whole.

Also, don't lie down for about 15 to 30 minutes after taking your dose. This helps to prevent irritation of your esophagus (food tube).

What to do if you miss a dose

Take it as soon as you remember. However, if it's almost time for your next dose, skip the missed dose and take your next dose on schedule. Never double the dose.

What to do about side effects

Check with your doctor if this medication makes you dizzy or if you develop a headache or rash. Also call him if you have ringing in your ears or changes in your vision.

Because diflunisal can irritate your digestive tract, call your doctor if you experience nausea, heartburn, stomach or abdominal pain, or diarrhea.

Call your doctor *at once* if you have any of the following warning signs of GI bleeding or ulcers: severe stomach or abdominal pain; black, tarry stools; and vomiting of blood or material that looks like coffee grounds.

What you must know about alcohol and other drugs

Don't drink alcoholic beverages while taking diflunisal because the combination increases the risk of stomach problems.

Tell the doctor about other medications you're taking. Don't take aspirin, acetaminophen (Tylenol), or other aspirin-related drugs together with diflunisal for more than a few days, unless your doctor gives you other directions, because doing so may cause unwanted side effects.

If you take blood thinners, be aware that diflunisal may increase your risk of bleeding. Antacids may decrease the effectiveness of this medication.

Special directions

• Tell your doctor if you have other medical problems, especially ulcers, a heart condition, or kidney disease. Also inform him if you're allergic to diflunisal, aspirin, or other medications.
• Before having any kind of surgery (including dental surgery), tell the doctor or dentist that you're taking diflunisal.
• Because this medication may make you dizzy, make sure you know how you react to it before you drive, use machines, or perform other activities that could be dangerous if you're not fully alert.

Important reminders

If you're pregnant or breast-feeding, don't take this medication unless you have your doctor's approval.

If you're an older adult, be aware that you may be especially sensitive to side effects from diflunisal.

Taking digoxin

Dear Patient:

Your doctor has prescribed digoxin to treat your heart condition. Digoxin helps to improve the strength and efficiency of the heart or to control an irregular heartbeat. Brand names for digoxin include Lanoxin and Lanoxicaps.

How to take digoxin

This medication is available as capsules, elixir, and tablets. Carefully check the label on your prescription bottle and follow the directions exactly as ordered. If you're taking the *elixir,* measure your dose only with the specially marked dropper.

Ask your doctor about checking your pulse rate. If he wants you to, you should check your pulse rate before each dose. If it's much slower or faster than your usual rate (or less than 50 beats per minute) or if it changes rhythm or force, check with your doctor. Such changes may mean side effects are occurring.

Don't stop taking digoxin without first checking with your doctor. Stopping suddenly may cause a serious change in your heart's function.

What to do if you miss a dose

If you remember the missed dose within 12 hours, take it as soon as you remember. However, if you don't remember until later, skip the missed dose and take your next dose on schedule. Don't double dose.

What to do abut side effects

Call your doctor *right away* if you develop any of the following symptoms:
• increased shortness of breath
• sudden weight gain (3 or more pounds in 1 week)
• swelling of your ankles or fingers
• visual changes: blurred vision, double vision, light flashes, or the appearance of yellow-green halos around images
• digestive problems: loss of appetite, nausea, vomiting, or diarrhea
• changes in your pulse rate
• hallucinations.

Check with your doctor if this medication makes you feel tired, weak, or agitated.

What you must know about other drugs

Tell your doctor about other medications you're taking because many prescription and nonprescription medications can interact with digoxin. For example, digoxin may become toxic if taken with many medications, including certain antibiotics, heart medications, steroids, and water pills.

Other medications can decrease the absorption of digoxin, including cholesterol-lowering drugs, antacids, and some diarrhea medications.

Special directions

• Tell your doctor if you have other medical problems, especially kidney, liver, or lung disease or a history of rheumatic fever.
• Before having any kind of surgery (including dental surgery) or emergency treatment, tell the doctor or dentist that you're taking digoxin.

Important reminders

If you're pregnant or breast-feeding, check with your doctor before using this medication. If you're an older adult, be aware that you may be especially prone to unwanted effects from digoxin.

Taking diltiazem

Dear Patient:

This medication is used to relieve and control angina (chest pain) and high blood pressure. If you're taking the *tablet* form of diltiazem, the label may read Cardizem. If you're taking the *sustained-release capsules,* the label may read Cardizem CD, Cardizem SR, or Dilacor XR.

How to take diltiazem
Carefully check the label on your prescription bottle, and follow the directions exactly as ordered.

If you're taking the *capsule* form, don't crush or chew it—swallow it whole.

If you're taking diltiazem regularly for several weeks, don't suddenly stop taking it. Your doctor may want to reduce your dose gradually before you stop completely.

If you have high blood pressure, you may not notice any symptoms of this disorder. Even so, it's essential that you take diltiazem exactly as directed.

What to do if you miss a dose
Take it as soon as possible. However, if it's almost time for your next dose, skip the missed dose and take your next dose on schedule. Don't double dose.

What to do about side effects
Check with your doctor if you feel nauseous, tired, or drowsy or have a headache or an irregular heartbeat. Also call if your feet and ankles become swollen or if you suddenly gain unexpected weight (more than 3 pounds in 1 week).

What you must know about other drugs
Tell your doctor about other medications you're taking, so harmful interactions can be avoided. For example, taking diltiazem with the ulcer medication cimetidine (Tagamet) can lead to toxic effects. If you take digoxin (Lanoxin) for a heart condition, diltiazem may cause an unwanted buildup of digoxin. Taking propranolol (Inderal) or other beta blockers (for high blood pressure) with diltiazem could lead to heart problems.

Special directions
• Tell your doctor if you have other medical problems, especially severe high blood pressure, heart disease, or a liver or kidney condition.
• Keep appointments for doctor's visits, so your doctor can check your progress and adjust your dosage, if needed.
• Talk to your doctor about how to exercise safely without overdoing it, to improve your condition.
• Ask your doctor how to count your pulse rate. While you're taking diltiazem, check your pulse rate regularly. If it's much slower than your usual rate or less than 50 beats per minute, check with your doctor. A pulse rate that is too slow may cause circulation problems.

Important reminders
If you're pregnant or breast-feeding, check with your doctor before using this medication. If you're an older adult, be aware that you may be especially sensitive to side effects from diltiazem.

Additional instructions

_____

_____

_____

Taking dimenhydrinate

Dear Patient:

Dimenhydrinate is used to relieve nausea and vomiting and to prevent or treat motion sickness. Brand names for this medication include Calm X, Dimetabs, Dinate, and Dramamine.

How to take dimenhydrinate

Dimenhydrinate comes in the form of tablets, chewable tablets, capsules, and syrup.

Carefully check the label on your prescription bottle, and follow the directions exactly as ordered.

If you're taking dimenhydrinate to prevent motion sickness, take it at least 1 to 2 hours before traveling. If this isn't possible, take it at least 30 minutes before traveling.

Take this medication with food or a glass of milk or water to lessen stomach irritation, if necessary.

What to do about side effects

Dimenhydrinate may make you feel drowsy. Occasionally, this medication causes headache, palpitations, blurred vision, and mouth dryness. If these side effects persist or become severe, call your doctor.

What you must know about alcohol and other drugs

Check with your doctor before drinking alcoholic beverages or taking other drugs because the combined effects may make you overly drowsy.

Special directions

• Check with your doctor before you take this medication if you have glaucoma, asthma, an enlarged prostate, or a seizure disorder.

• Don't take dimenhydrinate if you're allergic to it or to theophylline (Theo-Dur), an asthma medication.
• Tell your doctor that you're taking dimenhydrinate before you have any skin tests for allergies because it may affect the test results.
• Because this medication may make you drowsy, make sure you know how you react to it before you drive, use machines, or perform other activities that could be dangerous if you're not fully alert.
• If this medication makes your mouth feel dry, you may get temporary relief by using sugarless hard candy or gum, melting bits of ice in your mouth, or using a saliva substitute.
• If you're taking dimenhydrinate to control nausea and vomiting, make sure your doctor knows that you're taking this medication if you should suddenly develop symptoms of appendicitis, such as stomach or lower abdominal pain, cramping, and soreness.

Important reminders

If you're pregnant or breast-feeding, check with your doctor before using dimenhydrinate.

Be aware that children and older adults are especially sensitive to side effects from this medication.

Additional instructions

_____

_____

_____

_____

Taking diphenhydramine

Dear Patient:

Diphenhydramine is used to relieve symptoms of numerous conditions, including hay fever, stuffy nose, insomnia, motion sickness, and nonproductive cough. This medication has more than 45 brand names, but some of the more common ones are Benadryl, Compoz, and Sominex Formula 2.

How to take diphenhydramine
Diphenhydramine is available without a prescription in the form of capsules, tablets, elixir, and syrup. Carefully check the medication label, and follow the directions exactly. Take your dose with food or a glass of milk or water to lessen stomach irritation, if necessary.

If you're taking diphenhydramine to prevent motion sickness, take it at least 1 to 2 hours before traveling. If that's not possible, take it at least 30 minutes ahead of time.

What to do if you miss a dose
If you're taking this medication regularly and you miss a dose, take it as soon as possible. However, if it's almost time for your next dose, skip the missed dose and take your next dose on schedule. Don't double dose.

What to do about side effects
While taking this medication, you may feel drowsy or nauseous or experience dryness of your mouth. Check with your doctor if these side effects bother you or become severe.

What you must know about alcohol and other drugs
Avoid drinking alcoholic beverages while taking diphenhydramine because the combination may make you overly drowsy.

For the same reason, avoid concurrent use of other medications that slow down the nervous system, including narcotic painkillers, tranquilizers, and many cold and flu remedies. Also, if you take certain antidepressants, your doctor may not want you to take diphenhydramine because of the increased risk of unwanted effects.

If you regularly take large doses of aspirin for arthritis, be aware that diphenhydramine can cover up signs of an aspirin overdose, such as ringing in your ears.

Special directions
• Tell your doctor if you have other medical problems, especially asthma, glaucoma, bladder conditions, heart disease, high blood pressure, or an overactive thyroid.
• Inform the doctor that you're taking diphenhydramine before you have skin tests for allergies because the drug may affect the test results.
• Make sure you know how you react to this medication before you drive, use machines, or perform other activities that could be dangerous if you're not fully alert.
• If diphenhydramine makes your mouth or throat feel dry, use sugarless hard candy or gum, ice chips, or a saliva substitute.

Important reminders
If you're pregnant or breast-feeding, check with your doctor before taking diphenhydramine. Also, be aware that children and older adults are especially prone to side effects from this medication.

Taking diphenoxylate with atropine

Dear Patient:

This medication, commonly known as Lomotil, is used to treat diarrhea. It works by slowing down intestinal movements.

How to take diphenoxylate with atropine

This medication comes in tablet and liquid forms. Carefully read the label on the medication bottle to know how much to take and when.

If you're taking the *liquid* form, make sure to measure the correct amount by using a specially marked measuring spoon or dropper. Using a regular household teaspoon may give you an incorrect dose.

What to do if you miss a dose

If you're taking this medication on a regular schedule and you forget to take a dose, take it when you remember. However, if it's almost time for the next dose, skip the missed dose and take your next dose on schedule. Don't double dose.

What to do about side effects

Call your doctor if this medication causes bloating, constipation, loss of appetite, or stomach pain with nausea and vomiting.

This medication also may make you feel sleepy or dizzy and can cause dry mouth. If these symptoms persist or become bothersome, call your doctor.

Special directions

• Tell your doctor if you have other medical problems, especially liver disease or glaucoma.
• To help replace the fluid lost in your stool, follow these suggestions: drink clear liquids, such as apple juice, broth, ginger ale, or tea. During the next 24 hours, eat bland foods, such as plain bread or crackers, cooked cereals, and applesauce.
• Avoid citrus fruits, tomatoes, tomato sauce, caffeine, and alcoholic beverages because these foods can make diarrhea worse.
• Call your doctor if your diarrhea continues after 2 days or you develop a fever.
• Because this medication may make you drowsy, make sure you know how you respond to it before you drive a car or perform activities that require mental alertness.
• Don't use this medication for any bout of diarrhea other than the prescribed condition. This medication can make certain forms of diarrhea worse.

Important reminders

If you're pregnant or breast-feeding, check with your doctor before using this medication.

If you're an older adult, you may be especially prone to side effects from diphenoxylate with atropine.

Don't give this medication to a child age 2 or younger because of the high risk of side effects.

Additional instructions

_____

_____

_____

_____

_____

Taking dipyridamole

Dear Patient:

Your doctor has prescribed dipyridamole to treat your heart condition. This medication is used to prevent blood clots after surgery to replace a heart valve. But it's also prescribed for other heart and blood vessel problems. Brand names include Dipridacot and Persantine.

How to take dipyridamole
This medication comes in tablet form. Carefully check the label on your prescription bottle, and follow the directions exactly as ordered. Take this medication in regularly spaced doses, as directed by your doctor.

Take your dose with a full glass (8 ounces) of water at least 1 hour before or 2 hours after meals. However, to lessen stomach upset, your doctor may want you to take dipyridamole with food or milk.

What to do if you miss a dose
Take it as soon as possible. But if it's within 4 hours of your next scheduled dose, skip the missed dose and go back to your regular dosing schedule. Don't double dose.

What to do about side effects
Check with your doctor if this medication makes you dizzy or nauseous. Also call if you get a headache or a rash or have chest pain.

What you must know about other drugs
Tell your doctor if you're taking dipyridamole along with a blood thinner or aspirin because these combinations increase the risk of bleeding. To reduce

this risk, don't take aspirin or any product containing aspirin unless the same doctor who prescribed your dipyridamole specifically tells you to do so.

If you've been instructed to take aspirin together with dipyridamole, take only the amount of aspirin ordered by your doctor. If you need a medication to relieve pain or a fever, your doctor may not want you to take extra aspirin. You may want to discuss this issue with your doctor ahead of time.

Special directions
• Tell your doctor if you have other medical problems, especially chest pain or low blood pressure.
• Keep all appointments for follow-up visits, so your doctor can check your progress.
• If you visit a dentist or doctor other than the one who prescribed dipyridamole, be sure to tell him that you take this medication. Also mention whether or not you're taking it with a blood thinner or aspirin.
• This medication may make you feel dizzy, light-headed, or faint, especially when you get up from a lying or sitting position. Getting up slowly may help. If this problem continues or gets worse, check with your doctor.

Important reminder
If you're pregnant or breast-feeding, check with your doctor before taking dipyridamole.

Additional instructions

_____

_____

Taking disopyramide

Dear Patient:

Your doctor has prescribed disopyramide to treat your heart condition. This medication is used to correct irregular heartbeats or to slow an overactive heart. If you're taking the *capsule* form of disopyramide, the label may read Norpace. If you're taking the *extended-release capsules,* the label may read Norpace CR.

How to take disopyramide
Check the label on your prescription bottle. Follow the directions exactly.

If you're taking the *extended-release capsule,* swallow it whole without breaking, crushing, or chewing it.

Don't stop taking disopyramide without first checking with your doctor. Stopping suddenly may cause a serious change in heart function.

What to do if you miss a dose
Take it as soon as possible unless the next scheduled dose is in less than 4 hours. In that case, skip the missed dose and take your next dose on schedule. Don't double dose.

What to do about side effects
Call your doctor *right away* if you experience increasing shortness of breath, sudden weight gain (3 or more pounds in 1 week), or swelling of your ankles or fingers. Check with your doctor if you experience blurred vision, constipation, or dryness of your eyes, nose, or mouth—especially if these symptoms persist or become severe.

What you must know about alcohol and other drugs
Don't drink alcoholic beverages until you've checked with your doctor. When taken with disopyramide, alcohol may make your glucose level drop dangerously low and make you faint or dizzy.

Tell your doctor about other medications you're taking. Other medications used to correct irregular heartbeats or slow an overactive heart may alter the effects of disopyramide beyond a safe level. Phenytoin (Dilantin), a seizure medication, may reduce the effectiveness of disopyramide.

Special directions
• Tell your doctor if you have other medical problems, especially myasthenia gravis, glaucoma, difficulty urinating, other heart conditions, or liver or kidney disease.
• This medication may make you dizzy, light-headed, or faint, especially when you get up from a lying or sitting position. Getting up slowly may help.
• Know how you react to this medication before you drive, use machines, or perform other activities that could be dangerous if you're not fully alert.
• Disopyramide may make you sweat less. To prevent becoming overheated, don't overdo it during exercise or hot weather.

Important reminders
If you're pregnant or breast-feeding, check with your doctor before taking disopyramide.

If you have diabetes or congestive heart failure, be alert for symptoms of low blood glucose while taking this medication. Symptoms include headache, shakiness, cold sweats, excessive hunger, and weakness. If these occur, eat or drink a sugary food and call your doctor *right away.*

Taking docusate salts

Dear Patient:

This medication is a laxative used to treat constipation. Docusate salts may contain calcium, potassium, or sodium. If you're taking *docusate calcium,* the medication comes in capsule form and the label may read Pro-Cal-Sof or Sur-fak. If you're taking *docusate potassium,* which also comes in capsules, the label may read Dialose or Kasof. *Docusate sodium* is available in tablet, capsule, oral liquid, and syrup forms. The label may read Colace or Dioeze.

How to take docusate salts
If your doctor prescribed this medication, follow his directions exactly. If you bought this medication without a prescription, carefully read the package directions before taking your first dose.

What to do about side effects
Although side effects aren't common, this medication may irritate your throat or leave a bitter taste in your mouth. You may also have mild abdominal cramping or diarrhea. If these symptoms persist or become severe, call your doctor.

What you must know about other drugs
Don't take mineral oil while you're taking docusate salts because it may cause your body to absorb too much mineral oil, causing unwanted effects.

Don't take docusate salts within 2 hours of taking another medication because docusate salts may interfere with the desired actions of other medications.

Special directions
• Don't use docusate salts (or any other laxative) if you have signs of appendicitis or inflamed bowel, such as stomach or lower abdominal pain, cramping, bloating, soreness, nausea, or vomiting. Instead, check with your doctor as soon as possible.
• Drink at least 6 to 8 glasses of water or other liquids daily. This will help soften your stools and relieve constipation.
• Don't take docusate salts for more than 1 week unless your doctor has prescribed or ordered a special schedule for you. This is true even if you continue to have constipation.
• If you notice a sudden change in your bowel habits or function that lasts longer than 2 weeks, or that occurs from time to time, check with your doctor before using this medication. Your doctor will need to find the cause of your problem before it becomes more serious.
• Don't overuse docusate salts. Otherwise, you may become dependent on this medication to produce a bowel movement. In severe cases, overuse of laxatives can damage the nerves, muscles, and other tissues of the bowel.

Important reminders
If you're pregnant, check with your doctor before taking docusate salts.

Don't give this medication to children under age 6 unless prescribed by a doctor.

Additional instructions

Taking doxazosin

Dear Patient:

Your doctor has prescribed this medication to treat your high blood pressure. The label may read Cardura.

How to take doxazosin
This medication comes in tablet form. Carefully check the label on your prescription bottle, which tells you how much medication to take and when. Follow the directions exactly as ordered.

What to do if you miss a dose
Before you start taking doxazosin, ask your doctor for instructions on what you should do in case you forget a dose of your medication.

What to do about side effects
This medication may lower your blood pressure, causing you to feel dizzy, light-headed, or faint when you get up from a sitting or standing position. Usually, this effect begins to go away after the first dose, but it may recur if you stop taking your medication for a few days or if your dosage is adjusted. If this problem persists or becomes severe, call your doctor.

Check with your doctor if doxazosin makes you feel sleepy or gives you a headache. Also call if you develop a rash, muscle or joint pain, or an irregular heartbeat.

What you must know about other drugs
Don't take doxazosin with other medications to treat high blood pressure unless your doctor has directed you to do so. Taking this combination of medications may cause dangerously low blood pressure, possibly leading to loss of consciousness.

Special directions
• Tell your doctor if you have other medical problems, especially liver disease.
• Keep appointments for doctor's visits. You'll need to see your doctor at least every 2 weeks until your dosage is set properly, then at regular intervals so your progress can be checked.
• If this medication makes you feel dizzy, light-headed, or faint when you get up from a lying or sitting position, try to get up slowly.
• Because doxazosin can make you dizzy, make sure you know how you react to it before you drive, use machines, or perform other activities that could be dangerous if you're not fully alert.
• Your doctor may teach you how to take your blood pressure at home. If so, check your blood pressure at regular intervals and call your doctor if you detect any significant changes.

Important reminder
If you're pregnant or breast-feeding, check with your doctor before taking this medication.

Additional instructions

_____

_____

_____

_____

_____

_____

Taking doxepin

Dear Patient:

Your doctor has prescribed doxepin to help relieve your depression. The label may read Adapin or Sinequan.

How to take doxepin
This medication is available in capsules or as an oral solution. Follow your doctor's instructions exactly. Don't take more of it, and don't take it more often or longer than he directs. Take doxepin with food, even for a daily bedtime dose, unless your doctor has told you to take it on an empty stomach.

If you're using the *oral solution,* use the dropper provided to measure the dose accurately. Just before you take each dose, dilute it in about 4 ounces of water, milk, or juice. Don't use grape juice or carbonated beverages because these liquids may decrease doxepin's effectiveness.

Don't stop taking doxepin suddenly without first checking with your doctor.

What to do if you miss a dose
If you miss a dose, adjust your dosing schedule as follows.

If you take one dose a day at bedtime, check with your doctor. Don't take the missed dose in the morning because it may cause disturbing side effects during waking hours.

If you take more than one dose a day, take the missed dose as soon as possible. But if it's almost time for your next dose, skip the missed dose and take your next dose on schedule. Don't double dose.

What to do about side effects
Check with your doctor if this medication makes you feel drowsy, dizzy, or faint, especially when you get up suddenly from a sitting or lying position. Also call if you experience blurred vision, dryness of your mouth, a fast pulse rate, constipation, difficulty urinating, or unusual sweating.

What you must know about alcohol and other drugs
Don't drink alcoholic beverages while taking doxepin unless your doctor okays it. Also, your medication may not work well if taken with barbiturates (found in some sleeping pills and seizure medications). Taking doxepin with the ulcer drug cimetidine (Tagamet) may cause unwanted effects.

While you're taking doxepin, your doctor may want you to avoid certain medications used to treat psychological disorders.

Special directions
• Tell your doctor if you have other medical problems, especially heart disease.
• Because this medication may make you drowsy or dizzy, make sure you know how it affects you before you drive, use machines, or perform other activities that could be dangerous if you're not fully alert.
• Before you have medical tests, tell the doctor that you're taking doxepin because the drug may affect some test results.

Important reminders
If you're pregnant or breast-feeding, check with your doctor before taking doxepin. If you have diabetes, this medication may affect your glucose levels. If you notice a change in the results of your blood or urine glucose tests, call your doctor.

Taking doxycycline

Dear Patient:

Your doctor has prescribed this antibiotic medication to treat your bacterial infection. The label may read Doxy-Caps, Vibramycin, or Vibra-Tabs.

How to take doxycycline

This medication comes in capsule, delayed-release capsule, oral suspension, and tablet forms. Take your dose with food, milk, or a full glass (8 ounces) of water to prevent irritation of your esophagus (food tube) or stomach.

If you're taking the *oral suspension,* use a specially marked spoon to measure each dose accurately.

Continue to take your medication, even if you start to feel better after a few days. Stopping too soon may allow your infection to return. Also, try to take your doses at evenly spaced times day and night.

What to do if you miss a dose

Take it as soon as possible. But if it's almost time for your next dose, adjust your dosing schedule as follows.

If you take one dose a day, space the missed dose and the next dose 10 to 12 hours apart.

If you take two doses a day, space the missed dose and the next dose 5 to 6 hours apart.

If you take three or more doses a day, space the missed dose and the next dose 2 to 4 hours apart. Then resume your regular dosing schedule.

What to do about side effects

Call your doctor *right away* if you develop any of the following symptoms of an allergic reaction to doxycycline: severe headache, vision changes, difficulty breathing, wheezing, hives, or itching.

Also check with your doctor if you experience heartburn, nausea, diarrhea, rashes, or increased light sensitivity, especially if these symptoms persist or become severe.

What you must know about alcohol and other drugs

Avoid drinking alcoholic beverages because it may prevent doxycycline from working well. Other medications that may reduce the effectiveness of doxycycline are antacids, iron preparations (such as iron-containing vitamins), and some seizure medications. Also, if you use birth control pills, doxycycline may keep them from working effectively. Use another form of birth control.

Special directions

• Tell your doctor if you have other medical problems, especially kidney disease. Also inform him if you're allergic to a tetracycline antibiotic.

• If your medication has changed color, tastes or looks different, has become outdated, or has been stored incorrectly (in a place too warm or too damp), don't use it—it could cause serious side effects. Discard the bottle and obtain a fresh supply.

• This medication may make your skin more sensitive to sunlight, so limit your exposure to the sun.

Important reminder

If you're pregnant or breast-feeding, don't take doxycycline. It could stain your developing baby's teeth.

Taking enalapril

Dear Patient:

Your doctor has prescribed enalapril to treat your condition. This medication is used to lower high blood pressure. It's also prescribed to treat heart problems, when used along with other medications. Enalapril is also called Vasotec.

How to take enalapril

Enalapril comes in tablet form. Carefully check the label on your prescription bottle, and follow these directions exactly, unless your doctor changes your dosage. Don't suddenly stop taking this medication without checking first with your doctor.

What to do if you miss a dose

Take it as soon as possible. But if it's almost time for your next dose, skip the missed dose and take your next dose on schedule. Don't double dose.

What to do about side effects

Get emergency help *at once* and stop taking your medication if you have any of the following symptoms: difficulty swallowing, difficulty breathing, or swelling of your face, eyes, lips, hands, feet, or tongue.

Check with your doctor as soon as possible if you feel dizzy or light-headed. Headaches and unusual tiredness also may occur, but these symptoms usually go away as your body adjusts to enalapril. However, if these symptoms persist or bother you, check with your doctor.

A blood problem that can cause severe infections is a rare but serious complication. Report fever, chills, weakness, or a sore throat to your doctor *right away.*

What you must know about other drugs

Don't use salt substitutes or low-salt milk unless your doctor directs you to do so. It may alter your heart rhythm or cause other problems due to a buildup of potassium in your body.

Check with your doctor before taking any nonprescription medications, and be sure your doctor is aware of all prescription medications you're taking. If you're taking lithium (Lithane), your doctor will closely watch your lithium level and may adjust your lithium dosage. He may tell you to use certain painkillers cautiously because they can prevent enalapril from working well.

Special directions

• Tell your doctor about any medical conditions you have, especially kidney, liver, or collagen (immune) disease. Also tell him if you have diabetes or heart or blood vessel disease or if you've recently had a heart attack or stroke.
• Make sure you know how you react to enalapril before driving, using machines, or performing other activities that could be dangerous, in case you become dizzy.
• Your doctor may prescribe a low-salt diet for you. If so, you need to limit canned soups, pickles, and other salty foods. Check with your doctor first because too little salt in your body can also cause problems.

Important reminder

If you're pregnant or think you may be, check with your doctor before taking this medication.

Taking enalapril with hydrochlorothiazide

Dear Patient:

Your doctor has prescribed this combination medication to lower your high blood pressure. The label may read Vaseretic.

How to take this drug
This medication comes in tablet form. Carefully check the label on your prescription bottle to determine how much medication to take and when.

This medication usually increases urination. If you take one dose per day, take it in the morning after breakfast. If you take two or more doses per day, take the last dose no later than 6 p.m. to prevent you from awakening during the night to urinate.

What to do if you miss a dose
Take it as soon as possible. But if it's almost time for your next dose, skip the missed dose and take your next dose on schedule. Don't double dose.

What to do about side effects
Call your doctor *right away* and stop taking this medication if you have:
• a fever that persists
• sore throat
• joint pain
• easy bleeding or bruising
• swelling of your face, mouth, hands, ankles, or feet.

Check with your doctor if you feel dizzy or very tired or if you have a headache, muscle cramps, or low blood pressure, especially if these symptoms continue or bother you.

What you must know about other drugs
Don't take this medication with lithium (Lithane) because lithium toxicity may occur. You may also be instructed to avoid nonsteroidal anti-inflammatory drugs (certain pain relievers) because these medications can prevent enalapril from working well.

Potassium supplements used with this medication may lead to dangerously high potassium levels. Also, avoid using cholestyramine (Questran) or colestipol (Colestid) — cholesterol-lowering drugs — because they reduce the absorption of this medication. Taking diazoxide (Proglycem) with this medication may cause high blood glucose levels and other problems.

Special directions
• Tell your doctor if you have other medical problems, especially diabetes, collagen (immune) disease, pancreatitis, and kidney or liver disease.
• Your doctor may instruct you to eat a diet that is low in salt because too much dietary salt can increase blood pressure.
• Because this medication can make you dizzy, make sure you know how you respond to it before you drive, use machinery, or perform other activities that require alertness.
• If you become sick and have persistant diarrhea or vomiting, call your doctor *right away.* These problems can make you lose too much water, leading to low blood pressure.

Important reminders
If you're pregnant, check with your doctor before taking this medication. If you're an older adult, be aware that you may be especially prone to side effects from this medication.

Taking ergonovine

Dear Patient:

This medication is used after delivery or miscarriage to prevent or treat excessive bleeding from your uterus. The label may read Ergotrate.

How to take ergonovine
Ergonovine comes in tablet form. Carefully check the label on your prescription bottle, which tells you how much to take at each dose. Follow these directions exactly.

Don't take more ergonovine, don't take it more often, and don't take it for a longer time than ordered because doing so could cause unwanted effects.

What to do if you miss a dose
If you miss a dose, skip it. Take your next dose on schedule. Don't double dose.

What to do about side effects
If you develop a rash or itchy skin, start to wheeze, or feel short of breath, stop the medication and call your doctor *immediately*. These symptoms may be warning signs of an allergic reaction, which could be serious. If you have difficulty breathing, get emergency medical care *immediately.*

Check with your doctor if you experience dizziness, headaches, chest pain, ringing in your ears, or nausea and vomiting. Also be aware that this medication can increase your blood pressure.

You may experience menstrual-like cramps. That's because this medication causes the muscles of your uterus to tighten; this is how it controls bleeding. If your cramping becomes very uncomfortable, call your doctor.

What you must know about other drugs
Tell your doctor if you're taking other prescription or nonprescription medications. You may need to avoid certain medications, such as some anesthetics, because they can cause unwanted effects.

Special directions
• Tell your doctor if you have other medical problems, especially chest pain or other heart problems, blood vessel disease (such as Raynaud's phenomenon), high blood pressure (now or in the past), toxemia, and kidney or liver disease. Also report any new medical problems if they occur while taking this medication.
• Let your doctor know if you're allergic to this medication or you have other drug or food allergies.
• If you have an infection, check with your doctor because ergonovine may have stronger effects in this case.
• Don't smoke while taking ergonovine because smoking may increase the risk of harmful side effects.
• Make sure your doctor knows if you're on any special diet, such as a low-salt or low-sugar diet.
• If your bleeding doesn't slow down or if it becomes heavier, call your doctor as soon as possible.

Important reminder
If you're breast-feeding, check with your doctor before taking this medication.

Additional instructions

_____

_____

Taking ergotamine

Dear Patient:

Your doctor has prescribed ergotamine to relieve your headaches. The label may read Ergomar, Ergostat, or Medihaler Ergotamine.

How to take ergotamine
This medication comes in the form of tablets to melt under your tongue, an inhaler, and suppositories.

To use the *under-the-tongue tablets,* place the tablet under your tongue so it dissolves. Don't chew or swallow it because it works faster when absorbed into the lining of your mouth.

If you have the *inhaler,* read the directions that come with it before using the medication. The inhaler gives about 300 measured sprays.

If you're using a *suppository* and it's too soft to insert, run cold water over it or chill it in the refrigerator for about 30 minutes before removing the foil wrapper. To insert it, remove the foil wrapper and moisten the suppository with cold water. Then lie on your side. With your index finger, gently push the suppository into your rectum as far as you can.

Don't take more than the prescribed amount of ergotamine without checking with your doctor.

For best results, take ergotamine at the first sign of a headache. Also, lie down in a quiet, dark room for at least 2 hours after taking your medication.

What to do about side effects
Call your doctor *right away* if you have any of these symptoms of too much ergotamine in your body: confusion; fast or slow heartbeat; numbness and tingling of your fingers, toes, or face; red blisters on or coldness of your hands and feet; shortness of breath; chest or stomach pains; bloating; and weakness.

If you start having headaches more often or they're more severe than before or if you develop swelling in your legs or feet, check with your doctor as soon as possible.

You may experience diarrhea, dizziness, nausea, or vomiting, but these symptoms usually stop when your body adjusts to the medication. If they continue or become bothersome, check with your doctor. If you're using the inhaler and you get a cold or a sore throat or mouth, call your doctor.

What you must know about alcohol and other drugs
Avoid alcoholic beverages because they can make your headaches worse. Tell your doctor if you're taking other medications. Taking a beta blocker, such as propranolol (Inderal), for high blood pressure or a heart condition may cause unwanted side effects.

Special directions
Tell your doctor if you have other medical problems, especially diseases of the heart, blood vessels, kidney, liver, or thyroid. Also tell him if you have high blood pressure or a skin condition that causes severe itching. Your doctor also needs to know if you've recently had an angioplasty (to open a blocked blood vessel) or surgery on a blood vessel.

Important reminders
If you're pregnant or breast-feeding, check with your doctor before taking this medication. If you're an older adult, you may be especially prone to side effects from ergotamine.

Taking ergotamine with caffeine

Dear Patient:

Your doctor has prescribed this combination medication to relieve your headaches. Ergotamine narrows your blood vessels, and caffeine helps ergotamine to be absorbed by the body. This combination is known by several brand names, the most common of which is Cafergot.

How to take ergotamine with caffeine

This medication is available in tablet and suppository forms. Carefully read the label on your medication bottle and follow the directions exactly. Take no more than 6 tablets or 2 suppositories for each attack or 10 tablets or 5 suppositories a week. If your headache isn't relieved, call your doctor. Don't increase the dose.

To use the *suppository,* remove the foil wrapper and moisten it with cold water. Lie on your side and use your middle or index finger to push the suppository into your rectum. If the suppository is too soft to insert, place it in the refrigerator for 30 minutes before removing the foil wrapper.

For best results, take ergotamine with caffeine at the first sign of a headache. Rest in a dark, quiet room for about 2 hours after taking it.

Don't stop this medication abruptly. Doing so may increase the frequency and duration of headaches.

What you must know about alcohol and other drugs

Avoid drinking alcoholic beverages because they can worsen your headache.

Don't use this medication if you're also taking a beta blocker, such as propranolol (Inderal). This combination may be hazardous because it could cause too much narrowing of the blood vessels.

Special directions
• Tell your doctor if you have other medical problems, especially diseases of the blood vessels, kidney, or liver. Also tell your doctor if you have high blood pressure or severe skin itching.
• Ergotamine may make you sensitive to cold temperatures. Wear warm clothes during cold weather, and be careful if you participate in winter activities that prolong your exposure to cold.

Important reminders
If you're pregnant or breast-feeding, don't take this medication.

If you're an older adult, you may be especially prone to side effects from ergotamine with caffeine.

If you're an athlete, you should know that high levels of caffeine are banned and sometimes tested for by the National Collegiate Athletic Association and the U.S. Olympic Committee.

Additional instructions

_____

_____

_____

_____

_____

_____

Taking oral erythromycin

Dear Patient:

Your doctor has prescribed erythromycin to treat your infection. The label may read E-Mycin, Erythrocin, or Wyamycin-S.

How to take erythromycin

This medication is available in tablet, capsule, and oral liquid forms. Carefully check the label on your prescription bottle, and follow the directions exactly as ordered.

Take your medication with a full glass (8 ounces) of water 1 hour before or 2 hours after meals. If the tablets are coated or the medication upsets your stomach, you may take it with food. But don't take your medication with fruit juice.

If you're taking the *chewable tablets,* chew or crush them before swallowing. If you're taking the *delayed-release capsules,* swallow them whole.

If you're taking the *oral liquid* form, measure your dose with a special dropper or measuring spoon made especially for medications.

Continue to take your medication for the full treatment time, even if you feel better after a few days. Stopping too soon may allow your infection to return.

What to do if you miss a dose

Take it as soon as possible. But if it's almost time for your next dose, change your schedule as follows.

If you take two doses a day, space the missed dose and the next one 5 to 6 hours apart.

If you take three or more doses a day, space the missed dose and the next one 2 to 4 hours apart.

Then resume your regular dosing schedule.

What to do about side effects

If you develop a rash or itchy skin, stop taking the medication and call your doctor *immediately.* Sometimes, these symptoms are warning signs of a serious allergic reaction. If you feel unusually restless or have trouble breathing, get medical care *right away.*

Tell your doctor if you have stomach pain, diarrhea, nausea, or vomiting. These symptoms may go away as your body adjusts to erythromycin, but let your doctor know if they bother you.

What you must know about other drugs

Tell your doctor if you're taking other medications. Erythromycin may not work well if taken with certain other antibiotics. Taking erythromycin with blood thinners may increase your risk of bleeding. Your doctor also may caution you against taking erythromycin with theophylline (Theo-Dur), an asthma drug, because of possible unwanted effects.

Special directions

• Tell your doctor if you have other medical problems, especially liver disease. Also inform him if you're allergic to erythromycin, another medication, or any food.
• Before you have medical tests, tell the doctor that you're taking erythromycin because the drug may interfere with some test results.

Additional instructions

_____

_____

Applying topical erythromycin

Dear Patient:

Your doctor has prescribed erythromycin for your skin problem. The medication label may read Akne-mycin, Erycette, or EryDerm.

How to apply erythromycin
This medication is available as an ointment, a gel, a pledget (swab), and a solution. Before applying it, wash the area with warm water and soap, rinse well, and pat dry. After washing or shaving, try to wait 30 minutes before applying the pledget, gel, or liquid forms. Otherwise, the alcohol in your medication may sting.

Keep the medication away from your eyes, nose, and mouth. If you do get some in your eyes, wash them out immediately, but carefully, with cool tap water.

If you're using the *ointment* or *gel,* apply a thin film of medication to cover the area lightly. If you're using the *solution,* dab the medication on with an applicator tip or a moistened pad.

What to do if you miss an application
Apply the medication as soon as possible. But if it's almost time for your next application, skip the missed one and go back to your regular schedule.

What to do about side effects
Expect some mild stinging of your skin for a few minutes after you apply erythromycin. This is normal. However, check with your doctor if your skin continues to itch or burn. Also call if your skin breaks out in a rash or becomes dry or scaly. These symptoms may go away as your body adjusts to erythromycin, but let your doctor know about them, especially if they become bothersome or severe.

What you must know about other drugs
If you're using another medication on your skin along with erythromycin, wait at least 1 hour before you apply the second medication to prevent skin irritation.

Special directions
• Tell your doctor if you're allergic to erythromycin, another medication, or any food.
• If you have acne, don't wash the affected area too much. Doing so could dry your skin and make your acne worse. Wash the area with a mild, bland soap two or three times a day, unless you have oily skin. Check with your doctor for specific instructions.
• If you're using erythromycin for acne, you may wear cosmetics, but use only water-based products. Also, don't apply cosmetics heavily or use them too frequently because your acne could worsen.

Additional instructions

_____

_____

_____

_____

_____

_____

Taking erythromycin with sulfisoxazole

Dear Patient:

Your doctor has prescribed this combination medication to treat your ear infection. The label may read Eryzole, Pediazole, or Sulfimycin.

How to take this drug
This medication comes as an oral liquid. Follow your doctor's instructions exactly. Use a specially marked measuring spoon—not a household teaspoon—to measure your dose. Take your medication with food or extra water, if possible, to help prevent side effects.

Because this medication works best if you have a constant amount in your blood, take it in evenly spaced doses during the day and night. If you need to take four doses a day, schedule each dose 6 hours apart. Talk to your doctor, nurse, or pharmacist if this schedule disrupts your sleep or other activities.

Continue to take your medication, even if you start to feel better in a few days. Stopping too soon may allow your infection to return.

What to do if you miss a dose
Take it as soon as possible unless it's almost time for your next dose. In that case, if you take three or more doses a day, space the missed dose and the next dose 2 to 4 hours apart. Then return to your regular dosing schedule.

What to do about side effects
If you become short of breath or have difficulty breathing, stop taking this medication and get emergency medical care *at once.* You may be experiencing a serious allergic reaction.

If you have a persistent fever, sore throat, joint pain, or start to bruise or bleed easily, don't take any more of this medication. Call your doctor as soon as possible.

You may also experience some abdominal pain, nausea, vomiting, or diarrhea. Check with your doctor about these symptoms, especially if they continue or become bothersome.

What you must know about other drugs
Tell your doctor about other medications you're taking. Taking this medication with oral blood thinners could put you at risk for bleeding. Also, your doctor may not want you to use theophylline (Theo-Dur), an asthma medication, or terfenadine (Seldane), an allergy drug, with this medication because it could cause unwanted effects.

Erythromycin with sulfisoxazole can decrease the effectiveness of birth control pills. If necessary, switch to another form of birth control.

Special directions
• Tell your doctor if you're allergic to erythromycin or sulfisoxazole.
• Drink lots of extra water to prevent side effects, such as kidney stones, caused by the sulfa in this medication.

Important reminder
If you're pregnant or breast-feeding, don't take this medication without first checking with your doctor.

Additional instructions

_____

_____

_____

Taking estazolam

Dear Patient:

Your doctor has prescribed this medication to help you sleep. The label may read ProSom.

How to take estazolam
Estazolam comes in tablet form. Follow your doctor's directions exactly. Don't take more of it or take it more often or for a longer time than ordered. If too much is taken, estazolam can become habit-forming or may not help you sleep.

Check with your doctor if you think the medication isn't working well, especially if you've been taking it every night for several weeks.

What to do if you miss a dose
Skip the missed dose and go back to your regular dosing schedule. Don't double dose.

What to do about side effects
If this medication makes you drowsy in the daytime or dizzy, check with your doctor, especially if these symptoms continue or bother you.

If you think you've taken an overdose or you experience severe side effects, such as prolonged confusion, severe drowsiness, trouble breathing, slow heartbeat, continuing slurred speech, staggering, or severe weakness, call for emergency help *immediately.*

What you must know about alcohol and other drugs
Don't drink alcoholic beverages while taking this medication because the combination can cause oversedation. For the same reason, avoid other central nervous system depressants (medications that slow down the nervous system), such as tranquilizers, other sleep medications, muscle relaxers, and cold, allergy, and flu medications.

Other medications that can cause oversedation if taken with estazolam include the ulcer drug cimetidine (Tagamet); birth control pills; disulfiram (Antabuse), a medication for alcoholism; and isoniazid (Laniazid), a tuberculosis medication.

Estazolam may not work well if taken with certain medications, so be sure to tell your doctor about other medications you're taking.

Special directions
• Tell your doctor if you have other medical problems, such as a history of alcohol or drug dependence, brain disorders, asthma or other lung diseases, kidney or liver disease, depression, myasthenia gravis, seizures, porphyria, or breathing problems while sleeping.
• Check with your doctor at least every 4 months to see if you need to continue taking estazolam.
• After stopping this medication, your body may need time to adjust. Call your doctor if you experience any irritability, nervousness, or trouble sleeping.

Important reminders
If you're pregnant or breast-feeding, check with your doctor before taking this medication. If you're an older adult, you may be especially prone to daytime drowsiness, so take care to prevent falls.

Additional instructions

_____

_____

Taking estradiol

Dear Patient:

Your doctor has prescribed estradiol to treat your condition. This estrogen-like medication is used to treat menopausal symptoms, vaginal dryness, and certain cancers. The label may read Estrace or Estraderm.

How to take estradiol
Estradiol comes in tablet, vaginal cream, and skin patch forms. Follow your doctor's instructions exactly. If the tablets cause nausea, you may take them with food.

Before applying a *patch,* read the accompanying instructions. Wash and dry your hands. Apply the patch to a clean, dry, nonoily skin area, such as your abdomen or buttocks.

If you're using the *vaginal cream,* your doctor may want you to use it at bedtime so it will be absorbed better. If you don't use it at bedtime, lie down for 30 minutes after use.

What to do if you miss a dose
If you forget to take a *tablet* or change a *skin patch,* do it as soon as possible. But if it's almost time for your next dose, skip the missed dose. Take your next tablet or apply a new patch on schedule. Don't take double doses of tablets or use more than one patch at a time.

If you forget to apply a dose of *vaginal cream* and don't remember until the next day, skip the missed dose. Resume your regular dosing schedule.

What to do about side effects
Be alert for symptoms of blood clots, a rare but serious complication. Call for emergency help *immediately* if you have:
• sudden or severe headache
• sudden loss of coordination
• blurred vision or other vision changes
• numbness or stiffness in your legs
• pain in your chest, groin, or legs
• shortness of breath.

Call your doctor *right away* if you experience rapid weight gain; swelling in your feet and lower legs; breast enlargement, pain, or lumps; or unusual vaginal bleeding. Also call if you become nauseous, lose your appetite, or have stomach bloating or cramps.

If you're using the vaginal cream, call your doctor if you develop swelling, redness, or itching in the vaginal area.

What you must know about other drugs
Because many medications can interfere with estradiol, tell your doctor about other medications (nonprescription and prescription) you're taking.

Special directions
• Because estradiol can aggravate many medical conditions, tell your doctor about other medical problems you have. Also tell him if you have female relatives who have had cancer of the breast or female organs.
• Keep all appointments for follow-up visits so your doctor can check your progress and detect side effects early.
• Perform breast self-examinations regularly and report unusual changes.

Important reminders
Don't take estradiol if you're pregnant or breast-feeding. If you have diabetes, be aware that estradiol may affect your glucose levels.

Taking estrogen

Dear Patient:

Your doctor has prescribed estrogen to help your conditon. This female hormone is used to relieve menopausal symptoms, to treat certain breast cancers, and to help prevent brittle bone disease (osteoporosis). Brand names include Premarin, Estratab, and Estinyl.

How to take estrogen
Estrogen comes in the form of tablets, capsules, and vaginal cream. Follow your doctor's instructions exactly. For best results, take your medication at the same time each day.

If you take *tablets,* take them with food if you develop nausea.

If you're using the *vaginal cream,* your doctor may want you to apply it at bedtime so it will be absorbed better. If you're not using it at bedtime, lie down for 30 minutes after use.

What to do if you miss a dose
If you miss a *tablet,* take it as soon as possible. But if it's almost time for your next dose, skip the missed dose and take your next dose on schedule. Don't double dose.

If you forget to apply a dose of *vaginal cream* and don't remember until the next day, skip the missed dose. Go back to your regular dosing schedule.

What to do about side effects
Be alert for symptoms of blood clots, a rare but serious complication. Call for emergency help *immediately* if you have:
• sudden or severe headache
• sudden loss of coordination
• vision changes, such as loss of sight or blurred vision, or see flashing lights
• numbness or stiffness in your legs
• pain in your chest, groin, or legs
• shortness of breath.

Also call your doctor *right away* if you experience rapid weight gain; breast swelling, pain, or lumps; or unusual vaginal bleeding. If you're using the vaginal cream, call your doctor if you develop swelling, redness, or itching in the vaginal area.

Check with your doctor if you feel nauseous or lose your appetite or your stomach becomes cramped or bloated.

What you must know about other drugs
Because many medications can interfere with estrogen therapy, make sure your doctor is aware of all other medications (both nonprescription and prescription) that you're taking.

Special directions
• Tell your doctor about other medical problems you have, especially breast disease, cancer, diabetes, high blood pressure, porphyria, gynecologic problems, or diseases of the major organs. Mention if you've ever had blood clots or a stroke. Also tell him if you have female relatives who have had breast or female organ cancer.
• Keep all appointments for follow-up care so your doctor can check your progress and detect side effects early.
• Be sure to perform regular breast self-examinations and see your doctor for routine breast examinations.

Important reminders
If you're pregnant or breast-feeding, don't use estrogen. If you have diabetes, estrogen could affect your glucose level, so check with your doctor if you notice any changes.

Taking estrogen with progestin

Dear Patient:

Your doctor has prescribed estrogen with progestin. Also known as an oral contraceptive or birth control pill, this medication prevents pregnancy by changing your body's hormonal balance. This medication comes in various brand names, including Ortho-Novum, Ovcon, or Triphasil.

How to take this drug
The drug comes in variously colored tablets. The color indicates the tablet strength. Carefully read and follow the directions. Usually, you take a certain color tablet at the same time every day in the order the tablets are arranged in the container. Don't take a tablet out of order.

To prevent nausea, take the tablet with food or just after eating.

Based on your needs, the doctor will prescribe a certain dosing schedule called a *one-phase, two-phase,* or *three-phase* schedule. Here's how each works.

One-phase schedules
If you're on a 20- or 21-day schedule, take a tablet of the same strength for 20 or 21 days.

If you're on a 28-day schedule, take one tablet for 21 days and a different color tablet (containing inactive ingredients) for 7 or 8 more days.

Two-phase schedules
If you're on a 21-day schedule, take a tablet of one strength (first color) for 10 days, then a different tablet (second color) for the next 11 days.

If you're on a 24-day schedule, take a tablet of one strength (first color) for 17 days, then a different tablet (second color) for the next 7 days.

If you're on a 28-day schedule, take a tablet of one strength (first color) for 10 days of the cycle, a different tablet (second color) for the next 11 days, then a tablet with inactive ingredients (third color) for 7 days.

Three-phase schedules
If you're on a 21-day schedule, take a tablet in the order directed by your prescription. For example, you may take the first tablet (first color) for 6 or 7 days, a different tablet (second color) for the next 5 to 9 days, and another tablet (third color) for 5 to 10 days, for a total of 21 tablets.

If you're on a 28-day schedule, follow a 21-day schedule, then take a tablet with inactive ingredients (fourth color) for the next 7 days, for a total of 28 tablets.

What to do if you miss a dose
If you forget to take your medication, consult your doctor and review the following guide.

One-phase and two-phase schedules
If you're on a 20-, 21-, or 24-day one-phase or two-phase schedule and you miss one dose, take it when you remember. If you don't remember until the next day, take the missed dose and your scheduled dose; you can take two tablets on the same day. Then resume your normal schedule.

If you miss two doses in a row, take two tablets a day for the next 2 days, then resume your normal schedule. Use another birth control method to protect

(continued)

Taking estrogen with progestin *(continued)*

you for the rest of your cycle, and consult your doctor.

If you miss three or more doses in a row, stop taking the tablets, and use another birth control method until you have your period or the doctor tells you you're not pregnant. Resume your normal schedule with the next cycle.

If you're on a 28-day cycle and you miss any of the first 21 tablets (which contain active ingredients), follow the instructions for the 21-day schedule and the number of doses you missed.

Three-phase schedules
If you're on a three-phase schedule and miss a dose during the 21-day period, take the missed tablet when you remember. If you don't remember until the next day, take the missed dose and the regular dose for that day. In this case, you can take two doses in the same day; then resume your regular schedule. Use another birth control method for the rest of your cycle, and consult your doctor.

If you miss two doses in a row, take two doses for the next 2 days, then resume your normal schedule. Use another birth control method, and consult your doctor.

If you miss three doses in a row, don't take any tablets. Instead, use another birth control method until you have your period or your doctor confirms that you're not pregnant. Resume your normal schedule as directed.

If you're on a 28-day cycle and you miss any of the first 21 tablets, follow the directions for the 21-day schedule, depending on how many doses you missed. Pregnancy isn't a risk if you miss any of the last seven tablets. But you must take the first tablet of the next

month's cycle on your regularly scheduled day to prevent pregnancy.

What to do about side effects
Seek *emergency* care if you cough up blood or experience sudden shortness of breath, severe headache, vision changes, slurred speech, unexplained weakness in your arms or legs, or stomach, chest, groin, or leg pain.

When you begin taking this medication, you may experience some vaginal bleeding. If so, consult your doctor.

Special directions
• You may need to take this medication for about 1 month before it works effectively. During this time, you may need to use an additional birth control method.
• Before having any dental work or surgery, tell the dentist or doctor that you're taking this medication.

Important reminders
If you become pregnant, stop taking this medication at once and notify your doctor. Also consult your doctor if you're breast-feeding.

Additional instructions

_____

_____

_____

_____

_____

_____

_____

Taking ethambutol

Dear Patient:

Your doctor has prescribed ethambutol to treat your tuberculosis (TB). The medication label may read Myambutol.

How to take ethambutol
Take this medication exactly as your doctor directs. Take it at the same time each day to help you remember not to miss a dose. If the medication upsets your stomach, you can take it with food.

Keep taking ethambutol as your doctor directs, even after you feel better. Otherwise, your TB may not clear up completely. Keep in mind that you may need to take it for 1 year or more.

What to do about side effects
Call your doctor *immediately* if you experience blurred vision, blindness, eye pain, or trouble differentiating between red and green. Also call your doctor *at once* if you have chills or fever; pain or swelling in your joints (especially in your feet); or burning, numbness, tingling, or weakness in your hands or feet or if you cough up mucus tinged with blood.

Other possible side effects, such as an upset stomach, diarrhea, loss of appetite, severe fatigue, dizziness, itching, and rashes, may go away as your body adjusts to ethambutol. However, be sure to discuss them with your doctor also.

Special directions
• Before taking ethambutol, tell your doctor if you have optic neuritis (eye nerve damage), cataracts, recurrent eye infections, or vision problems related to diabetes, gout, or kidney disease. That's because ethambutol may aggravate these conditions.

• Your doctor may order you to have regular blood tests to monitor you for certain disorders, such as gout.
• Your doctor may ask you to schedule regular eye examinations while you're taking ethambutol.
• Until you know how your body responds to ethambutol, don't drive or perform activities requiring alertness and clear vision.
• Notify your doctor if your symptoms don't disappear or if you feel worse after 2 to 3 weeks of ethambutol therapy.

Important reminders
If you're breast-feeding, check with your doctor before taking this medication.

Ethambutol isn't recommended for children under age 13.

Additional instructions

_____

_____

_____

_____

_____

_____

_____

_____

_____

Taking famotidine

Dear Patient:

This medication helps treat ulcers. (It's also used to treat Zollinger-Ellison disease, in which the stomach produces too much acid). The medication label may read Pepcid.

How to take famotidine

This medication comes in tablets and powder for oral suspension. Carefully follow the prescription directions.

If you're taking this medication once a day, take it at bedtime unless your doctor directs otherwise. If you're taking it twice a day, take one dose in the morning and one at bedtime. If you're taking it more than twice a day, take your dose with meals and at bedtime for best results.

What to do if you miss a dose

Take a missed dose as soon as possible. If it's almost time for your next regular dose, skip the missed dose and take your next dose on your regular schedule. Don't take a double dose.

What to do about side effects

If you have a headache (a common side effect) that persists or becomes severe, contact your doctor.

Special directions

• Be sure to tell your doctor if you have other medical problems, especially kidney or liver disease, because certain disorders may affect the way famotidine works for you.
• This medication may not begin to relieve your stomach pain for several days. Unless your doctor directs otherwise, you may take antacids to help relieve the pain. However, wait 30 minutes to 1 hour after taking the antacid before taking famotidine.
• Tell your doctor that you're taking famotidine before you undergo any skin tests for allergies or tests to determine how much acid your stomach produces.
• If you smoke, stop smoking—or at least try not to smoke after taking the last dose of this medication each day. That's because cigarette smoking tends to decrease famotidine's effects, especially at night.
• Contact your doctor if your ulcer pain continues or gets worse.

Important reminders

If you're pregnant or breast-feeding, check with your doctor before taking this medication.

If you're an older adult, you may be especially sensitive to famotidine's side effects.

Additional instructions

_____

_____

_____

_____

_____

_____

_____

_____

Taking fenoprofen

Dear Patient:

Fenoprofen helps relieve the inflammation, swelling, stiffness, and joint pain of rheumatoid arthritis or osteoarthritis. The label may read Nalfon.

How to take fenoprofen
Take the drug with food or an antacid and a full glass of water. Avoid lying down for 15 to 30 minutes after taking this medication. Doing so will help prevent swallowing problems.

What to do if you miss a dose
Take a missed dose as soon as you remember if it's within 2 hours of your regular time. If it's later than that, skip the missed dose and take your next dose at the regular time. Don't take two doses at once.

What to do about side effects
Serious side effects, including ulcers or bleeding, can occur with or without warning. As a result, you should stop taking fenoprofen and call your doctor *right away* if you notice any of these warning signs: severe stomach cramps, pain, or burning; severe, continuing nausea, heartburn, or indigestion; or vomit tinged with blood or material that looks like coffee grounds.

You may experience dizziness, headache, drowsiness, heartburn, nausea, vomiting, itching, and black, tarry stools while taking fenoprofen. If these symptoms persist or become severe, call your doctor.

What you must know about alcohol and other drugs
Avoid alcoholic beverages; they increase your risk of stomach problems.

Also, don't take aspirin or acetaminophen (Tylenol) with fenoprofen for more than a few days (unless your doctor directs otherwise) because this may increase your risk of serious side effects.

Because some other drugs interfere with fenoprofen's effects, be sure to tell your doctor about other medications you're taking, particularly anticoagulants (blood thinners) and sulfonylureas (drugs for diabetes).

Special directions
• If you have other medical problems, let your doctor know. They may affect the use of this medication.
• Be sure you know how you react to fenoprofen before driving or performing other activities that require alertness.
• If fenoprofen makes you more sensitive to sunlight than normal, wear a hat and sunglasses and use a sunblock outdoors.

Important reminders
If you're pregnant or breast-feeding, consult your doctor about taking fenoprofen.

If you're an older adult, you may be especially prone to side effects.

Additional instructions

_____

_____

_____

_____

_____

Applying a fentanyl patch

Dear Patient:

Your doctor has prescribed the fentanyl transdermal patch to help relieve your pain. The label may read Duragesic-25, Duragesic-50, Duragesic-75, or Duragesic-100.

How to apply a fentanyl patch

Apply a new patch to a new site every 72 hours or as ordered by your doctor. First, clip excess hair at the patch site. Don't use a razor because shaving may irritate or scratch your skin.

Wash your skin with clear water if necessary, but don't use soap, oil, lotion, alcohol, or any other substance that may irritate your skin or interfere with the patch's stickiness.

Make sure your skin is completely dry. Then put the patch on your skin and hold it in place for 10 to 20 seconds to make sure it stays on.

What to do if you miss an application

If you don't apply a new patch when scheduled, do so as soon as you can. Don't apply more than one patch at a time. Doing so may cause serious side effects.

What to do about side effects

Seek medical care *at once* if you have trouble breathing.

Fentanyl also may make you feel drowsy and lethargic. It may lower your blood pressure, causing you to feel dizzy or light-headed. You may also experience constipation and problems with urination. If these side effects persist or become severe, contact your doctor.

What you must know about alcohol and other drugs

Don't drink alcoholic beverages or take medications that affect your nervous system (such as many allergy or cold medications, narcotics, muscle relaxants, sleeping pills, and seizure medications). Combined with fentanyl, these medications may produce serious side effects.

Special directions

• Before taking fentanyl, inform your doctor of other medical problems you may have. They may affect the use of this medication.
• Don't stop taking fentanyl suddenly. Doing so may cause undesirable withdrawal effects. Consult your doctor, who may reduce your dosage gradually before stopping the medication completely.
• Don't drive or perform activities requiring alertness until you know how fentanyl affects you.

Important reminders

If you're breast-feeding, consult your doctor before taking fentanyl.

Young children and older adults are especially sensitive to fentanyl.

If you're an athlete, you should know that the U.S. Olympic Committee tests for and bans fentanyl's use.

Additional instructions

_____

_____

_____

_____

Taking flecainide

Dear Patient:

Your doctor has prescribed flecainide to help stabilize your heart rhythm. The label on your medication may read Tambocor.

How to take flecainide
This medication comes in tablet form. Take two daily doses 12 hours apart in the morning and evening unless your doctor orders otherwise.

What to do if you miss a dose
Take a missed dose of flecainide as soon as you remember within 6 hours of your regularly scheduled time. If it's later than that, skip the missed dose and resume your normal dosing schedule. Don't take double doses.

What to do about side effects
Seek medical treatment *right away* if you experience any of these side effects: chest pain, irregular heartbeat, shortness of breath, swelling in your feet or lower legs, and trembling or shaking.

Flecainide may also cause dizziness, headache, and vision problems. If these symptoms persist or become severe, consult your doctor.

What you must know about other drugs
Tell your doctor if you're taking other drugs—particularly other heart medications. These may produce unpredictable effects when taken with flecainide.

Special directions
• Before taking flecainide, discuss other medical problems you have with your doctor, especially kidney or liver disease, a recent heart attack, or a pacemaker.
• See your doctor regularly so he can check your progress and adjust your dosage as needed.
• Carry medical identification with you or wear a medical identification bracelet stating that you're taking flecainide.
• If possible, before you undergo any dental or surgical procedure or emergency treatment, tell the dentist or doctor that you're taking flecainide.
• Because flecainide may make you feel dizzy, light-headed, or sluggish, don't drive a car or perform activities requiring alertness until you know how this medication affects you.
• If you've been taking this medication regularly for several weeks, don't suddenly stop taking it. Check with your doctor, who can help you reduce the dosage gradually.

Important reminders
If you're pregnant or breast-feeding, check with your doctor before taking flecainide.

If you're an older adult, you may be especially susceptible to flecainide's side effects.

Additional instructions

_____

_____

_____

_____

_____

_____

Taking fluconazole

Dear Patient:

Your doctor has prescribed fluconazole to treat your fungal infection. Your prescription label may read Diflucan.

How to take fluconazole

Take fluconazole exactly as prescribed. To help clear up your infection completely, take it for the full course of treatment even if your symptoms subside. A fungal infection may require many months of treatment even after your symptoms are no longer bothersome.

What to do if you miss a dose

Take a missed dose of medication as soon as you remember. If it's almost time for your next dose, skip the missed dose and take your next dose as scheduled. Don't take double doses.

What to do about side effects

Fluconazole causes nausea in some people. If you experience persistent or severe nausea, contact your doctor.

What you must know about other drugs

Combined with other medications, fluconazole may produce unwanted side effects. Be sure to tell your doctor about all the medications you take, especially cyclosporine (Sandimmune), phenytoin (Dilantin), isoniazid (Laniazid), rifampin (Rifadin), valproic acid (Depakene), warfarin (Coumadin), and some oral medications used to lower blood glucose levels.

Special directions

• Before taking fluconazole, tell your doctor about other medical problems you have, especially kidney or liver disease. They may affect the use of this medication.
• See your doctor regularly so he can monitor your progress and check for unwanted effects.
• Check with your doctor if your symptoms don't disappear within a few weeks or if you feel worse.

Important reminders

Consult your doctor if you become pregnant while taking fluconazole.

If you're breast-feeding, check with your doctor before taking fluconazole.

Additional instructions

_____

_____

_____

_____

_____

_____

_____

_____

_____

_____

Applying fluocinolone

Dear Patient:

Your doctor has prescribed fluocinolone cream, ointment, or solution to help relieve redness, swelling, itching, and other skin discomfort. The label may read Bio-Syn, Fluonid, or Synalar.

How to apply fluocinolone
Follow your doctor's directions exactly to apply fluocinolone. Use your finger to apply it to your skin. Then wash your hands. Don't bandage or wrap the area being treated unless your doctor directs you to do so.

What to do if you miss an application
If you miss a dose of this medication, apply it as soon as possible. But if it's almost time for your next dose, skip the missed dose and apply the next dose on your regular schedule.

What to do about side effects
Although side effects from using fluocinolone are uncommon, the drug may produce such skin reactions as burning, itching, dryness, changes in color or texture, or a rash and inflammation (dermatitis). Consult your doctor if you have these side effects.

Special directions
• If you have other medical problems, be sure to let your doctor know. A change in your medication may be necessary.
• Don't get fluocinolone in your eyes. If you do, flush your eyes with water.
• If the doctor tells you to apply an occlusive dressing (an airtight covering, such as plastic wrap or a special patch) over fluocinolone, be sure to get complete directions for doing so.

• Don't use leftover medication for other skin problems without first consulting your doctor.
• If you're applying fluocinolone to a child's diaper area, avoid using tight-fitting diapers or plastic pants, which could increase absorption of the medication through the skin and possibly cause side effects.

Important reminders
If you become pregnant while using fluocinolone, consult your doctor.

Don't apply this medication to your breasts before breast-feeding.

Children and adolescents using this medication should be checked closely. Fluocinolone can affect growth and cause other unwanted effects.

If you're an older adult, you may be especially susceptible to certain side effects, such as skin tearing and blood blisters.

Additional instructions

_____

_____

_____

_____

_____

_____

_____

_____

Applying fluocinonide

Dear Patient:

Your doctor has prescribed fluocinonide to help relieve redness, swelling, itching, and other skin discomfort. The prescription label may read Lidex, Lidex-E, or Fluocin.

How to apply fluocinonide
This medication comes in cream, ointment, gel, and solution forms. Apply it exactly as your doctor directs. Wash your hands after using your finger to apply it. Don't bandage or wrap the skin being treated unless your doctor directs you to do so.

What to do if you miss an application
Apply a missed dose as soon as possible. If it's almost time for your next dose, skip the missed dose and apply the next dose on schedule.

What to do about side effects
Although side effects are uncommon, fluocinonide can cause such skin reactions as burning, itching, dryness, changes in color or texture, or a rash and inflammation (dermatitis). Tell your doctor if such effects occur.

Special directions
• If you have other medical problems, be sure to let your doctor know. They may affect the use of this medication.
• Don't get fluocinonide in your eyes. If you do, flush your eyes with water.
• If your doctor instructs you to use an occlusive dressing (an airtight covering, such as plastic wrap or a special patch) over fluocinonide, make sure you understand how to apply it.

• Don't use leftover medication for other skin problems without first consulting your doctor.
• If you're applying fluocinonide to a child's diaper area, avoid using tight-fitting diapers or plastic pants. They may cause unwanted side effects.

Important reminders
Consult your doctor if you become pregnant while using fluocinonide.

Don't apply this medication to your breasts before breast-feeding.

Children and adolescents who use fluocinonide should have frequent medical checkups because this medication can affect growth and cause other unwanted effects.

If you're an older adult, you may be especially susceptible to certain side effects, such as skin tearing and blood blisters.

Additional instructions

_____

_____

_____

_____

_____

_____

_____

_____

Taking fluoxetine

Dear Patient:

This medication is prescribed to help relieve depression. The label may read Prozac.

How to take fluoxetine

Take fluoxetine exactly as prescribed. You may need to take it for 4 weeks or longer before you begin to feel better.

What to do if you miss a dose

Skip a missed dose and take your next regular dose as scheduled. Never take a double dose.

What to do about side effects

If you develop a rash or hives, stop taking this medication and call your doctor *immediately*—you may be having an allergic reaction.

This medication may cause nervousness, anxiety, insomnia, headache, drowsiness, shakiness, dizziness, nausea, diarrhea, dry mouth, loss of appetite, stomach upset, weight loss, itching, and weakness. If you have any of these symptoms and they persist or worsen, contact your doctor.

What you must know about alcohol and other drugs

Avoid drinking alcoholic beverages while taking fluoxetine. Also avoid taking other medications that affect the nervous system (such as cough, cold, and allergy medications; narcotics; muscle relaxants; sleeping pills; and seizure medications).

Tell your doctor about other medications you're taking. For example, taking fluoxetine with diazepam (Valium), warfarin (Coumadin), or digitoxin (Crystodigin) may cause serious side effects.

Special directions

• Before taking fluoxetine, tell your doctor if you have other medical problems, especially diabetes, kidney or liver disease, or a seizure disorder.
• Schedule regular checkups so your doctor can monitor your progress, check for side effects, and adjust your dosage as needed.
• Because fluoxetine may cause drowsiness, don't drive or perform activities requiring alertness until you know how the medication affects you.
• If you feel dizzy, light-headed, or faint when getting up from a bed or chair, rise slowly. If the problem persists or worsens, consult your doctor.
• To relieve a dry mouth, use sugarless gum or hard candy, ice chips, or a saliva substitute. Dryness that persists for longer than 2 weeks increases your chance for dental problems. Consult your doctor or dentist.

Important reminders

If you have diabetes, fluoxetine may affect your glucose levels. Report changes in your home blood or urine glucose tests to your doctor.

If you're breast-feeding, check with your doctor before taking fluoxetine.

Additional instructions

_____

_____

_____

_____

_____

Taking fluphenazine

Dear Patient:

Fluphenazine is prescribed to treat emotional problems. The label may read Permitil or Prolixin.

How to take fluphenazine
Take fluphenazine exactly as your doctor directs. You may take it with food or a full glass (8 ounces) of water or milk to minimize possible stomach upset.

If your medication comes in a dropper bottle, measure each dose with the special dropper. Dilute the medication in one-half glass (4 ounces) of orange juice, grapefruit juice, or water. Avoid spilling liquid medication on your skin because it may cause irritation and a rash.

What to do if you miss a dose
If you take one dose a day and miss the dose, take it as soon as possible. Then take your next dose at the regular time. But if you don't remember the missed dose until the next day, skip it and take your next scheduled dose.

If you take more than one dose a day and miss a dose, take the missed dose as soon as you remember if it's within an hour or so of the scheduled time. But if you don't remember until later, skip the missed dose and take your next dose as scheduled. Don't double dose.

What to do about side effects
Contact your doctor *immediately* if you learn that your blood count is abnormal or if you develop an infection or fever, rapid heartbeat, rapid breathing, and profuse sweating.

Also call your doctor *immediately* if you have these uncontrollable movements: lip smacking, mouth puckering, cheek puffing, wormlike tongue movements, chewing motions, and arm or leg movements.

Fluphenazine also may cause dizziness, light-headedness, or faintness when arising from a bed or a chair; blurred vision; dry mouth; constipation; urine retention; and mild sensitivity to sunlight. Contact your doctor if these side effects are persistent or bothersome.

What you must know about alcohol and other drugs
Avoid alcoholic beverages and other medications that affect your nervous system. Tell your doctor about all other prescription and nonprescription medications you're taking. They may interact with fluphenazine and cause problems.

Special directions
• Before taking fluphenazine, tell your doctor about other medical problems you have. They may affect the use of this medication.
• Know how you react to fluphenazine before driving or performing activities requiring alertness and clear vision.
• Relieve a dry mouth with sugarless hard candy or gum, ice chips, or a saliva substitute.
• Protect yourself against overexposure to sunlight.

Important reminders
If you're pregnant or breast-feeding, check with your doctor before taking this medication. Children and older adults are especially sensitive to this medication. If you're an athlete, be aware that the National Collegiate Athletic Association and the U.S. Olympic Committee ban the use of fluphenazine.

Applying flurandrenolide

Dear Patient:

Your doctor has prescribed flurandrenolide to help relieve redness, swelling, itching, and other skin discomfort. Your prescription label may read Cordran.

How to apply flurandrenolide
This medication is available as cream, lotion, ointment, and tape. Carefully check the medication directions. Apply flurandrenolide exactly as prescribed. Wash your hands after using your finger to apply it. Don't bandage or wrap the skin being treated unless your doctor directs you to do so.

What to do if you miss an application
Apply a missed dose as soon as possible. But if it's almost time for your next dose, skip the missed dose and apply the next scheduled dose.

What to do about side effects
Although side effects are uncommon, flurandrenolide can cause such skin reactions as burning, itching, dryness, changes in color or texture, or a rash and inflammation (dermatitis). Tell your doctor if these effects occur.

Special directions
• If you have other medical problems, let your doctor know. They may affect the use of this medication.
• Don't get flurandrenolide in your eyes. If you do, flush your eyes with water.
• If your doctor orders an occlusive dressing (an airtight covering, such as plastic wrap or a special patch) to be applied over this medication, make sure you understand how to apply it.
• Don't use leftover medication for other skin problems without first checking with your doctor.
• If you're applying flurandrenolide to a child's diaper area, avoid using tight-fitting diapers or plastic pants. They could cause unwanted side effects.

Important reminders
Consult your doctor if you become pregnant while using flurandrenolide.

Don't apply this medication to your breasts before breast-feeding.

Children and adolescents using this medication should have frequent medical checkups because this medication can affect growth and cause other unwanted effects.

If you're an older adult, you may be especially susceptible to certain side effects, such as skin tearing and blood blisters.

Additional instructions

_____

_____

_____

_____

_____

_____

_____

_____

_____

Taking flurazepam

Dear Patient:

Your doctor has prescribed flurazepam to help you sleep. Your medication label may read Dalmane or Durapam.

How to take flurazepam
Take flurazepam capsules exactly as directed. Don't increase your dose because overuse may lead to mental or physical dependence.

What to do if you miss a dose
Take a missed dose as soon as you remember if it's within 1 hour of the scheduled time. If it's later than that, skip the missed dose and take your next dose as scheduled. Don't take a double dose.

What to do about side effects
Flurazepam may cause drowsiness, dizziness, headache, and poor coordination. If these symptoms persist or become severe, consult your doctor.

If you think you may have taken an overdose, seek emergency help *at once.* Overdose symptoms include continuing slurred speech or confusion, severe drowsiness, and staggering.

What you must know about alcohol and other drugs
Avoid alcoholic beverages, cimetidine (Tagamet), and medications that depress the nervous system (such as many allergy and cold remedies, narcotics, muscle relaxants, sleeping pills, and seizure medications). The combination of flurazepam and these medications may cause excessive drowsiness.

Special directions
• Tell your doctor about other medical problems you have. They may affect the use of this medication.
• See your doctor regularly to monitor your progress and check for side effects.
• Because flurazepam can affect some diagnostic test results, tell the doctor that you're taking this medication before you undergo any tests.
• Before you have dental work that requires an anesthetic, tell the dentist you're taking flurazepam.
• Don't drive or perform activities requiring alertness until you know how the medication affects you.
• Don't stop taking flurazepam suddenly; doing so may cause unpleasant withdrawal symptoms. Consult your doctor about gradually reducing your dosage before stopping the medication completely.

Important reminders
If you're pregnant or breast-feeding, consult your doctor before taking this medication.

Children and older adults are especially prone to flurazepam's side effects.

If you're an athlete, be aware that the National Collegiate Athletic Association and the U.S. Olympic Committee ban the use of flurazepam.

Additional instructions

_____

_____

_____

_____

Taking flurbiprofen

Dear Patient:

Your doctor has prescribed flurbiprofen to relieve the inflammation, swelling, stiffness, and joint pain of arthritis. The label may read Ansaid.

How to take flurbiprofen
Take your medication exactly as directed. Take flurbiprofen tablets with food or an antacid and a full glass (8 ounces) of water. To prevent possible swallowing problems, don't lie down for 15 to 30 minutes after taking it.

What to do if you miss a dose
Take a missed dose as soon as you remember if it's within 1 to 2 hours of the scheduled time. If it's later than that, skip the missed dose and take your next regularly scheduled dose. Don't take a double dose.

What to do about side effects
Sometimes serious side effects, including ulcers and bleeding, may occur with or without warning. Stop taking flurbiprofen and seek medical attention *at once* if you experience severe abdominal cramps, pain, or burning; have severe, continuing nausea, heartburn, or indigestion; or vomit blood or material that looks like coffee grounds.

Flurbiprofen also may cause headache, fluid retention, heartburn, nausea, diarrhea, stomach pain, burning and frequent urination, drowsiness, and dark, tarry stools. If these symptoms persist or become severe, tell your doctor.

What you must know about alcohol and other drugs
Don't drink alcoholic beverages while taking flurbiprofen; stomach problems are more likely to occur. Also, don't take acetaminophen (Tylenol) or aspirin or another salicylate together with flurbiprofen for more than a few days because this increases your risk for unwanted effects. And aspirin may decrease flurbiprofen's effectiveness.

Taking flurbiprofen with anticoagulants (blood thinners) may increase your risk for bleeding. And diuretics (water pills) may be less effective with flurbiprofen.

Special directions
• Be sure to tell your doctor about other medical problems you have. They may affect the use of this medication.
• Schedule regular medical checkups so your doctor can monitor your progress and check for unwanted side effects.
• Before undergoing a dental or surgical procedure, tell the dentist or doctor that you're taking flurbiprofen.
• Don't drive or perform activities requiring alertness until you know how you react to flurbiprofen.
• Protect yourself from excessive sun.

Important reminders
Consult your doctor if you're breastfeeding or become pregnant while taking flurbiprofen.

If you're an older adult, you may be especially prone to side effects from flurbiprofen.

Additional instructions

_____

_____

_____

Taking flutamide

Dear Patient:

Your doctor has prescribed flutamide to treat prostate cancer. The label may read Eulexin.

How to take flutamide

Take flutamide exactly as directed. Continue taking it for the full course of treatment, even after you begin to feel better. Don't stop taking the drug without first talking to your doctor.

When you take flutamide, you usually take other medications also. If you do, follow your doctor's instructions on their use.

What to do if you miss a dose

Take a missed dose of flutamide as soon as possible. If it's almost time for your next dose, skip the missed dose and take your next dose as scheduled. Don't take double doses.

What to do about side effects

Flutamide may diminish your sexual desire and ability. It can also cause diarrhea, nausea, vomiting, and hot flashes. If these symptoms persist or become severe, call your doctor.

Special directions

• If you vomit shortly after taking a dose of this medication, check with your doctor. He may tell you to take the dose again or to wait until the next scheduled dose.
• Schedule regular medical checkups so your doctor can monitor your progress.

Important reminder

If you want to have children, talk to your doctor about it. That's because flutamide lowers your sperm count. And the medication it's used with causes sterility, which may be permanent.

Additional instructions

_____

_____

_____

_____

_____

_____

_____

_____

_____

_____

_____

_____

_____

_____

_____

_____

_____

_____

_____

Taking folic acid

Dear Patient:

Your doctor has instructed you to take folic acid, a B vitamin, to help prevent or treat anemia. The label may read Folvite.

How to take folic acid
Follow your doctor's instructions exactly. Don't take more than he prescribes.

What to do if you miss a dose
Although you should try to remember to take folic acid every day, don't worry if you forget to take it, even for a few days. Don't make up missed doses, and never increase your dosage.

What to do about side effects
If you experience wheezing and difficulty breathing, stop taking folic acid and call your doctor *immediately.*

What you must know about other drugs
Be aware that chloramphenicol (Chloromycetin), an antibiotic, may decrease folic acid's effects.

Special directions
• Because certain medical problems may affect the use of folic acid, be sure to tell your doctor about other medical problems you have, especially a blood disorder known as pernicious anemia. Taking folic acid while you have pernicious anemia may cause serious side effects.
• Eat plenty of foods high in folic acid content. Such foods include green vegetables, potatoes, fruits, grains, and organ meats. Eat fresh foods when possible; cooking may reduce a food's folic acid content.

Important reminder
If you're pregnant or breast-feeding, ask your doctor whether you should continue taking folic acid.

Additional instructions

_____

_____

_____

_____

_____

_____

_____

_____

_____

_____

_____

_____

_____

_____

_____

Taking furosemide

Dear Patient:

Your doctor has prescribed furosemide to help reduce the amount of water in your body. The label may read Lasix or Myrosemide.

How to take furosemide
Furosemide comes in tablet and liquid forms. Take a single dose in the morning after breakfast or, if you're taking more than one dose a day, take the last dose no later than 6 p.m., unless your doctor instructs otherwise. This schedule will avoid having your sleep interrupted by the need to urinate.

If you're taking the *liquid* form, use a special measuring spoon (not a household teaspoon) to measure each dose accurately. To reduce stomach upset, take furosemide with food or milk.

What to do if you miss a dose
Take it as soon as possible. But if it's almost time for your next dose, skip the missed dose and take your next dose at its scheduled time. Don't double dose.

What to do about side effects
Contact your doctor *immediately* if you've been told that you have an abnormal complete blood count and you develop an infection or a fever.

Furosemide may cause dehydration and lower your body's levels of potassium, chloride, sodium, calcium, or magnesium. As a result, your doctor may tell you to have your blood tested regularly.

Furosemide commonly causes dizziness, fatigue, and increased urination, particularly when you first start taking it. If any of these effects persists or becomes severe, tell your doctor.

What you must know about alcohol and other drugs
Limit your intake of alcoholic beverages. Taking an aminoglycoside antibiotic with furosemide increases the risk of hearing problems. Indomethacin (Indocin) can decrease furosemide's effects, and clofibrate (Atromid-S) can enhance its effects.

Special directions
• Tell your doctor about other medical problems you have. They may affect the use of this medication.
• Because furosemide may lower your body's potassium level, eat plenty of foods with high potassium content (for example, oranges or other citrus fruits).
• To prevent excessive water and potassium loss, call your doctor if you become ill and experience continuing vomiting or diarrhea.
• Minimize dizziness by getting up slowly after lying down or sitting. Also avoid overexertion and standing for long periods.
• When exposed to sunlight, wear a hat and sunglasses and use a sunblocker.

Important reminders
If you're pregnant or breast-feeding, check with your doctor before taking furosemide.

If you're an older adult, you may be especially prone to side effects.

If you have diabetes, furosemide may affect your blood glucose levels. Report any consistent change in your home test results.

If you're an athlete, be aware that furosemide is banned by the National Collegiate Athletic Association and the U.S. Olympic Committee.

Taking gemfibrozil

Dear Patient:

Your doctor has prescribed gemfibrozil to reduce cholesterol and triglyceride (fat) levels in your blood. The label may read Lopid.

How to take gemfibrozil
Gemfibrozil is available in tablets and capsules. Take the drug exactly as prescribed. Don't take more or less of it, don't take it more or less often, and don't take it for a longer or shorter period than your doctor has ordered.

If your doctor tells you to take two doses a day, take one dose 30 minutes before breakfast and take the second dose 30 minutes before your evening meal.

What to do if you miss a dose
Take it as soon as you remember. But if it's almost time for your next dose, skip the missed dose and take your next dose as scheduled. Never take two doses at once.

What to do about side effects
While taking gemfibrozil, you may have stomach pain, heartburn, nausea, and diarrhea. If these symptoms persist or become severe, tell your doctor.

What you must know about other drugs
Because gemfibrozil may increase the effects of blood thinners (such as Coumadin), don't take these two medications together.

Special directions
• Carefully follow the special diet your doctor has ordered for you, so that this medication can work properly.
• Don't stop taking gemfibrozil without first asking your doctor. That's because if you stop taking it, your cholesterol and triglyceride levels could rise again.

Important reminder
If you're pregnant or breast-feeding, check with your doctor before taking this medication.

Additional instructions

_____

_____

_____

_____

_____

_____

_____

_____

_____

_____

_____

_____

_____

Using gentamicin

Dear Patient:

Your doctor has prescribed gentamicin to treat your eye infection. The label may read Garamycin.

How to use gentamicin

Gentamicin is available as eyedrops and as ointment. Carefully read the instructions on the medication label, which tell you how much to use for each dose.

If you're using *eyedrops,* follow these steps:
• Wash your hands.
• Tilt your head back and pull the lower eyelid away from the eye to form a pouch.
• Squeeze the correct number of drops into the pouch and gently close your eye. Don't blink.
• Keep your eye closed for 1 to 2 minutes to allow the medication to come into contact with the infection. If you think you didn't get a drop into your eye, use another drop.
• Repeat on the other eye, if directed.

If you're applying *ointment,* follow these steps:
• Wash your hands.
• Pull the lower eyelid away from the eye to form a pouch.
• Squeeze a thin strip of ointment into the pouch, and gently close your eye. Keep your eye closed for 1 to 2 minutes to allow the medication to come into contact with the infection.
• Repeat on the other eye, if directed.

What to do if you miss a dose

Use the eyedrops or apply the ointment as soon as possible. But if it's almost time for the next dose, skip the missed dose and take your next dose on schedule.

What to do about side effects

Your eyes may temporarily feel irritated if you're using the eyedrops.

If you're applying the ointment, expect your eyes to burn or sting; you may also have blurred vision.

If these side effects persist or become bothersome, tell your doctor.

Special directions

Tell your doctor if you're allergic to this medication or to related antibiotics, such as amikacin (Amikin), kanamycin (Kantrex), neomycin (Mycifradin), streptomycin, or tobramycin (Tobrex).

Additional instructions

_____

_____

_____

_____

_____

_____

_____

_____

_____

Taking glipizide

Dear Patient:

Your doctor has prescribed glipizide, in combination with a special diet and exercise program, to control your blood glucose level. The label may read Glucotrol.

How to take glipizide
Take glipizide exactly as prescribed. Take it at the same time each day, about 30 minutes before a meal, to ensure the best blood glucose control. If you take one dose a day, take it in the morning.

What to do if you miss a dose
Take it as soon as possible. But if it's almost time for your next dose, skip the missed dose and take the next dose as scheduled.

What to do about side effects
Glipizide may cause nervousness, increased sweating, fast heartbeat, headache, and yellowing of your skin and the whites of your eyes. If these symptoms persist or worsen, tell your doctor.

What you must know about alcohol and other drugs
Avoid alcoholic beverages; they can lower blood glucose levels and also cause stomach pain, nausea, vomiting, dizziness, and excessive sweating.

Glipizide can change the effects of many drugs, and other drugs can reduce glipizide's effects. Check with your doctor before taking other medications, either prescription or nonprescription.

Special directions
• Tell your doctor about other medical conditions you have, especially heart, kidney, liver, or thyroid disease.
• If you develop new medical problems, especially infections, tell your doctor.
• Follow your prescribed diet and exercise plan carefully.
• Test your blood glucose level as your doctor instructs.
• If you experience increased sensitivity to sunlight, wear protective clothing, use a sun-blocking agent, and limit sun exposure.
• Wear medical identification at all times and carry an identification card indicating your medical problems and medications.
• Tell family members how to treat the symptoms of hyperglycemia and hypoglycemia in case you can't direct them.

Important reminders
If you're pregnant or think you may be, tell your doctor, who will change your medication to insulin. If you plan to breast-feed, check with your doctor first.

If you're an older adult, you may be especially sensitive to this medication.

Additional instructions

_____

_____

_____

_____

_____

_____

_____

Taking glyburide

Dear Patient:

Your doctor has prescribed glyburide, in combination with a special diet and exercise program, to control your blood glucose level. The label may read Dia-Beta or Micronase.

How to take glyburide
Take glyburide exactly as prescribed. Take it at the same time each day to ensure the best blood glucose control. If you take one dose a day, take it in the morning with breakfast. If you're taking more than one dose a day, you may need to take the doses before breakfast and dinner or with meals. Check with your doctor.

What to do if you miss a dose
Take it as soon as possible. But if it's almost time for your next dose, skip the missed dose and take the next dose as scheduled.

What to do about side effects
Glyburide may cause nervousness, increased sweating, fast heartbeat, headache, and yellowing of your skin and the whites of your eyes. If these symptoms persist or worsen, tell your doctor.

What you must know about alcohol and other drugs
Avoid alcoholic beverages; they can lower blood glucose levels and also cause stomach pain, nausea, vomiting, dizziness, and excessive sweating.

Glyburide can change the effects of many drugs, and other drugs can reduce glyburide's effects. Check with your doctor before taking other medications, either prescription or nonprescription.

Special directions
• Tell your doctor about other medical conditions you have, especially heart, kidney, liver, or thyroid disease.
• If you develop new medical problems, particularly infections, tell your doctor.
• Follow your prescribed diet and exercise plan carefully.
• Test your blood glucose level as your doctor instructs.
• If you experience increased sensitivity to sunlight, wear protective clothing, use a sun-blocking agent, and limit sun exposure.
• Wear medical identification at all times and carry an identification card indicating that you're taking this medication.

Important reminders
If you're pregnant or think you may be, tell your doctor, who will change your medication to insulin. If you plan to breast-feed, check with your doctor.

If you're an older adult, be aware that you may be especially sensitive to this medication.

Additional instructions

_____

_____

_____

_____

_____

_____

_____

Taking griseofulvin

Dear Patient:

Your doctor has prescribed griseofulvin to treat your fungal infection. Brand names include Fulvicin P/G, Fulvicin-U/F, Grifulvin V, and Grisactin.

How to take griseofulvin
Take griseofulvin tablets, capsules, or liquid exactly as prescribed. To help clear up your infection completely, take the medication for the full length of time ordered by your doctor, even if you begin to feel better after a few days.

Take griseofulvin with or after meals, preferably with fatty foods (for example, whole milk or ice cream), which reduces stomach upset and helps your body absorb the medication.

What to do if you miss a dose
Take it as soon as possible unless it's almost time for your next dose. If so, skip the missed dose and take the next dose as scheduled. Don't double dose.

What to do about side effects
If you develop a rash or itchy skin, stop taking griseofulvin and *immediately* call your doctor. Sometimes an allergic reaction such as this can be serious. If you become restless or have difficulty breathing, get emergency care *immediately.*

Griseofulvin may cause a blood problem that can increase your risk of infection. This side effect can become serious, especially when you take the medication for a long period. Promptly report fever, weakness, sore throat, or mouth sores to your doctor.

Griseofulvin may cause a headache, which usually goes away as your body adjusts to the medication. If it persists or worsens, call your doctor.

What you must know about alcohol and other drugs
Avoid alcoholic beverages; they could cause a fast heartbeat, sweating, and skin flushing.

Because griseofulvin may interfere with the action of birth control pills, consider using another birth control method while you're taking griseofulvin and for 1 month after stopping it.

Don't take barbiturates when using griseofulvin because barbiturates can decrease griseofulvin's effects. Also, oral blood thinners may not work as well when taken with griseofulvin.

Special directions
• Tell the doctor about other medical conditions you have, particularly liver disease, lupus or lupus-like disease, or porphyria.
• Because griseofulvin may make you dizzy or less alert than usual, don't drive or perform other activities requiring alertness until you know how you respond to this medication.
• To protect light-sensitive skin, wear sunglasses and a wide-brimmed hat and use a sun-blocking agent when in the sun.

Important reminder
If you're pregnant, stop the medication and check with your doctor.

Additional instructions

_____

_____

Taking guaifenesin

Dear Patient:

This medication will help relieve your cough by loosening mucus or phlegm in your lungs. It's helpful for coughs due to colds but not for long-term coughs, such as those associated with asthma, emphysema, or smoking. Among the many brand names are Anti-Tuss, Glycotuss, and Robitussin.

How to take guaifenesin

Guaifenesin is available without a prescription; however, your doctor may suggest the proper dosage for your specific condition. It comes in tablets, capsules, extended-release tablets and capsules, an oral liquid, and a syrup.

Carefully read and follow the directions and precautions on the medication label. You may take a dose every 4 hours. Don't take more than the recommended total daily dosage.

Drink a full glass (8 ounces) of water with each dose to help loosen phlegm. Also, drink at least eight full glasses during the day unless your doctor orders otherwise.

If you're taking an *extended-release tablet or capsule,* swallow it whole. Don't crush, break, or chew it.

Don't use this medication for longer than the directions recommend, unless your doctor directs otherwise.

What to do if you miss a dose

If you're taking this medication regularly, take a missed dose as soon as possible. But if it's almost time for the next dose, skip the missed dose and take the next dose at its scheduled time. Don't take double doses.

What you must know about other drugs

If you're also taking heparin (Liquamin), your doctor may need to adjust the dosage. Watch for unusual bruising or bleeding; if it occurs, tell your doctor promptly.

Check with your doctor before using other medications—especially nonprescription cough or cold medications—because they can increase guaifenesin's effects and cause an overdose.

Special directions

• If your cough doesn't improve within 7 days or if you develop a fever, rash, persistent headache, or sore throat, check with your doctor.
• Because this medication may cause dizziness or drowsiness, don't drive or perform other activities requiring alertness until you know how you respond.
• Occasionally throughout the day, take several deep breaths and then cough to help bring up phlegm.
• Avoid fumes, smoke, and dust because they can irritate your lungs.

Important reminder

If you're pregnant or think you may be, check with your doctor before taking this medication.

Additional instructions

_____

_____

_____

_____

_____

Taking halazepam

Dear Patient:

Your doctor has prescribed halazepam to relieve your tension and anxiety. The label may read Paxipam.

How to take halazepam
Take halazepam tablets exactly as your doctor prescribes. Overuse could lead to dependency and increased risk of overdose.

What to do if you miss a dose
Take it as soon as you remember if it's within an hour or so after the scheduled time. Otherwise, skip the missed dose and take the next dose as scheduled. Don't take two doses at once.

What to do about side effects
If you think you've taken an overdose or if you experience severe side effects, such as prolonged confusion, severe drowsiness, difficulty breathing, slow heartbeat, slurred speech, staggering, or severe weakness, get emergency care *immediately*.

Halazepam may cause drowsiness, dizziness, difficulty thinking clearly, a hangover-type feeling, nausea, vomiting, and mouth dryness. These side effects commonly disappear as your body adjusts to the medication; if they continue or are bothersome, notify your doctor.

What you must know about alcohol and other drugs
Don't drink alcoholic beverages while taking halazepam—this combination could cause an overdose. Also, tell your doctor about other prescription or non-prescription medications you're taking. They can add to halazepam's effects and lead to overdose.

Special directions
• Because many medical problems can affect halazepam use, tell your doctor about your medical history.
• Because halazepam can cause drowsiness or dizziness, don't drive or perform other activities requiring alertness until you know how your body responds.
• To minimize dizziness, rise slowly after sitting or lying down.
• Relieve mouth dryness with sugarless hard candy or gum, ice chips, mouthwash, or a saliva substitute. If dryness continues for more than 2 weeks, tell your doctor or dentist because this increases your risk of tooth and gum problems.
• Don't suddenly stop taking halazepam. Rather, follow your doctor's instructions for gradually decreasing your doses to minimize withdrawal effects.
• After stopping this medication, your body may need time to adjust. Call your doctor if you experience irritability, nervousness, or trouble sleeping.

Important reminders
If you're pregnant or breast-feeding, check with your doctor before taking halazepam.

Children and older adults may be especially prone to halazepam's side effects.

If you're an athlete, be aware that halazepam is banned by the U.S. Olympic Committee and the National Collegiate Athletic Association.

Additional instructions

_____

_____

Taking haloperidol

Dear Patient:

Your doctor has prescribed haloperidol to treat your condition. Brand names include Haldol and Halperon.

How to take haloperidol
Take this medication exactly as prescribed. To prevent stomach upset, take it with food or milk.

If you're using the *liquid* form, take it by mouth even if it comes with a dropper. If it doesn't come in a dropper bottle, use a specially marked measuring spoon.

What to do if you miss a dose
Take it as soon as possible, and space any doses remaining for that day at regular intervals. Then resume your regular dosage schedule. Don't double dose.

What to do about side effects
If you develop a fever, fast heartbeat, difficult or rapid breathing, profuse sweating, or seizures, stop taking haloperidol and get emergency care *immediately.*

Haloperidol may cause blurred vision and mouth dryness, which usually disappear as your body adjusts to the drug. If they persist or are bothersome, tell your doctor. Also call if you notice fine, shaky movements of your tongue or any uncontrollable movements of your mouth, face, arms, or legs.

After you stop taking haloperidol, sometimes such side effects as trembling or uncontrolled movements, nausea, or vomiting may occur. If they do, call your doctor promptly.

What you must know about alcohol and other drugs
Don't drink alcoholic beverages while taking haloperidol because the combination could cause an overdose. Also, check with your doctor before taking any prescription or nonprescription medications.

Special directions
• Tell your doctor about other medical problems you have because they may affect the use of this medication.
• Don't drive or perform other activities requiring alertness until you know how you react to this medication.
• Don't stop taking this medication without first consulting your doctor.
• Because haloperidol may make you sweat less, which raises your body temperature and increases the chance of heatstroke, be careful not to become overheated.
• Relieve mouth dryness with sugarless hard candy or gum, ice chips, mouthwash, or a saliva substitute. If this dryness continues for more than 2 weeks, tell your doctor or dentist.
• Because haloperidol may make your skin more sensitive to light, wear protective clothing and sunglasses and use a sun-blocking agent when outdoors.

Important reminders
If you're pregnant or think you may be, check with your doctor before taking haloperidol. And don't breast-feed while taking this medication. Children and older adults are especially sensitive to haloperidol's side effects. If you're an athlete, be aware that haloperidol use is banned by the U.S. Olympic Committee and the National Collegiate Athletic Association.

Taking hydralazine

Dear Patient:

Your doctor has prescribed hydralazine to lower your blood pressure or to treat your heart condition. The label may read Alazine or Apresoline.

How to take hydralazine

Take hydralazine exactly as prescribed at the same time each day, preferably at mealtimes. Take it for as long as your doctor orders, even after you begin to feel better. That's because hydralazine doesn't cure high blood pressure. You must continue using it to control your blood pressure and reduce the risk of complications of high blood pressure.

What to do if you miss a dose

Take it as soon as possible. But if it's almost time for your next regular dose, skip the missed dose and resume your normal dosing schedule. Don't take double doses.

What to do about side effects

A rare but possibly serious side effect of hydralazine is an irregular heartbeat. If this occurs, call your doctor *immediately*. Also call him if you develop chest pain, swelling of the feet or lower legs, weight gain, sore throat, fever, muscle and joint pain, or a rash.

Hydralazine may cause headaches, dizziness, fast heartbeat, nausea, vomiting, diarrhea, or loss of appetite. These effects may go away as your body adjusts to the medication; check with your doctor if they continue or are bothersome. But don't suddenly stop taking hydralazine.

What you must know about other drugs

Check with your doctor before taking nonprescription or prescription medications because some medications can interfere with hydralazine's action or can cause side effects.

Special directions

• Tell your doctor about other medical problems you have, especially kidney, heart, or blood vessel disease, including stroke.
• Because hydralazine can cause dizziness, make sure you know how you react to this medication before driving or performing other activities requiring alertness.
• To minimize dizziness, rise slowly from a sitting or lying position.
• Follow a low-salt diet if your doctor has prescribed it.
• If your doctor has instructed you to take your blood pressure at home, follow directions closely and notify your doctor of any significant change.

Important reminders

If you're pregnant or think you may be, check with your doctor before taking hydralazine.

Older adults may be especially sensitive to side effects.

Additional instructions

_____

_____

_____

_____

_____

Taking hydrochlorothiazide

Dear Patient:

Your doctor has prescribed this thiazide diuretic to lower your blood pressure. It works by reducing the amount of water in your body. Brand names include HydroDIURIL, Mictrin, and Oretic.

How to take hydrochlorothiazide
This medication comes in tablet and liquid forms. If you're taking one dose a day, take it in the morning after breakfast. If you're taking more than one dose a day, take the last dose before 6 p.m. so you won't awaken to urinate.

If you're taking the oral liquid form, use a specially marked dropper or measuring spoon.

What to do if you miss a dose
Take it as soon as you remember unless it's almost time for your next regular dose. If so, skip the missed dose and take your next dose as scheduled. Never double dose.

What to do about side effects
If you experience persistent fever, sore throat, joint pain, or easy bruising and bleeding, stop taking this medication and call your doctor *immediately.*

This medication may cause dehydration, low blood glucose level, fatigue, muscle cramps, numbness, "pins and needles" sensation, and weakness. If these side effects persist, tell your doctor.

What you must know about other drugs
Cholestyramine (Cholybar, Questran), colestipol (Colestid), and nonsteroidal anti-inflammatory drugs decrease hydrochlorothiazide's effects. If you're taking any of these medications along with hydrochlorothiazide, follow your dosage schedule exactly to minimize drug interactions. Avoid taking diazoxide (Proglycem), which may worsen hydrochlorothiazide's side effects.

Special directions
• Before taking hydrochlorothiazide, tell your doctor if you're allergic to sulfa drugs or other medications.
• Because this medication may decrease your body's potassium level, the doctor may instruct you to eat foods high in potassium, such as uncooked dried fruits and fresh orange juice, take a potassium supplement, and decrease your salt intake.
• Inform your doctor if you're already on a special diet, such as one for diabetes.
• Contact your doctor if you experience persistent or severe diarrhea or vomiting, which can cause excessive potassium and water loss and decrease blood pressure too much.
• Because hydrochlorothiazide may increase your sensitivity to sunlight, limit sun exposure, wear protective clothing and sunglasses, and use a sunblocker.

Important reminders
If you're pregnant or breast-feeding, check with your doctor before taking this medication. If you have diabetes, this medication can interfere with blood or urine glucose tests. If you're an older adult, you may be especially sensitive to side effects. If you're an athlete, be aware that diuretics are banned and tested for by the National Collegiate Athletic Association and the U.S. Olympic Committee.

Taking hydrochlorothiazide with spironolactone

Dear Patient:

The doctor has prescribed this medication to treat your high blood pressure. It works by decreasing the amount of water in your body. Brand names include Aldactazide and Spirozide.

How to take this drug
Take this medication exactly as prescribed. If you're taking one dose a day, take it in the morning after breakfast. If you're taking more than one dose a day, take the last dose before 6 p.m. so the need to urinate won't disturb your sleep. If necessary, take the medication with milk or meals to prevent stomach upset.

What to do if you miss a dose
Take it as soon as possible unless it's almost time for the next dose. If so, skip the missed dose and take your next dose as scheduled. Don't double dose.

What to do about side effects
If you develop persistent fever, sore throat, joint pain, or easy bleeding or bruising, stop taking this medication and call your doctor *immediately.*

This medication may cause dehydration, low blood glucose level, fatigue, anxiety, irritability, muscle cramps, numbness, "pins and needles" sensation, weakness, increased urination and thirst, and weak, irregular pulse. If these effects persist, call your doctor.

What you must know about other drugs
Check with your doctor before taking prescription or nonprescription drugs while taking this medication. Other medications may increase or decrease this medication's effects.

Special directions
• Before taking this medication, inform your doctor if you're allergic to sulfa drugs or other medications.
• Because this medication may decrease your body's potassium level, your doctor may tell you to eat foods high in potassium, such as uncooked dried fruits and fresh orange juice, take a potassium supplement, and cut down on salt.
• Inform your doctor if you're already on a special diet, such as one for diabetes.
• Contact your doctor if you experience persistent or severe diarrhea or vomiting, which can cause excessive potassium and water loss and decrease blood pressure too much.
• Because this medication may make you sensitive to sunlight, limit sun exposure, wear protective clothing and sunglasses, and use a sun-blocking agent.

Important reminders
If you're pregnant or breast-feeding, check with your doctor before taking this medication.

Older adults are especially sensitive to this medication's effects.

If you're an athlete, be aware that the National Collegiate Athletic Association and the U.S. Olympic Committee ban the use of diuretics.

Additional instructions

_____

_____

_____

_____

Taking hydrochlorothiazide with triamterene

Dear Patient:

Your doctor has prescribed this medication to control your blood pressure. It works by reducing the amount of water in your body. The label may read Dyazide or Maxzide.

How to take this drug
Take this drug exactly as prescribed. If you're taking one dose a day, take it in the morning after breakfast. If you're taking more than one dose a day, take your last dose before 6 p.m. so the need to urinate won't disturb your sleep. To prevent stomach upset, take this medication with milk or meals.

What to do if you miss a dose
Take it as soon as you remember unless it's almost time for your next dose. If so, skip the missed dose and take your next dose as scheduled. Never take two doses at once.

What to do about side effects
If you feel like your throat is closing and you have trouble breathing, stop taking this medication and get emergency care *at once.* Also stop taking this medication and call your doctor if you experience persistent fever, sore throat, joint pain, or easy bleeding or bruising.

Common side effects include dehydration, low blood glucose level, chronic fatigue, anxiety, irritability, muscle cramps, numbness, pain, "pins and needles" sensation, weakness, increased urination and thirst, and weak, irregular pulse. If these symptoms persist, tell your doctor.

What you must know about other drugs
Tell your doctor if you're taking other prescription or nonprescription drugs. For example, taking this medication with angiotensin-converting enzyme inhibitors (such as Captopril) or potassium supplements can raise blood potassium levels, possibly leading to kidney and heart problems.

Special directions
• Because this medication may decrease your body's potassium level, your doctor may instruct you to eat foods high in potassium, such as uncooked dried fruits and fresh orange juice, take a potassium supplement, and cut down on salt.
• Contact your doctor if you develop persistent or severe diarrhea or vomiting, which can cause excessive potassium and water loss and decrease blood pressure too much.
• This medication may make you sensitive to sunlight, so limit sun exposure.

Important reminders
If you're pregnant or breast-feeding, check with your doctor before taking this medication.

Older adults are especially sensitive to this medication.

If you're an athlete, be aware that the National Collegiate Athletic Association and the U.S. Olympic Committee ban the use of this medication.

Additional instructions

_____

_____

_____

Applying hydrocortisone

Dear Patient:

This medication is used to help relieve the itching, redness, swelling, and discomfort of your skin problem. The label may read Cortaid, Cort-Dome, or Cortizone.

How to apply hydrocortisone

Hydrocortisone is available as an aerosol, cream, gel, lotion, ointment, or topical solution. Carefully read and follow the instructions on the medication container. Wash your hands and skin before applying the medication. When applying the medication to hairy areas, part the hair and apply directly to the skin.

If your doctor has prescribed an occlusive dressing (an airtight covering, such as plastic wrap or a special patch), apply a heavy layer of medication, cover the area with the occlusive dressing, then secure the dressing to your skin with hypoallergenic tape.

If you're using the *aerosol* form, shake the can well. Direct the spray onto the area from a distance of 6 inches. To avoid freezing the tissues, spray for no more than 3 seconds. Apply to a dry scalp after shampooing; don't rub the medication into your scalp after spraying.

Avoid breathing in the spray and getting it in your eyes. If the medication accidently gets in your eyes, promptly flush them with water.

What to do if you miss an application

Apply it as soon as you can. But if it's almost time for your next regular dose, skip the missed dose and apply the next dose as scheduled.

What to do about side effects

Fever, skin tearing, painful reddened and inflamed skin with pus-filled blisters, thinning skin, reddish purple lines on the skin, or burning and itching skin with pinhead-size blisters may occur with the use of an occlusive dressing. If any of these problems occurs, remove the dressing and contact your doctor.

Special directions

• Before using hydrocortisone, tell your doctor if you're allergic to any medications or foods.
• For safety reasons, don't apply topical hydrocortisone near heat or open flame or while smoking.
• Don't use topical hydrocortisone more often or for a longer time than your doctor has instructed. Doing so increases the risk of side effects.
• Don't share your medication with others. Also, don't use any remaining medication to treat other skin problems without first consulting your doctor.

Important reminders

If you're pregnant or breast-feeding, check with your doctor before using this medication.

Don't use hydrocortisone for a child under age 2 without a doctor's order.

Children, adolescents, and older adults are especially prone to side effects and should be closely monitored by a doctor.

Additional instructions

_____

_____

_____

Using hydrocortisone with neomycin and polymyxin B

Dear Patient:

This medication helps to treat ear infections. It may also be used to relieve discomfort, irritation, and redness from other ear problems. Common brand names for this medication include Cortisporin, Otocort, and Pediotic.

How to use this drug
Insert the eardrops, following the instructions you received from the nurse or doctor.

Before inserting the eardrops, warm them to body temperature (98.6° F) by holding the bottle in your hand for a few minutes. Don't heat the bottle on the stove or in the microwave—the medication won't work if it gets too warm.

Continue using this medication as ordered by your doctor even after you feel better. Complete the full treatment to make sure the infection is completely cleared up.

What to do if you miss a dose
Insert the eardrops as soon as you remember unless it's almost time for your next regular dose. If so, skip the missed dose and insert the drops when next scheduled.

What to do about side effects
If you have itching, redness, swelling, or other signs of irritation, tell your doctor.

Special instructions
• Before using this medication, tell your doctor if you have other ear problems because using this medication could make some problems worse.
• Inform your doctor if you're allergic to this medication or other medications, particularly related antibiotics, such as gentamicin (Garamycin), streptomycin, or tobramycin (Nebcin).
• If your symptoms persist for more than 1 week or become worse, contact your doctor.
• Don't use this medication for more than 10 days in a row unless your doctor prescribes a longer course of treatment.

Additional instructions

_____

_____

_____

_____

_____

_____

_____

_____

_____

_____

_____

_____

Taking hydromorphone

Dear Patient:

This medication is prescribed to relieve pain or cough. The label may read Dilaudid.

How to take hydromorphone

Hydromorphone comes in tablet, suppository, and injection forms. Take it only as prescribed. Overuse could lead to dependency and risk of overdose.

To insert a *suppository,* follow these steps: If the suppository is too soft to insert, run cold water over it or chill it in the refrigerator for about 30 minutes before removing the foil wrapper. Then remove the wrapper and moisten the suppository with cold water. Lie down on your side. Using your index finger, gently push the suppository into your rectum as far as possible.

If you're using the *injectable* form, follow your doctor's instructions for performing injections. Alternate among several injection sites to help prevent complications.

What to do if you miss a dose

Take it as soon as you remember. However, if it's almost time for your next regular dose, skip the missed dose and take the next one at the regular time. Don't take two doses at once.

What to do about side effects

If you think you've taken an overdose or develop symptoms of an overdose, get emergency medical care *immediately.* Symptoms of overdose include seizures, cold and clammy skin, confusion, severe drowsiness or dizziness, slow or troubled breathing, slow heartbeat, extreme nervousness or restlessness, severe weakness, and very small pupils.

Hydromorphone may cause drowsiness, dizziness, difficulty thinking clearly, nausea, vomiting, constipation, difficulty urinating, or a false sense of well-being. These problems may go away as your body adjusts to the medication; if they continue, tell your doctor.

What you must know about alcohol and other drugs

Don't drink alcoholic beverages while taking hydromorphone—the combination can cause an overdose. Check with your doctor before taking other prescription or nonprescription medications. Some can add to hydromorphone's effects.

Special directions

• Let your doctor know if you have other medical problems. They may affect the use of this medication.
• Don't drive or perform other activities requiring alertness until you know how you respond to this medication.
• To help prevent or relieve constipation, drink plenty of fluids and eat high-fiber foods.
• If you've taken hydromorphone regularly for several weeks or more, don't stop taking it without first checking with your doctor. He'll want to decrease your dosage gradually to minimize withdrawal side effects.

Important reminders

If you're pregnant or think you may be, check with your doctor before taking this medication.

Children and older adults are especially sensitive to this medication.

Taking hydroxyzine

Dear Patient:

Hydroxyzine helps to treat many problems. For instance, it helps relieve anxiety and tension. It also treats a rash and itching. It may even be given to treat hyperactivity in children. Its brand names include Anxanil, Atarax, and Vistaril.

How to take hydroxyzine
This medication comes in tablets, capsules, a syrup, and an oral liquid. Follow your doctor's instructions exactly for taking hydroxyzine.

Take this medication with food or a glass of water or milk to reduce stomach upset.

What to do if you miss a dose
Take it as soon as possible unless it's almost time for the next regular dose. If so, skip the missed dose and take the next dose at the scheduled time. Never take two doses at once.

What to do about side effects
If you think you've taken an overdose or experience symptoms of an overdose—including seizures, clumsiness or unsteadiness, severe drowsiness, trouble breathing, extreme mouth dryness, and hallucinations—get emergency medical care *immediately*.

Common side effects include drowsiness and dry mouth. These problems should subside as your body adjusts to the medication; if they persist or worsen, tell your doctor.

What you must know about alcohol and other drugs
Don't drink alcoholic beverages while taking hydroxyzine. This combination can cause an overdose. Check with your doctor before taking other prescription or nonprescription medications while you're taking hydroxyzine.

Special directions
• Tell your doctor about other medical conditions you have. Also tell him if you're on a special diet, such as low-salt or low-sugar.
• Make sure you know how you react to hydroxyzine before you drive or perform other activities requiring alertness.
• Relieve mouth dryness with sugarless hard candy or gum, ice chips, mouthwash, or a saliva substitute. If dryness continues for more than 2 weeks, tell your doctor or dentist; it increases your risk of tooth and gum problems.
• This medication may mask the signs of appendicitis or overdose of other medications. If you develop symptoms of appendicitis (such as stomach pain, cramping, or tenderness) or you think you may have taken an overdose of another medication, be sure your doctor knows that you're taking hydroxyzine.

Important reminders
If you're pregnant or think you may be, check with your doctor before starting this medication. Don't take this medication while breast-feeding.

Children and older adults are especially sensitive to hydroxyzine's side effects.

Additional instructions

_____

_____

_____

Taking ibuprofen

Dear Patient:

Also called Advil, Motrin, and Nuprin, ibuprofen relieves mild to moderate pain and reduces fever.

How to take ibuprofen

Ibuprofen comes in tablets, caplets, and an oral liquid. Although you can get its 200-mg strength without a prescription, only a doctor can prescribe stronger doses.

If your doctor has prescribed ibuprofen, follow his instructions. If you're taking ibuprofen without a prescription, follow the package instructions.

To reduce stomach upset, take ibuprofen with food or an antacid. However, your doctor may instruct you to take the first few doses of ibuprofen either 30 minutes before or 2 hours after meals. That's because taking it on an empty stomach helps the medication work faster when you first start taking it.

When taking the tablet or caplet form, drink a full glass (8 ounces) of water. To prevent irritation that may cause trouble swallowing, avoid lying down for 15 to 30 minutes after taking the medication.

What to do if you miss a dose

Take it as soon as you remember. But if it's almost time for your next regular dose, skip the missed dose and take the next one at the regular time.

What to do about side effects

If your throat feels like it's closing and you have trouble breathing, get emergency medical care *immediately.*

Ibuprofen may also cause dizziness, drowsiness, headache, heartburn, and nausea. Other, less common effects include swelling of your ankles and feet or ringing in your ears. If these problems persist or worsen, tell your doctor.

What you must know about other drugs

Avoid taking furosemide (Lasix) or thiazide diuretics (water pills) with ibuprofen because ibuprofen can reduce these drugs' effects. Because ibuprofen increases the effects of oral anticoagulants (blood thinners) and lithium (Lithane), don't take these medications together.

Special directions

• Don't take ibuprofen if you're allergic to aspirin. If you have other allergies, check with your doctor before taking ibuprofen.
• Tell your doctor if you're on a special low-salt or diabetic diet before taking ibuprofen oral liquid.
• If you're using nonprescription ibuprofen and your symptoms don't disappear or if they worsen, contact your doctor.
• If you're taking ibuprofen to reduce fever, call your doctor if your fever lasts for more than 3 days. If you're taking it for pain, call the doctor if the injured area becomes or stays red or swollen.
• Before undergoing surgery or dental work, tell the doctor or dentist that you're taking ibuprofen.
• Be sure you know how you respond to ibuprofen before driving or performing other activities requiring alertness.

Important reminders

If you're pregnant, check with your doctor before taking ibuprofen. If you're an older adult, you may be especially susceptible to ibuprofen's side effects.

Using idoxuridine

Dear Patient:

Your doctor has prescribed idoxuridine eyedrops or eye ointment to treat your viral eye infection. The label may read Herplex Liquifilm or Stoxil.

How to use idoxuridine

Use the medication exactly as prescribed. Follow these steps.
• Wash your hands, then gently clean away any crusting around your eyes. If it's dried, moisten it with warm water.
• Gently pull down your lower lid, creating a pocket.
• If you're using *eyedrops,* tilt your head back and carefully squeeze the prescribed number of drops into the pocket.
• If you're using the *ointment,* squeeze a thin strip into the pocket.
• Close your eyes gently. Don't blink. Hold your finger lightly on the innermost part of your eye (near the bridge of your nose) for 1 minute. Keep your eyes closed for 1 to 2 minutes so the medicine can come into contact with the infection.

To keep the medication as germfree as possible, don't touch the dropper, don't lay it down, and don't let it touch anything else, including your eye. After using the ointment, wipe the tip of the tube with a clean tissue. Keep the container tightly closed.

Use idoxuridine for the entire time prescribed, even if your symptoms disappear, to help clear up your infection completely. But don't use it more often or for a longer time than prescribed; overuse could cause eye problems.

What to do if you miss a dose

Take it as soon as possible unless it's almost time for your next regular dose. If so, skip the missed dose and take your next dose as scheduled.

What to do about side effects

Stop taking idoxuridine and call your doctor if you develop itching, swelling, redness, pain, or persistent burning in your eyes. Also tell him if you experience blurred or dimmed vision.

What you must know about other drugs

Don't use other eye medications, especially those that contain boric acid, along with idoxuridine. Boric acid can interfere with idoxuridine or cause side effects.

Special directions

• Before using idoxuridine, tell your doctor if you have other medical conditions or if you've ever had an unusual reaction to this medication, any iodine-containing preparation, or another medication or food.
• If this medication makes your eyes more sensitive to light, wear sunglasses and avoid bright lights.
• Don't share your medication with family members; also, use separate washcloths and towels to help prevent the spread of infection.
• Never use old medication because it can cause your eyes to burn. Also, old medication may have lost its ability to fight infection.
• If your symptoms don't get better within 1 week or if they worsen, tell your doctor.

Important reminder

If you're pregnant or think you may be, check with your doctor before using this medication.

Taking imipramine

Dear Patient:

This medication is used to treat depression and to relieve severe, chronic pain. It may also be prescribed to treat childhood bed-wetting. The label may read Janimine, Tipramine, or Tofranil.

How to take imipramine
Unless your doctor instructs otherwise, take imipramine with food (even at bedtime) to reduce stomach upset.

What to do if you miss a dose
If you take your medication once a day at bedtime, check with your doctor.

If you take more than one dose a day, take the missed dose as soon as possible. But if it's almost time for your next dose, skip the missed dose and resume your schedule. Don't double dose.

What to do about side effects
If you develop blurred vision, constipation, a fast heartbeat, or trouble urinating, call your doctor *immediately.*

Dizziness, drowsiness, dry mouth, headache, and increased sweating may occur but go away as your body adjusts to the medication. If they persist, tell your doctor.

If you think you've taken an overdose or experience symptoms of overdose—such as seizures, confusion, severe drowsiness, or fast, slow, or irregular heartbeat—stop taking imipramine and get emergency care *immediately.*

Call your doctor if you can't sleep or have uncontrolled lip, arm, or leg movements after you stop taking imipramine.

What you must know about alcohol and other drugs
Don't drink alcoholic beverages while taking imipramine. Check with your doctor if you're taking other prescription or nonprescription medications. They can interact with imipramine and possibly cause problems.

Special directions
• Tell your doctor about other medical conditions you have. They may affect the use of imipramine.
• Make sure you know how you react to imipramine before you drive or perform other activities requiring alertness and the ability to see clearly.
• If you feel dizzy or faint when arising from a sitting or lying position, get up slowly.
• Relieve mouth dryness with sugarless hard candy or gum, ice chips, mouthwash, or a saliva substitute. If dryness continues for more than 2 weeks, tell your doctor or dentist because it puts you at risk for tooth or gum problems.
• To protect light-sensitive skin, limit sun exposure; when outdoors, wear protective clothing and sunglasses and use a sun-blocking agent.
• Unless your doctor instructs otherwise, drink plenty of liquids and eat a high-fiber diet to prevent constipation.
• Don't stop taking imipramine without first consulting your doctor, who may decrease your dosage gradually to minimize withdrawal effects.

Important reminders
If you're pregnant or breast-feeding, check with your doctor before starting this medication.

Children and older adults are at special risk for side effects.

If you have diabetes, imipramine can affect your glucose levels. If it does, call your doctor.

Taking indomethacin

Dear Patient:

Indomethacin is prescribed to relieve fever, pain, swelling, or joint stiffness. The label may read Indocin or Indomed.

How to take indomethacin

Take *capsules* or *oral liquid* on a full stomach or with an antacid unless your doctor instructs otherwise. Don't mix the *liquid* form with the antacid or any other liquid before taking it; take the antacid first. Take *capsules* with a full glass (8 ounces) of water, and don't lie down for 15 to 30 minutes afterward. If you're taking the *sustained-release capsule,* swallow it whole. Don't crush, break, or chew it.

To use a *suppository,* follow these steps.
• If the suppository is too soft to insert, run cold water over it or chill it in the refrigerator for about 30 minutes.
• Remove the foil wrapper and moisten the suppository with cold water.
• Lie on your side. With your index finger, gently push the suppository into your rectum as far as possible.
• Keep the suppository in place for at least 1 hour.

What to do if you miss a dose

If you're using the *regular capsules, liquid,* or *suppositories,* take a missed dose when you remember it. But if it's almost time for your next dose, skip the missed dose and take the next one as scheduled. If you're taking *sustained-release capsules* once or twice a day, take a missed dose if it's within 1 to 2 hours after the scheduled time. But if it's later, skip the missed dose and take the next dose at its scheduled time.

What to do about side effects

If you develop a hive-like rash or itching, stop taking indomethacin and call your doctor *immediately.* If you become restless, wheeze, and have difficulty breathing or have puffiness around your eyes, seek emergency care *immediately.*

Stop taking the medication and call your doctor *at once* if you have stomach pain; pass black, tarry stools; have severe nausea, heartburn, or indigestion; or vomit coffee ground–like matter.

Also tell your doctor about other side effects, including weakness, sore throat, or swelling of your face, feet, or lower legs.

What you must know about alcohol and other drugs

Don't drink alcoholic beverages while taking indomethacin. Tell your doctor if you're taking other medications because many drugs can interact with indomethacin. In particular, mention blood pressure medications, diflunisal (Dolobid), probenecid (Benemid), and lithium (Eskalith).

Special directions

• Tell the doctor if you have other medical problems. They may affect the use of this medication.
• Don't drive or perform other activities requiring alertness until you know how you react to this medication.

Important reminders

If you're pregnant or think you may be, check with your doctor before taking this medication. Don't breast-feed while taking indomethacin. If you're an older adult, you may be especially sensitive to side effects.

Injecting insulin

Dear Patient:

Your doctor has prescribed insulin injections to control your blood glucose level.

How to inject insulin

You've been given instructions on the kind of insulin to use, the correct dose, the number of injections you need each day, and the times to perform them. Follow these instructions exactly—they're tailored especially for you.

Use the guidelines below to help you prepare and administer your insulin injection.

Drawing up insulin into the syringe

To draw up insulin into the syringe correctly, follow these steps.

1 Before you do anything else, wash your hands.

2 If your insulin is the intermediate- or long-acting kind (cloudy), mix it by slowly rolling the bottle between your hands or gently tipping it over a few times. Never shake the bottle vigorously.

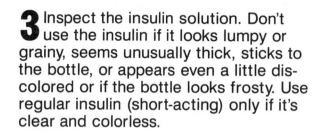

3 Inspect the insulin solution. Don't use the insulin if it looks lumpy or grainy, seems unusually thick, sticks to the bottle, or appears even a little discolored or if the bottle looks frosty. Use regular insulin (short-acting) only if it's clear and colorless.

4 Remove the colored protective cap on the bottle. Don't remove the rubber stopper.

5 Wipe the top of the bottle with an alcohol swab.

6 Remove the needle cover of the insulin syringe.

7 Draw air into the syringe by pulling back on the plunger. The amount of air that you draw into the syringe should be equal to your insulin dose.

8 Gently push the needle through the top of the rubber stopper.

9 Push the plunger in all the way to inject the air from the syringe into the bottle.

10 Turn the bottle with syringe upside down in one hand. Be sure the tip of the needle is covered by the insulin.

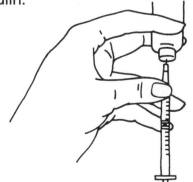

(continued)

Injecting insulin *(continued)*

With your other hand, pull the plunger back slowly to draw the correct dose of insulin into the syringe.

11 Check the insulin in the syringe for air bubbles. To remove air bubbles, push the insulin slowly back into the bottle and draw up your dose again.

12 Check your dose again, then remove the needle from the bottle and recover the needle.

Mixing two types of insulin
If you're mixing more than one type of insulin in the same syringe, you also need to know the following.
• When mixing two types of insulin, first draw into the syringe the same amount of air as the amount of insulin you'll be withdrawing from each bottle.
• If you're mixing regular insulin with another type of insulin, *always* draw up the regular insulin into the syringe first. When mixing two types of insulin other than regular insulin, you can draw them in any order, but use the same order each time.
• Some insulin mixtures must be injected immediately. Others may be stable for a while, which means you can draw up the mixture into the syringe ahead of time. Check with your doctor, nurse, or pharmacist to find out which type you have.
• If your mixture is stable and you mixed it ahead of time, gently turn the filled syringe back and forth to remix the insulins before you inject them. Don't shake the syringe.

Giving the injection
Inject the insulin into fatty tissue. Injection sites include the thighs, abdomen, upper arms, and buttocks. The abdomen is the preferred site because insulin is absorbed into the bloodstream most evenly from the abdomen. Rotate among injections sites within the same anatomic area as you've been instructed, such as moving from left to right in rows, from the top to the bottom of the area. Remember, inject each new dose at least 1 inch from the previously used site.

After you've prepared your syringe, inject the insulin, following these steps.

1 Clean the site for the injection with an alcohol swab, and let the area dry.

2 Remove the protective covering from the needle. Pinch up a large area of skin and hold it firmly. With your other hand, push the needle straight into the pinched-up skin at a 90-degree angle. Be sure the needle is all the way in.

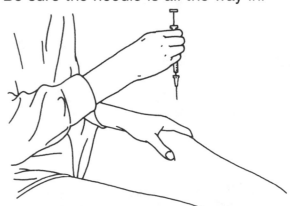

Note: If you're thin or greatly overweight, you may be given special instructions for giving yourself insulin injections.

3 Push the plunger all the way down to inject the dose quickly (in less than 5 seconds).

(continued)

Injecting insulin (continued)

4 Then hold an alcohol swab near the needle, and pull the needle straight out of the skin.

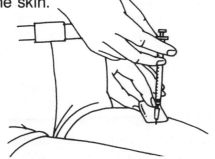

5 Press the swab against the injection site for several seconds. Don't rub.

If you're using an insulin pump for continuous insulin infusion, follow your doctor's and the pump manufacturer's instructions exactly.

What to do if you miss a dose
Follow your doctor's instructions. What you must do depends on the type and amount of insulin you're taking as well as how much time has elapsed since your last insulin injection.

What to do about side effects
Contact your doctor *immediately* if you develop itching, hives, a rash, difficulty breathing, or wheezing after your insulin injection. You may be having an allergic reaction; your doctor will need to change your type of insulin.

Insulin may cause low blood glucose, especially if you delay or miss a meal or snack, exercise much more than usual, or drink alcoholic beverages. Watch for cool pale skin, difficulty concentrating, shakiness, headache, cold sweats, or anxiety—but keep in mind that everyone has different symptoms. Be sure to learn your own early symptoms so you can take quick action.

If you have symptoms of low blood glucose, eat or drink something containing sugar, such as glucose tablets or gel or fruit juice. If possible, check your blood glucose level to confirm that it's low. If symptoms don't go away in 15 minutes, again eat or drink something containing sugar and wait another 15 minutes. If symptoms still don't go away, seek emergency medical care *immediately.*

Notify your doctor if you have frequent or severe low blood glucose reactions—your insulin dosage or type may need to be changed.

Also tell your doctor if you note skin changes at injection sites, such as pitting or thickening.

What you must know about alcohol and other drugs
Because alcohol can cause severe low blood glucose, ask your doctor whether you can safely drink alcoholic beverages and, if so, how much.

Beta blockers (Inderal), clofibrate (Atromid-S), fenfluramine (Pondimin), monoamine oxidase (MAO) inhibitors (drugs for depression), salicylates, or tetracycline (Achromycin) can prolong a low blood glucose reaction when taken with insulin. Corticosteroids (prednisone) and thiazide diuretics (water pills) can decrease insulin's ability to lower your blood glucose level. Check with your doctor before taking any of these drugs.

Special directions
• Tell your doctor if you have other medical problems, especially infections or kidney, liver, or thyroid disease. Other medical problems may affect the use of insulin.
• Although disposable syringes are usu-

(continued)

Injecting insulin *(continued)*

ally used only once, you may wish to reuse a syringe until its needle becomes dull. If you reuse the syringe, check with your nurse, doctor, or pharmacist for cleaning instructions. Make sure you recap the needle after each use. Throw away the syringe when the needle becomes dull or bent or comes into contact with any surface other than the cleaned and swabbed area of skin.

• Don't use insulin after the expiration date on the package, even if the bottle has never been opened. Instead, check with your pharmacist about the possibility of exchanging bottles.

• Keep unopened bottles of insulin refrigerated until needed. Never freeze insulin. Remove the insulin from the refrigerator and allow it to reach room temperature before injecting it.

• You may keep an insulin bottle in use at room temperature for up to 1 month. Throw away any insulin that has been kept at room temperature for longer than 1 month.

• Don't expose insulin to extremely hot temperatures or to sunlight. Extreme heat will reduce its effectiveness.

• See your doctor regularly so he can check your condition and adjust your insulin therapy as needed.

• If you've been smoking for a long time and suddenly stop, tell your doctor, who will probably reduce your insulin dosage.

• Follow your prescribed diet and exercise plan strictly. Don't miss or delay any meals.

• When you become sick with a cold, fever, or the flu, make sure you take your insulin, but check with the doctor to determine the dose. Take your insulin even if you feel too sick to eat. This is especially true if you have nausea, vomiting, or diarrhea.

• Learn how to check your own blood glucose level and urine for ketones (an acid that may be released from your bloodstream into your urine when your blood glucose level is too high).

• You'll develop high blood glucose if you're not getting enough insulin. Contact your doctor if you experience excessive thirst, hunger, and urination or if your blood glucose levels are high even without symptoms. If left untreated, high blood glucose can cause diabetic coma, an emergency condition.

• Wear a medical identification bracelet or necklace and carry an identification card indicating that you have diabetes and listing your insulin type and dosage.

• Keep a glucagon kit and a syringe and needle available, and teach your family how to prepare and use it if you develop severe low blood glucose. Keep some kind of quick-acting sugar handy to treat low blood glucose symptoms.

• Discuss any travel plans with your doctor, especially if you're changing time zones. You may need to make some temporary adjustments to your insulin dosage.

Important reminder
If you become pregnant, tell your doctor, who will adjust your insulin therapy.

Additional instructions

_____

_____

_____

_____

Taking oral iron supplements

Dear Patient:

Iron supplements are used to help correct iron deficiency. Your body needs enough iron to produce the number of red blood cells that you need to stay healthy. Brand names for iron supplements may include Feostat, Ferranol, Feosol, and Fumerin.

How to take oral iron supplements

Iron supplements come in many forms—for example, tablets, capsules, and elixir. Carefully follow your doctor's instructions. For best results, take the supplement on an empty stomach either 1 hour before or 2 hours after meals. Take the supplement with water or, even better, orange juice because vitamin C increases iron absorption into your blood.

If necessary, take iron supplements with food or immediately after meals to reduce stomach upset.

If you're taking the *elixir,* sip it through a narrow straw to keep it from staining your teeth.

What to do if you miss a dose

Skip the missed dose and take your next dose as scheduled. Don't double your dose.

What to do about side effects

Constipation, nausea, and black stools are common. If these problems become bothersome or severe, tell your doctor.

What you must know about other drugs

Don't take iron supplements at the same time as antacids (such as Maalox or Mylanta), cholestyramine (Questran), chloramphenicol (Chloromycetin), or vitamin E. Ask a nurse, pharmacist, or doctor to help you schedule these medications to minimize interactions.

Special directions

• Tell your doctor if you're allergic to any iron medication or to another drug, food, or chemical.

• Don't take high doses of iron for longer than 6 months without consulting your doctor. Prolonged overuse could lead to iron poisoning. Also, unabsorbed iron could hide blood in your stool, possibly delaying discovery of a serious disorder.

• To help prevent constipation, drink plenty of fluids, exercise regularly, and eat foods high in fiber, such as fresh fruits and vegetables and foods containing bran and oats.

• Remove tooth stains caused by liquid iron supplements with baking soda or hydrogen peroxide solution (3%).

Important reminders

If you're pregnant or breast-feeding, check with your doctor before taking an iron supplement.

Carefully follow the directions for giving an iron supplement to a child. Overdose and iron poisoning are especially dangerous in children.

If you're an older adult, check with your doctor before taking an iron supplement.

Additional instructions

_____

_____

_____

Taking isoetharine

Dear Patient:

Isoetharine is prescribed to relieve the symptoms of asthma, bronchitis, and emphysema and to prevent wheezing and troubled breathing resulting from exercising. The label may read Bronko-meter or Bronkosol.

How to take isoetharine
Isoetharine comes as an aerosol spray and a solution used with a nebulizer. Take isoetharine exactly as your doctor has prescribed. Overuse can cause serious side effects or decrease the medication's effectiveness.

To use the *aerosol spray,* first clear your nose and throat. Then breathe out, exhaling as much air as you can. Put the mouthpiece in your mouth, release the spray, and inhale deeply. Hold your breath in for a few seconds, then remove the mouthpiece and exhale slowly.

Wait 1 to 2 minutes before using it again. You may not need another spray.

If you're also taking another inhaled medication, take isoetharine first and wait 5 minutes before taking the other medication.

If you're using the *solution form in a nebulizer,* follow your doctor's, nurse's, or pharmacist's instructions exactly.

What to do if you miss a dose
Take it as soon as you can. Then evenly space your remaining doses for the day. Never take a double dose.

What to do about side effects
If you think you may have taken an overdose or if you develop symptoms of an overdose—chest pain, seizures, chills, fever, severe muscle cramps, nausea, vomiting, fast or slow heartbeat, shortness of breath, and severe trembling or weakness—seek emergency care *immediately.*

Also seek emergency care if your skin develops a bluish color and you experience severe dizziness, continuing facial flushing, increased difficulty breathing, a rash, and swelling of your face or eyelids.

Isoetharine may cause tremor, headache, or fast or pounding heartbeat. These side effects should disappear after you use the medication for a while. If they don't, tell your doctor.

What you must know about other drugs
Tell your doctor about other prescription and nonprescription medications you're taking, especially beta blockers, such as propranolol, atenolol, metoprolol, or nadolol.

Special directions
• Tell your doctor if you have other medical problems. They may affect the use of this medication.
• Don't use medication that's cloudy or discolored.
• If you don't breathe easier after using this medication, call your doctor immediately.
• Avoid caffeine-containing food and drink—coffee, tea, cola, and chocolate.

Important reminders
If you're pregnant or think you may be or if you're breast-feeding, check with your doctor before taking isoetharine.

If you're an athlete, be aware that isoetharine is banned and tested for by the U.S. Olympic Committee.

Taking isoniazid

Dear Patient:

Your doctor has prescribed isoniazid to treat your tuberculosis (TB). The label may read Laniazid, Nydrazid, or Tubizid.

How to take isoniazid
Take this medication exactly as your doctor has prescribed. Take it at the same time each day to help you avoid missed doses. If the medication upsets your stomach, take it with food or an antacid.

Keep taking isoniazid as your doctor directs, even after you feel better. Otherwise, your TB may not clear up completely. You may need to take this medication for 1 or more years.

What to do about side effects
Call your doctor *right away* if you experience any of the following side effects:
• nausea, vomiting, diarrhea, or loss of appetite
• blurred vision, loss of vision, or eye pain
• clumsiness or unsteadiness
• burning, numbness, tingling, or weakness in your hands or feet (which may signal peripheral neuritis)
• fever, hives, itching, or rash—signs of hypersensitivity that may herald an allergic reaction to the medication
• abdominal pain, yellowing of the skin or whites of the eyes, dark urine, or light-colored stools (which may signal liver inflammation)
• behavioral changes, hallucinations, or seizures.

What you must know about alcohol and other drugs
Avoid drinking alcoholic beverages while taking isoniazid because doing so increases the risk of liver problems.

Tell your doctor about prescription and nonprescription drugs you're taking because some drugs interact with isoniazid. For example, you should avoid taking any antacid that contains aluminum within 1 hour of the time you take isoniazid because the antacid will decrease isoniazid's effectiveness. Also, isoniazid increases the blood levels and potential side effects of phenytoin (Dilantin).

Special directions
• Don't drive or perform other activities requiring alertness and clear vision until you know how your body responds to this medication.
• Avoid Swiss cheese and tuna. Coupled with isoniazid, these foods can cause chills, headache, light-headedness, red and itchy skin, increased sweating, and rapid or pounding heartbeat. If these symptoms occur, call your doctor.

Important reminders
If you're pregnant or breast-feeding, check with your doctor before taking isoniazid.

If you're an older adult, you may be especially sensitive to isoniazid's side effects.

Additional instructions

_____

_____

_____

_____

_____

_____

Taking isoproterenol

Dear Patient:

Isoproterenol is prescribed to relieve the wheezing and shortness of breath caused by asthma, bronchitis, or emphysema or to treat heart rhythm problems. Brand names include Aerolone, Isuprel, and Medihaler-Iso.

How to take isoproterenol
Isoproterenol comes as an aerosol inhaler, a solution used with a nebulizer inhaler, and as sublingual tablets. Follow your doctor's instructions closely.

To use the *aerosol inhaler* or *nebulizer solution,* first clear your nose and throat. Then breathe out, exhaling as much air as you can. Put the mouthpiece in your mouth, release the spray, and inhale deeply. Hold your breath in for a few seconds, then remove the mouthpiece and exhale slowly.

Wait 1 to 2 minutes before using it again. You may not need another spray.

If you're also taking another inhaled medication, take isoproterenol first and wait 5 minutes before taking the other medication.

To take a *sublingual tablet,* place the tablet under your tongue and let it dissolve. Don't chew or swallow it, and don't swallow saliva until it dissolves completely.

Avoid taking isoproterenol at bedtime, if possible. It may disturb your sleep.

What to do if you miss a dose
Take it as soon as you can. Then evenly space your remaining doses for the day. Never take a double dose.

What to do about side effects
If you think you may have taken an overdose or if you develop symptoms of an overdose—chest pain, seizures, chills, fever, severe muscle cramps, nausea, vomiting, shortness of breath, severe trembling or weakness, and fast, slow, or fluttering heartbeat—seek emergency care *immediately.*

Also seek emergency care if your skin develops a bluish color and you experience severe dizziness, facial flushing, increased difficulty breathing, a rash, and swelling of your face or eyelids.

Isoproterenol may cause headache and rapid or pounding heartbeat. These side effects should disappear after you use the medication for a while. If they persist, call your doctor.

What you must know about other drugs
Tell your doctor about other prescription or nonprescription medications you're taking, especially a beta blocker (such as propranolol), epinephrine (Adrenalin), or digitalis glycosides (heart medication).

Special directions
• Tell your doctor about other medical problems you have. They may affect the use of this medication.
• If you don't breathe easier after taking the medication, call your doctor right away.
• Avoid caffeine-containing food and drink—coffee, tea, cola, and chocolate.

Important reminders
If you're pregnant or think you may be or if you're breast-feeding, check with your doctor before taking this medication. If you're an athlete, be aware that isoproterenol is banned and tested for by the U.S. Olympic Committee.

Taking isosorbide dinitrate

Dear Patient:

This medication is used to treat angina attacks and certain other heart conditions. Brand names may include Dilatrate-SR, Isonate, and Isorbid.

How to take isosorbide dinitrate

For best results, take this medication exactly as your doctor has instructed.

Regular or extended-release tablets or capsules are used to prevent angina attacks. Take a regular or an extended-release tablet or capsule with a full glass (8 ounces) of water on an empty stomach (30 minutes before or 1 to 2 hours after meals). Swallow the extended-release tablet or capsule whole; don't crush, break or chew it.

Sublingual or chewable tablets are used to relieve the pain of an attack that's occurring. Place a sublingual tablet under your tongue and let it dissolve. Don't chew or swallow it, and don't swallow saliva until the tablet dissolves completely. Chew a chewable tablet well and hold it in your mouth for about 2 minutes before swallowing.

If you still have chest pain after taking three sublingual or chewable tablets in 15 minutes, get emergency medical care.

What to do if you miss a dose

Take it as soon as possible. But if it's within 2 hours of your next scheduled dose (or within 6 hours if you're taking an extended-release form), skip the missed dose and take the next one as scheduled. Never take two doses at once.

What to do about side effects

If you think you may have taken an overdose or if you develop signs and symptoms of an overdose—bluish lips, nails, or palms; extreme dizziness or fainting; extreme head pressure; shortness of breath; severe tiredness or weakness; weak and fast heartbeat; fever; or seizures—seek emergency medical care *immediately.*

More common side effects—dizziness, rapid or pounding heartbeat, skin redness, headache, nausea, or vomiting—should go away after you've been taking the medication for a while. If they don't, consult your doctor.

What you must know about other drugs

If you're also taking a blood pressure medication or another heart medication, your blood pressure may decrease even more. Check with your doctor.

Special directions

• Tell your doctor about other medical conditions you have. They may affect the use of this medication.
• Don't suddenly stop using this medication if you've been taking it regularly. This could trigger an angina attack.
• To minimize dizziness or fainting, get up slowly from a lying or sitting position.
• If you're taking extended-release tablets or capsules, call your doctor if you find any partially dissolved tablets in your stool.

Important reminders

If you're pregnant or think you may be, check with your doctor before taking this medication. If you're an older adult, you may be especially susceptible to side effects.

Taking isotretinoin

Dear Patient:

Isotretinoin is prescribed to treat acne. The label may read Accutane.

How to take isotretinoin
Take isotretinoin capsules exactly as prescribed. Take each dose either with a meal or shortly afterward. This will help your body absorb the medication.

What to do if you miss a dose
Take it as soon as you can. But if it's almost time for your next dose, skip the missed dose and take the next one at the scheduled time. Don't double dose.

What to do about side effects
Call your doctor if you develop headache, nausea, vomiting, vision problems, or burning, redness, and itching of your eyes.

Dry, itchy skin or pain, soreness, or stiffness in your muscles, bones, or joints should go away after you've taken this medication for a while. If they don't, check with your doctor.

What you must know about alcohol and other drugs
Limit alcoholic beverages when taking isotretinoin because alcohol can increase the triglyceride (fat) level in your blood. Using drying skin preparations, medicated soaps, acne preparations that contain skin peeling agents, and alcohol preparations (such as cosmetics, after-shave lotion, and cologne) can increase skin drying and irritation. Vitamin A and tetracycline antibiotics can aggravate isotretinoin's side effects. Check with your doctor before taking these medications.

Special directions
• Before taking isotretinoin, tell your doctor about other medical problems you have. They may affect the use of this medication.
• When you start this medication, your acne may worsen temporarily. If it becomes severe, check with your doctor.
• If this medication interferes with night vision, don't drive or perform other activities that could be dangerous if you can't see clearly. Notify your doctor.
• When you first start taking this medication, limit sun exposure to protect light-sensitive skin.
• Relieve mouth dryness with sugarless hard candy or gum, ice chips, mouthwash, or a saliva substitute. If the dryness continues for more than 2 weeks, check with your doctor or dentist.
• Don't donate blood for at least 30 days after you stop taking isotretinoin, so that no pregnant woman receives blood containing this medication.

Important reminders
Don't take isotretinoin if you're pregnant or think you may be or if you're breast-feeding.

Children are especially susceptible to side effects.

If you have diabetes, this medication can alter your blood glucose level. If you notice any change, tell your doctor.

Additional instructions

_____

_____

_____

Taking kaolin with pectin

Dear Patient:

This combination medication of kaolin with pectin is used to treat diarrhea. Brand names include Kaopectate, K-P, and K-Pek.

How to take kaolin with pectin

Carefully read and follow all instructions and precautions on the medication bottle. Also follow any special directions your doctor may have given you. Shake the bottle vigorously before pouring your dose.

Special directions

• Avoid using this medication if you have a bowel obstruction because it may aggravate the problem.
• If you still have diarrhea after taking this medication for more than 48 hours, don't take any more and contact your doctor promptly.
• Besides using this medication to treat your diarrhea, you also need to replace lost body fluids and comply with an appropriate diet. During the first 24 hours, drink plenty of clear liquids, such as apple juice, broth, plain gelatin, and decaffeinated tea. Eat bland foods, such as applesauce, bread, cooked cereals, and crackers. Avoid bran, alcoholic beverages, caffeine, candy, fried or spicy foods, fruits, and vegetables. These foods can worsen your diarrhea.
• If your body loses too much fluid from diarrhea, you will become severely dehydrated. Call your doctor if you have the following symptoms: dizziness, dry mouth, increased thirst, decreased urination, and wrinkled skin.

Important reminders

Don't give this medication to a child age 3 or younger because the fluid loss caused by diarrhea may lead to severe health problems.

If you give this medication to a child over age 3, make sure the child drinks at least 3 to 4 quarts of liquid each day to replace lost body fluids and prevent dehydration.

If you're an older adult, you may develop severe health problems from the fluid loss caused by diarrhea. Drink extra fluids to offset this loss.

Additional instructions

_____

_____

_____

_____

_____

_____

_____

_____

_____

_____

_____

_____

Taking oral ketoconazole

Dear Patient:

Your doctor has prescribed ketoconazole to treat your fungal infection. The label may read Nizoral.

How to take oral ketoconazole
Take ketoconazole exactly as prescribed. Take it for the full time prescribed even if your symptoms disappear. If you don't, your symptoms may return.

If necessary, take the tablets with food to decrease stomach upset. If you have achlorhydria (absence of stomach acid), your doctor may have you dissolve each tablet in a weak acid solution so your body can absorb it. A pharmacist will prepare the solution for you. After dissolving the tablet, add it to 1 to 2 teaspoons of water in a glass. Drink it through a straw placed far back in your mouth and away from your teeth. Then swish about half a glass (4 ounces) of water around in your mouth and swallow it.

What to do if you miss a dose
Take a missed dose as soon as possible. But if it's almost time for your next dose, space the missed dose and the next dose 10 to 12 hours apart. Then resume your normal dosing schedule.

What to do about side effects
If you develop dark urine, pale stools, severe weakness, yellowing of your skin or the whites of your eyes, or loss of appetite, contact your doctor *immediately.*

Nausea, vomiting, and diarrhea may occur when you first start taking the tablets but should disappear as your body adjusts to the medication. If these symptoms are bothersome, tell your doctor.

What you must know about alcohol and other drugs
Don't drink alcoholic beverages while you're taking ketoconazole and for at least 1 day after stopping it because alcohol may aggravate liver or stomach problems. Because many medications can interact with ketoconazole, tell your doctor about other medications you're taking.

Special directions
• Tell your doctor about other medical problems you have. They may affect the use of this medication.
• If your symptoms don't improve in a few weeks or if they get worse, tell your doctor.
• Don't drive or perform other activities requiring alertness until you know how you react to this medication.

Important reminders
If you're pregnant or think you may be, check with your doctor before taking this medication. Don't breast-feed while you're taking ketoconazole and for 24 to 48 hours after stopping it.

Additional instructions

_____

_____

_____

_____

_____

Applying topical ketoconazole

Dear Patient:

Your doctor has prescribed ketoconazole to treat your fungal infection. The label may read Nizoral.

How to apply topical ketoconazole
Apply ketoconazole exactly as prescribed. Apply it for the full time prescribed even if your symptoms disappear. If you don't, your symptoms may return.

To apply the cream, first wash your hands. Then apply enough to cover the affected area and surrounding skin. Rub it in gently. Keep the medication away from your eyes. Wash your hands again after applying the cream.

What to do if you miss an application
Skip the missed dose and apply the cream at the next scheduled time.

What to do about side effects
Ketoconazole cream may cause skin irritation, itching, and stinging. Call your doctor if these effects persist.

Special directions
• Tell your doctor if you're allergic to this or another antifungal medication or to other medications, foods, dyes, or preservatives.
• If you're using this medication for *skin infection,* keep your skin clean and dry.
• If you're using the cream to treat *ringworm of the groin (jock itch),* wear loose-fitting cotton underwear and use a bland, absorbent powder (such as talcum) on your skin between the times you apply ketoconazole.
• If you're using the cream to treat *athlete's foot,* wear clean cotton socks and change them often to keep your feet dry. Wear sandals or shoes with lots of air holes. Remember to apply talcum or another absorbent powder between your toes, on your feet, and in your socks and shoes once or twice a day, between the times you apply ketoconazole.

Important reminders
If you're pregnant or think you may be or if you're breast-feeding, check with your doctor before using this medication.

Additional instructions

_____

_____

_____

_____

_____

_____

_____

_____

_____

_____

_____

Taking ketoprofen

Dear Patient:

Your doctor has prescribed ketoprofen to relieve fever, pain, swelling, and joint stiffness. The label may read Orudis.

How to take ketoprofen
Take ketoprofen exactly as your doctor has prescribed. Overuse can aggravate side effects.

Continue taking the medication regularly for best results. You may not feel its full effects for several weeks.

Take the capsules with a full glass (8 ounces) of water either 30 minutes before or 2 hours after meals. Avoid lying down for 15 to 30 minutes after you take it. If stomach upset occurs, take the capsules with food or milk.

What to do if you miss a dose
Take it as soon as you remember. But if it's almost time for your next dose, skip the missed dose and take the next one as scheduled.

What to do about side effects
If you develop a hivelike rash or itching, stop taking ketoprofen and call your doctor *immediately*—you may be experiencing an allergic reaction. Although rare, an allergic reaction can be serious. If you become restless, wheeze, and have difficulty breathing or get puffy around your eyes, get emergency medical care *immediately.*

Ketoprofen may cause ulcers and internal bleeding. Stop taking the medication and call your doctor *at once* if you have stomach pain; pass black, tarry stools; have severe nausea, heartburn, or indigestion; or vomit coffee ground–like matter.

Abdominal cramps, nausea, diarrhea, constipation, gas, headache, nervousness, dizziness, and drowsiness can occur but usually disappear as your body adjusts to the medication. Tell your doctor if these side effects persist or are bothersome.

What you must know about alcohol and other drugs
Don't drink alcoholic beverages while taking ketoprofen because doing so could increase stomach problems. Tell your doctor about other drugs you're taking, especially probenecid (Benemid) and blood thinners.

Special directions
• Tell the doctor if you have other medical problems. They may affect the use of this medication.
• If you're on a special diet, let your doctor know because this medication may contain sugar or sodium.
• Because ketoprofen makes some people dizzy or drowsy, don't drive or perform other activities requiring alertness until you know how you react to this medication.

Important reminders
If you're pregnant or breast-feeding, check with your doctor before taking ketoprofen.

If you're an older adult, you may be especially susceptible to side effects.

Additional instructions

_____

_____

_____

Taking labetalol

Dear Patient:

Your doctor has prescribed labetalol to control your blood pressure. Labetalol is one of a group of medications commonly called beta blockers. Brand names may include Normodyne and Trandate.

How to take labetalol
Take your medication exactly as prescribed, either with food or on an empty stomach, as you prefer. Swallow the tablets whole; don't break, crush, or chew them.

What to do if you miss a dose
Take it as soon as you remember unless it's within 8 hours of your next dose. If so, skip the missed dose and take the next one at the scheduled time. Never take two doses at once.

What to do about side effects
Labetalol may cause dizziness and a sudden blood pressure drop when you stand up quickly. If these side effects become bothersome, tell your doctor.

What you must know about alcohol and other drugs
Avoid alcoholic beverages, which in combination with labetalol may cause an excessive drop in blood pressure. Check with your doctor before taking cimetidine (Tagamet), insulin, or oral antidiabetic drugs with labetalol.

Special directions
• Tell your doctor about other medical problems you have. They may affect the use of this medication.
• Keep in mind that labetalol controls high blood pressure but doesn't cure it. For this reason, keep taking it as prescribed even if you think you don't need it anymore.
• Make sure you always have enough labetalol on hand, even when you're away from home, so you don't have to interrupt your dosing schedule because you run out.
• Carry medical identification stating that you're taking labetalol.
• If your doctor has also instructed you to reduce your intake of salt, follow his directions.
• To minimize dizziness, get up slowly from a sitting or lying position.
• Because labetalol may make some people dizzy, don't drive or perform other activities requiring alertness until you know how you respond to this medication.

Important reminders
If you're pregnant or breast-feeding, check with your doctor before taking labetalol.

If you're an older adult, you may be especially sensitive to side effects.

If you have diabetes, be aware that labetalol may cause your blood glucose level to drop and also may mask signs of low blood glucose (hypoglycemia), such as altered pulse rate.

If you're an athlete, be aware that the National Collegiate Athletic Association and the U.S. Olympic Committee ban beta blockers.

Additional instructions

_____

_____

Taking lactulose

Dear Patient:

Your doctor has prescribed this laxative to relieve your constipation. Lactulose promotes bowel movements by drawing water into the bowel from surrounding body tissues. Brand names for lactulose include Cephulac, Cholac, and Chronulac.

How to take lactulose
Take each dose of lactulose in or with a full glass (8 ounces) of cold water or fruit juice. For the best effect, your doctor may recommend that you then drink another glass of water by itself.

What to do if you miss a dose
Take it as soon as you remember unless it's almost time for your next dose. If so, skip the missed dose and take the next dose at its scheduled time.

Special directions
• Before taking lactulose, tell your doctor if you're allergic to laxatives or to another medication or substance.
• Don't use this or any other laxative if you have symptoms of appendicitis or an inflamed bowel—lower abdominal or stomach pain, bloating, cramping, soreness, nausea, or vomiting. Instead, call your doctor *immediately.*
• If you notice a sudden change in your bowel habits or function that lasts longer than 2 weeks or that keeps returning on and off, contact your doctor before taking lactulose.
• Keep in mind that you may have to wait 24 to 48 hours before lactulose starts working.
• Because lactulose contains large amounts of carbohydrates, sodium, and sugar, don't take this medication if you're on a low-calorie, low-sodium, or low-sugar diet. Instead, check with your doctor or pharmacist.

Important reminder
Don't give this or any other laxative to a child under age 6 unless your doctor prescribes it.

Additional instructions

_____

_____

_____

_____

_____

_____

_____

_____

_____

_____

_____

_____

_____

Taking levodopa

Dear Patient:

This medication is usually given to treat Parkinson's disease. Brand names include Dopar and Larodopa.

How to take levodopa
Carefully check the label on your prescription bottle, which tells you how much to take at each dose. Take only the amount prescribed by your doctor.

What to do if you miss a dose
Take the missed dose as soon as possible. However, if your next scheduled dose is within 2 hours, skip the missed one and resume your regular dosage schedule. Never take a double dose.

What to do about side effects
Call your doctor if you have fatigue, headache, shortness of breath, insomnia, depression, mood or behavior changes, or unusual and uncontrolled body movements. Also tell him if you feel faint, dizzy, or light-headed when rising from a lying or sitting position.

Anxiety, confusion, or nervousness may occur. If these symptoms persist or are bothersome, call your doctor.

This drug may turn your urine and sweat red or black. This is normal and doesn't require medical attention.

What you must know about other drugs
Check with your doctor or pharmacist before taking other prescription or non-prescription drugs. Other drugs can change the way levodopa works.

Monoamine oxidase (MAO) inhibitors (drugs for depression) can cause very high blood pressure when taken within 14 days of levodopa. Check with your doctor about stopping treatment.

Special directions
• Be sure your doctor knows your medical history before you take levodopa.
• Avoid hazardous activities, such as driving a car, until you know how the drug affects you. Levodopa may make you drowsy or less alert.
• If levodopa upsets your stomach, take it with food. Don't take it with high-protein foods, such as poultry and eggs; they can make the drug less effective.
• When getting out of bed, change positions slowly and dangle your legs for a few moments to reduce dizziness.
• If your diet usually includes avocados, bacon, beans, liver, oatmeal, peas, pork, sweet potatoes, or tuna, check with your doctor to find out if you should cut down on these foods. They contain large amounts of vitamin B_6 (pyridoxine), which can make levodopa less effective. Also, don't take supplements containing vitamin B_6 unless your doctor approves them.
• Contact your doctor if you believe your behavior or mental status is changing.
• You may not notice levodopa's effects for several weeks. If you don't think the drug is working, don't stop taking it; call your doctor. Also, if your symptoms persist or get worse, check with the doctor.

Important reminders
If you're breast-feeding, check with your doctor before taking levodopa.

If you have diabetes, the doctor may need to adjust your dosage of insulin or other diabetes medication. Also, you may need to switch to another type of urine glucose test.

Taking levodopa with carbidopa

Dear Patient:

This medication is usually given to treat Parkinson's disease. The brand name for this medication is Sinemet.

How to take this drug
This medication is available in tablets. Carefully check the label on your prescription bottle, which tells you how much to take. The doctor may prescribe three to six tablets daily. Take only the amount prescribed.

What to do if you miss a dose
Take the missed dose as soon as possible. However, if your next scheduled dose is within 2 hours, skip the missed one and resume your regular dosage schedule. Never take a double dose.

What to do about side effects
Call your doctor if you experience fatigue, headache, shortness of breath, insomnia, depression, mood or behavior changes, or unusual and uncontrolled body movements.

This medication may make you dizzy, especially when you first start taking it. Tell your doctor if you feel dizzy or lightheaded when you get up from a lying or sitting position.

What you must know about other drugs
Check with your doctor or pharmacist before taking other prescription or nonprescription drugs. Other drugs can change the way levodopa works.

Monoamine oxidase (MAO) inhibitors (drugs for depression) can cause very high blood pressure when taken within 14 days of levodopa. Check with your doctor or pharmacist about stopping treatment.

Special directions
• Be sure your doctor knows about your medical history before you take this medication.
• Avoid hazardous activities, such as driving a car or using dangerous tools, until you know how this medication affects you. The medication may make you drowsy or less alert.
• The doctor may need to change your dosage—possibly several times—to find the right amount for you to take.
• If this drug upsets your stomach, you may take it with food.
• Before getting out of bed, change position slowly and dangle your legs for a few moments to avoid dizziness.
• Contact your doctor if you believe your behavior or mood is changing.
• Increase your physical activities gradually so your body can adjust to your changing balance, coordination, and circulation.
• You may not notice this drug's effects for several weeks. If you don't think it's working, don't stop taking it; call your doctor. Also, don't increase the dosage if your symptoms continue or get worse; check with the doctor.

Important reminders
If you're breast-feeding, check with your doctor before taking this drug.

If you have diabetes, the doctor may need to adjust your dosage of insulin or other diabetes medication. Also, you may need to switch to another type of urine glucose test.

Using levonorgestrel

Dear Patient:

This contraceptive prevents pregnancy. It's commonly called the Norplant System.

How to use levonorgestrel
The doctor will make a small cut in your upper arm, put six tablets there, and close the skin over them. The tablets will start to work and won't require any action on your part. Their contraceptive effect lasts for 5 years.

What to do about side effects
Call your doctor if you have pain in your stomach or muscles or discharge from your breasts or vagina.

You should expect changes in your menstrual bleeding pattern. For instance, your menstrual period may stop or it may last longer than usual. You may have spotting, scanty or irregular bleeding, or frequent bleeding episodes. These changes usually go away over time. If they don't, call your doctor.

What you must know about other drugs
Check with your doctor before taking carbamazepine (Tegretol) or phenytoin (Dilantin) because these drugs may make your contraceptive less effective.

Special directions
• Before you get the implants, be sure your doctor knows about your medical history, especially if you've had thrombophlebitis or a thromboembolic disorder; seizures; liver, kidney, or heart disease; breast cancer; or unusual genital bleeding that hasn't been diagnosed. Also, if you've ever had depression or an emotional disorder, tell your doctor because levonorgestrel may make these conditions worse.
• Because your contraceptive can cause you to retain fluid, the doctor may want you to limit salt in your diet if you've had heart or kidney disease. Follow any specially prescribed diet.
• Don't assume you're pregnant if you miss a menstrual period. However, if your period still doesn't come after 6 or more weeks (after a pattern of regular periods), tell your doctor because this could mean you're pregnant.
• Call the doctor right away if one of the tablets falls out because this could reduce the contraceptive effect.
• Have a physical examination at least every year so the doctor can check for any problems caused by levonorgestrel.
• Your implants must be removed if you become pregnant, develop phlebitis or a thromboembolism, have jaundice, or must stay in bed for a long time.
• Call your doctor if you notice a change in vision—for instance, if you wear contact lenses and suddenly have vision changes or can't tolerate your lenses.

Important reminders
If you're breast-feeding, inform your doctor before getting these implants.

If you suspect you're pregnant—either before or after receiving the implants—make sure to tell your doctor right away.

Additional instructions

_____

_____

_____

_____

Taking levorphanol

Dear Patient:

This drug is usually prescribed to treat moderate to severe pain. The label may read Levo-Dromoran.

How to take levorphanol
This drug is available in tablet and injection forms.

Carefully check the label on your prescription bottle, which tells you how much to take at each dose. Take only the amount prescribed by your doctor.

If you're taking the *injection* form of levorphanol at home, make sure you fully understand your doctor's instructions and follow them carefully.

What to do if you miss a dose
Take the missed dose as soon as you remember. However, if it's almost time for your next dose, skip the missed dose and resume your regular schedule. Don't double dose.

What to do about side effects
Get emergency help *immediately* if you think you may have taken an overdose. Symptoms of an overdose include slow or troubled breathing, seizures, confusion, severe drowsiness, weakness, dizziness, restlessness, and nervousness.

You may experience milder forms of dizziness or drowsiness, as well as light-headedness, fainting, an unusual feeling of well-being, nausea, vomiting, or constipation. These side effects usually go away over time as your body adjusts to the medication. But you should check with your doctor if they persist or become bothersome.

What you must know about alcohol and other drugs
Avoid alcoholic beverages, sedatives (such as drugs that relax you and make you feel sleepy), antihistamines (such as diphenhydramine [Benadryl]), and other depressant drugs while taking levorphanol because of the risk of additive sedative effects.

Special directions
• Don't take levorphanol if you're allergic to it or to similar medications (such as codeine and morphine).
• Be sure your doctor knows about your medical history, especially if you've had an abnormal heart rhythm, a head injury, liver or kidney problems, seizures, or a respiratory disorder, because this medication could cause serious problems. Also tell your doctor if you've ever been addicted to any drug.
• Avoid hazardous activities, such as driving a car or using dangerous tools, because levorphanol may make you drowsy or less alert.
• Don't stop taking this drug suddenly without first checking with your doctor. Levorphanol is a narcotic. If you use it for a long time, you may become dependent on it and have withdrawal side effects when you stop taking it.

Important reminders
If you're pregnant or breast-feeding, be sure to tell your doctor before taking this medication.

If you're an older adult, you may be especially sensitive to side effects, particularly breathing problems, when taking levorphanol.

Applying lindane

Dear Patient:

This medication is prescribed to treat scabies and lice infestations. Brand names of the medication include Kwell and Scabene.

How to apply lindane

This medication is available as a cream, lotion, and shampoo. The cream and lotion forms are used to treat scabies. The shampoo form is used to treat lice.

Don't exceed the amount your doctor has ordered, and don't use the medication more often or for a longer time than ordered because this could cause poisoning.

To use the *cream* or *lotion,* apply a thin layer to your freshly washed and dried skin. Use enough medication to cover the entire skin surface from the neck down, including your soles. Rub in the cream or lotion well, then leave it on. After the prescribed number of hours (usually 8 to 12 hours), wash yourself thoroughly. If you need a second application, wait 1 week before repeating.

To use the *shampoo,* apply it undiluted to freshly washed and dried hair. Apply enough to your dry hair to thoroughly wet both the affected areas and surrounding hair-covered areas. Rub the shampoo into your hair and scalp. If you're applying it while taking a bath, make sure the shampoo doesn't drip onto other parts of your body or into the bath water. Leave it on for 4 to 5 minutes, then add enough water to create a lather. Rinse your hair thoroughly, then dry it with a clean towel. When your hair is dry, comb it with a fine-toothed comb dipped in white vinegar to remove any remaining lice eggs.

What to do about side effects

Call your doctor *right away* if you have symptoms of lindane poisoning, such as seizures, dizziness, nervousness, restlessness, clumsiness, a fast heartbeat, muscle cramps, or vomiting.

If you use lindane repeatedly, your skin may become irritated and you may have toxic drug effects. Report skin irritation to your doctor.

Special directions

• Don't swallow lindane. This medication is poisonous and can be fatal.
• Keep the medication away from your eyes, nose, mouth, and lips. If some gets in your eyes, *immediately* flush your eyes with water and notify the doctor.
• Don't use lindane on open cuts, sores, or inflamed areas of your skin.
• Don't inhale vapors from this medication.
• Your sexual partner and members of your household may need to be treated with lindane because scabies and lice spread through close contact.
• After you wash the medication off your body, change and sterilize (dry-clean or wash in very hot water) all your clothing and bed linens.
• After using lindane shampoo, clean your combs and brushes with lindane shampoo, then wash them thoroughly. Don't use as a regular shampoo.

Important reminder

If you're pregnant or breast-feeding, tell your doctor before using lindane.

Additional instructions

_____

_____

Taking lisinopril

Dear Patient:

This medication treats high blood pressure. The label for this medication may read Prinivil or Zestril.

How to take lisinopril
This medication is available in tablets. Carefully check the label on your prescription bottle. Take only the amount prescribed by your doctor.

What to do if you miss a dose
Take it as soon as you remember. However, if it's almost time for your next dose, skip the missed one and resume your regular schedule. Don't double dose.

What to do about side effects
Call the doctor *right away* if you suddenly have trouble breathing or swallowing or if you experience dizziness, light-headedness, nausea, vomiting, diarrhea, loss of taste, fever, chills, hoarseness, or swelling of the face, mouth, hands, or feet.

This drug may make you cough. If coughing continues or becomes bothersome, call your doctor.

What you must know about other drugs
Check with your doctor or pharmacist before taking other drugs, especially nonprescription medications (such as remedies for colds, asthma, cough, hay fever, or appetite control). These drugs may change the way lisinopril works or cause high blood pressure and other medical problems.

Diuretics (water pills) or indomethacin (Indocin), an arthritis drug, may cause your blood pressure to drop too low or your potassium level to rise too high if you take them with lisinopril.

Drugs and nutritional supplements that contain potassium or salt substitutes may cause your potassium level to rise too high. This could make your heart beat abnormally.

Special directions
• You shouldn't take lisinopril if you're allergic to it.
• Be sure your doctor knows about your medical history, especially if you have diabetes; heart, kidney, or liver disease; a kidney transplant; or lupus.
• Call your doctor *right away* if severe nausea, vomiting, or diarrhea occurs after you start taking this medication. These symptoms may cause you to lose too much water and lead to low blood pressure.
• Avoid hazardous activities, such as driving a car or using dangerous tools, until you know how the medication makes you feel. That's because lisinopril makes some people feel dizzy.
• Follow any special diet the doctor has prescribed.
• You may not notice the effects of this medication for several weeks. However, don't suddenly stop taking it if you don't think it's working or if you have unpleasant side effects. Instead, check with your doctor.
• Continue to take this medication as directed even if you feel well. You may have to take this or another blood pressure medication for the rest of your life.

Important reminder
If you're pregnant or breast-feeding, check with your doctor before taking lisinopril.

Taking lithium

Dear Patient:

Your doctor has prescribed lithium to treat your condition. This medication acts on the central nervous system to help you control your emotions and cope better with everyday problems.

Other names for the medication include Eskalith, Lithane, and Lithobid.

How to take lithium

This medication is available in regular and sustained-release tablets, regular capsules, and a syrup. You may need to take up to four doses a day.

Carefully check the label on your prescription bottle, which tells you how much to take at each dose. Take only the amount prescribed by your doctor.

Take doses of lithium every day at regularly spaced intervals to keep a constant amount of the drug in your blood.

If you're taking the *sustained-release tablets,* swallow the tablet whole. Don't crush, chew, or break it before swallowing.

If you're taking the *syrup,* dilute it in fruit juice or another flavored beverage.

What to do if you miss a dose

Take the missed dose as soon as you remember. However, if your next scheduled dose is within 2 hours (or 6 hours for sustained-release tablets), skip the missed dose and resume your regular dosage schedule. Never take a double dose.

What to do about side effects

If you have symptoms of lithium toxicity, withhold one dose and contact your doctor *immediately.* These symptoms include diarrhea, nausea, vomiting, drowsiness, muscle weakness, and clumsiness.

Contact your doctor *at once* if you feel faint or have a fast or slow heartbeat, seizures, an irregular pulse rate, troubled breathing, unusual weakness or fatigue, or weight gain.

Inform your doctor if you start to lose hair, become hoarse, experience depression or unusual excitement, notice your skin getting dry, or become more sensitive to cold temperatures. Also report any swelling of the neck, feet, or lower legs. These symptoms mean that lithium is affecting your thyroid function.

You may become thirstier, urinate more often, lose bladder control, and have mild nausea and slight hand trembling while taking lithium. These side effects usually go away over time as your body adjusts to the medication. But you should check with your doctor if they persist or become bothersome.

What you must know about other drugs

Check with your doctor or pharmacist before taking diuretics (water pills) or nonnarcotic medications for pain or inflammation (such as indomethacin [Indocin]). These medications can increase the level of lithium in your blood and cause serious side effects.

Tell your doctor or pharmacist if you're taking medications for psychosis (mental illness). When taken with lithium, these medications can increase your chance for side effects and may cause lethargy, tremor, and other symptoms.

(continued)

Taking lithium *(continued)*

Check with your doctor or pharmacist before taking aminophylline (Aminophyllin), an asthma medication; sodium bicarbonate (baking soda), which is used to treat indigestion; or sodium chloride. These medications may make lithium less effective in treating your condition.

Special directions
• You shouldn't take lithium if you're allergic to it.
• Be sure your doctor knows about your medical history, especially schizophrenia, brain or kidney disease, diabetes, difficult urination, severe infection, seizures, heart problems, psoriasis, Parkinson's disease, thyroid disease, or leukemia.
• Avoid hazardous activities, such as driving a car or using dangerous tools, until you know how the drug affects you. Lithium can make you drowsy or less alert.
• To reduce stomach upset, take lithium after meals with plenty of water.
• You probably won't get the full benefits of lithium for several weeks. However, don't stop taking it if you think you're not getting better. Instead, call your doctor.
• Drink 2 to 3 quarts of water or other fluids daily and salt your food as you normally do unless your doctor tells you otherwise.
• If you usually drink large amounts of caffeine-containing beverages (such as coffee, tea, or colas), you may need to cut down on these beverages to get the full benefits of lithium.
• During hot weather and activities that make you sweat heavily, take extra precautions because you could get serious side effects if you lose too much water and salt. For instance, if you start sweating too much, drink more fluids and increase your salt intake.
• Don't switch lithium brands without your doctor's approval.
• Don't stop taking lithium even if you start to feel better, unless your doctor approves.
• Check with your doctor if you get an illness that causes vomiting, diarrhea, or heavy sweating. These conditions can make you lose too much water and salt.
• Call your doctor before going on a weight-loss diet or making major changes in your diet. If you lose too much water and salt while dieting, serious side effects could occur.
• Make sure to have your lithium blood levels checked regularly because even a slightly increased level can be dangerous.
• Have regular medical checkups so your doctor can make sure lithium is working properly and detect any side effects.
• Carry an identification card (available at drugstores) that tells others how to respond in case of lithium toxicity or another emergency.

Important reminders
If you become pregnant while taking lithium, check with your doctor.

If you're breast-feeding, don't take lithium without your doctor's approval. Lithium may be harmful to your baby.

If you're an older adult, you may be especially sensitive to the effects of this medication.

Additional instructions

_____

_____

Taking loperamide

Dear Patient:

This drug is usually used to treat diarrhea. Brand names include Imodium and Imodium A-D.

How to take loperamide
This medication is available in tablet, capsule, and liquid forms.

If you buy this medication without a prescription and are treating yourself, carefully follow the instructions on the package. Don't take more than the recommended amount.

If you're taking loperamide by prescription, follow your doctor's instructions carefully.

What to do if you miss a dose
If you're taking loperamide on a regular schedule, skip the missed dose and resume your regular dosage schedule. Never take a double dose.

What to do about side effects
Constipation may occur. If it's severe and occurs suddenly, check with your doctor *immediately.*

What you must know about other drugs
Check with your doctor or pharmacist if you're taking an antibiotic (a drug used to treat infection). Some antibiotics cause diarrhea. Taking loperamide at the same time may worsen or prolong the diarrhea.

Before taking a narcotic pain reliever, check with your doctor or pharmacist. Combining a narcotic with loperamide may increase your chance for severe constipation.

Special directions
• Don't take loperamide if you're allergic to it or if you have colitis.
• Be sure your doctor knows about your medical history. Especially mention a history of liver disease, a severely enlarged prostate, or dependence on narcotics because loperamide can make these conditions worse.
• After the initial dose, take the medication after each unformed stool until your diarrhea goes away (unless the doctor tells you otherwise).
• Replace the fluid your body has lost from diarrhea. For the first 24 hours of your illness, drink plenty of clear liquids that don't contain caffeine (such as caffeine-free cola and tea, ginger ale, gelatin, and broth). After that, you may eat bread, crackers, hot cereal, and other bland foods. Avoid caffeine, spicy or fried foods, vegetables, fruits, bran, candy, and alcoholic beverages because these could make your diarrhea worse.
• If you lose a great deal of fluid from diarrhea, you may suffer dehydration, a serious condition. Call your doctor *right away* if you have any of the following symptoms: dry mouth, increased thirst, decreased urination, dizziness, lightheadedness, or wrinkled skin.
• If your diarrhea doesn't go away after 2 days or if you develop a fever, stop taking loperamide and contact your doctor.

Important reminders
If you're breast-feeding or pregnant, check with the doctor before using loperamide.

Check with the doctor before giving loperamide to children.

If you're an older adult, losing fluid from diarrhea can be especially dangerous. Call your doctor or pharmacist for instructions on how to replace lost fluid.

Taking lorazepam

Dear Patient:

This medication may be prescribed to treat anxiety, tension, agitation, irritability, or insomnia (difficulty sleeping). Brand names include Alzapam, Ativan, and Loraz.

How to take lorazepam
This medication is available in tablets. Carefully check the prescription label. Take only the amount prescribed.

What to do if you miss a dose
If you're taking this medication on a regular schedule, take the missed dose right away if you remember within an hour or so. If you remember more than 1 hour later, skip the missed dose and resume your regular dosage schedule. Never take a double dose.

What to do about side effects
If you think you've taken an overdose, get emergency help *immediately.* Symptoms of an overdose include confusion, staggering, slurred speech, extreme drowsiness, and weakness.

Drowsiness, light-headedness, dizziness, and clumsiness may occur. These side effects usually go away over time as your body adjusts to the medication. But you should check with your doctor if they persist or become bothersome.

What you must know about alcohol and other drugs
Avoid alcoholic beverages, sedatives (such as drugs that relax you and make you feel sleepy), antihistamines (such as diphenhydramine [Benadryl]), and other depressants while taking this medication because of the risk of additive sedation.

Special directions
• You shouldn't take lorazepam if you're allergic to it or if you have glaucoma.
• Be sure your doctor knows your medical history, especially psychosis (mental illness), myasthenia gravis, Parkinson's disease, respiratory problems, liver problems, drug addiction, or drug abuse.
• Avoid hazardous activities, such as driving a car or using dangerous tools, until you know how the drug affects you. Lorazepam can make you drowsy or less alert.
• Take the medication only as directed. Don't take it longer than directed because this may cause drug dependence and withdrawal symptoms.
• Don't stop taking this medication without your doctor's approval.

Important reminders
If you're pregnant or breast-feeding, be sure to tell your doctor before taking lorazepam.

Older adults are especially likely to become dizzy, drowsy, light-headed, clumsy, and less alert when taking lorazepam.

If you're an athlete, you should know that lorazepam is banned by the U.S. Olympic Committee and the National Collegiate Athletic Association for athletes participating in shooting events.

Additional instructions

_____

_____

_____

_____

Taking lovastatin

Dear Patient:

This medication is prescribed to lower the levels of cholesterol and other fats in the blood. Lovastatin works by blocking an enzyme that the body needs to make cholesterol. The label may read Mevacor.

How to take lovastatin
This medication is available in tablets.

Carefully check the prescription label, Take only the amount prescribed by your doctor.

Taking this medication with food makes it work better. If the doctor has prescribed one dose a day, take it with your evening meal. If he has prescribed several daily doses, take them with meals or snacks.

What to do if you miss a dose
Take the missed dose as soon as possible. However, if it's almost time for your next scheduled dose, skip the missed dose and resume your regular dosage schedule. Never take a double dose.

What to do about side effects
Contact the doctor *right away* if you have blurred vision, fever, unusual weakness or fatigue, or muscle aches or cramps.

What you must know about other drugs
Check with your doctor or pharmacist if you're taking niacin, an immunosuppressive drug (such as cyclosporine [Sandimmune]), or gemfibrozil (Lopid). These drugs increase the risk of side effects from lovastatin.

Special directions
• You shouldn't take this medication if you're allergic to it or if you have liver disease.
• Be sure your doctor knows your medical history, especially if you've had an organ transplant, if you're about to have major surgery, or if you have low blood pressure, uncontrolled seizures, or a severe metabolic or endocrine disorder.
• Also tell the doctor if you drink large amounts of alcoholic beverages, which can affect your cholesterol level.
• Follow any special diet the doctor has prescribed, such as a low-fat, low-cholesterol diet.
• Have regular medical checkups so the doctor can make sure lovastatin is working properly and detect any side effects.
• Make sure to have regular liver function tests, if the doctor orders this.
• Have regular eye examinations because this medication can cause blurred vision.
• Don't stop taking lovastatin unless the doctor approves. Stopping treatment could make your blood cholesterol level rise again.
• Before having surgery (including dental surgery), tell the doctor or dentist you're taking lovastatin.

Important reminder
If you're pregnant or breast-feeding, check with your doctor. Lovastatin may cause serious problems in a fetus or breast-feeding baby.

Additional instructions

_____

_____

Taking magaldrate

Dear Patient:

This medication is used to relieve heartburn or acid indigestion or to treat symptoms of a stomach or duodenal ulcer. The label may read Lowsium or Riopan.

How to take magaldrate
This medication is available in regular and chewable tablets and an oral suspension.

If you buy magaldrate without a prescription and are treating yourself, carefully follow the instructions on the label. If your doctor prescribed this medication or gave you special instructions on how to use it and how much to take, follow those instructions carefully.

If you're using the *chewable tablets,* chew them completely before swallowing. Drink a glass of milk or water afterward.

If you're using the *oral suspension,* shake it well. Sip water or juice after taking it.

What to do if you miss a dose
If you're taking this medication on a regular schedule, take the missed dose as soon as possible. However, if it's almost time for your next dose, skip the missed dose and resume your regular dosage schedule. Never take a double dose.

What to do about side effects
Constipation or diarrhea may occur. If these symptoms persist or are bothersome, call your doctor.

What you must know about other drugs
Check with your doctor or pharmacist before taking other medications. Magaldrate may change the way other drugs work, or other drugs may change the way magaldrate works.

As a general rule, don't take magaldrate within 1 to 2 hours of taking another medication by mouth (such as a tablet, capsule, or liquid). Magaldrate may make the other medication less effective.

If you're taking tetracycline (Achromycin), ketoconazole (Nizoral), or methenamine (Urex), wait 3 hours after a dose before you take magaldrate.

If you're taking mecamylamine (Inversine), check with your doctor before taking magaldrate because magaldrate may increase the risk of side effects.

Special directions
• You shouldn't take magaldrate if you have a colostomy or an ileostomy, ulcerative colitis, diverticulitis, chronic diarrhea, kidney problems, a low blood phosphate level, appendicitis, Alzheimer's disease, or unexplained bleeding from the rectum or GI tract.
• Check with your doctor if magaldrate doesn't improve your stomach problem.
• If you have cramping, bloating, nausea, vomiting, or pain in your stomach or lower abdomen, stop taking magaldrate and call your doctor promptly.
• Don't take this medication for more than 2 weeks unless your doctor tells you to.
• Be aware that the chewable tablets contain sugar.

Important reminder
If you're an older adult, check with your doctor before taking magaldrate.

Taking magnesium hydroxide (milk of magnesia)

Dear Patient:

This medication is used to relieve constipation. The label may read Phillips' Milk of Magnesia.

How to take magnesium hydroxide

This medication is available in an oral solution, an oral suspension, and granules.

You can buy magnesium hydroxide without a prescription. If you're treating yourself, carefully follow the instructions on the label, which tell you how much to take at each dose. If your doctor prescribed this drug or gave you special instructions on how to use it and how much to take, follow those instructions carefully.

If you're taking the *oral suspension,* shake it well and take it with a full glass (8 ounces) of fruit juice or water. To prevent dehydration, you may take the dose with another full glass of water or juice.

What to do about side effects

Call your doctor as soon as possible if you become confused, dizzy, or lightheaded; if you develop an irregular heartbeat; or if you experience muscle cramps or unusual tiredness or fatigue.

Diarrhea, abdominal cramps, gas, nausea, and increased thirst may occur. These side effects usually subside as your body adjusts to the medication. But you should check with your doctor if they persist or become bothersome.

What you must know about other drugs

Check with your doctor or pharmacist if you're taking tetracycline (Achromycin) because magnesium hydroxide may make tetracycline less effective.

Don't take magnesium hydroxide within 1 to 2 hours of taking another medication by mouth (such as a tablet, capsule, or liquid) because it may make the other medication less effective.

Special directions

• You shouldn't take this medication if you have kidney failure, a colostomy or an ileostomy, abdominal pain, nausea, vomiting, fecal impaction, or intestinal obstruction. Magnesium hydroxide may make these conditions worse.
• Schedule the dose so that the bowel movement it produces won't interfere with your sleep or activities. Magnesium hydroxide usually produces a watery stool in 3 to 6 hours. However, it may take longer if you take a small dose with food.
• Don't take this or any other laxative regularly. Laxatives are meant only for short-term relief of constipation. Don't take this drug if you don't need it or if you miss a bowel movement merely for 1 or 2 days.
• To help prevent the need for a laxative, eat a high-fiber diet, exercise regularly, and increase your fluid intake. Good sources of dietary fiber include bran and other cereals and fresh fruits and vegetables.
• Don't take this medication for more than 1 week unless ordered by your doctor.
• If you have a sudden change in bowel habits that lasts for more than 2 weeks or returns every now and then, contact your doctor before using this medication. You may have a more serious problem.

Important reminder

Don't give laxatives to children unless prescribed by the doctor.

Taking mebendazole

Dear Patient:

This medication is usually prescribed to treat worm infections, such as pinworm, roundworm, whipworm, and hookworm. A brand name for the medication is Vermox.

How to take mebendazole
This medication is available in tablets and an oral suspension.

Carefully check the prescription label. Take only the prescribed amount.

If you're taking the *tablets,* you may chew them, swallow them whole, or crush them and mix them with food.

If the doctor has prescribed high doses of this medication, take the doses with meals. Fatty foods, such as ice cream and whole milk, help the medication work better. However, if you're on a low-fat diet, check with your doctor before taking the drug with fatty foods.

What to do if you miss a dose
Take the missed dose as soon as possible. However, if it's almost time for your next scheduled dose and the doctor has prescribed two doses a day, space the missed dose and the next dose 4 to 5 hours apart. If the doctor has prescribed eight doses a day, space the missed dose and the next dose 1½ hours apart. Then resume your normal dosage schedule.

What to do about side effects
Contact your doctor *immediately* if you have a fever, itching, a rash, a sore throat, or unusual weakness or fatigue.

Special directions
• You shouldn't take this medication if you're allergic to it.

• Wash your hands often and thoroughly to avoid spreading the infection. Be sure to wash your hands and clean your fingernails before meals and after bowel movements.
• Don't prepare food as long as your infection lasts.
• If your symptoms don't improve within a few days or if they get worse, notify your doctor.
• If you have anemia caused by whipworm or hookworm, the doctor may prescribe an iron supplement in addition to mebendazole. Make sure to take the supplement every day and to take all prescribed doses of it. You may need to take the iron supplement for several months after you've finished mebendazole treatment.
• To prevent reinfection, the doctor may want members of your household to take mebendazole while you're being treated with it. To eliminate the infection completely, they may require a second treatment 2 to 3 weeks after the first treatment.
• If you're being treated for pinworm but the infection returns after mebendazole treatment, wash all bedding and pajamas to help prevent a recurrence after a second treatment.
• See your doctor regularly to make sure the infection has gone away and to check for any side effects of this medication.

Important reminder
If you're pregnant, check with your doctor before taking this medication.

Taking meclizine

Dear Patient:

This medication is usually prescribed to prevent and treat nausea, vomiting, and dizziness caused by motion sickness. The doctor sometimes prescribes it to treat dizziness caused by other medical problems. Brand names include Antivert, Bonine, and Ru-Vert M.

How to take meclizine
This medication is available in regular and chewable tablets and in capsules.

Some preparations of this medication are available only by prescription. Others are available without a prescription. If you're treating yourself, carefully follow the instructions on the label, which tell you how much to take at each dose. If your doctor prescribed this drug or gave you special instructions on how to use it and how much to take, follow those instructions carefully.

What to do if you miss a dose
If you're taking meclizine on a regular schedule, take the missed dose as soon as possible. However, if it's almost time for your next dose, skip the missed dose and resume your regular dosage schedule. Never take a double dose.

What to do about side effects
Drowsiness may occur. If it persists or becomes bothersome, call your doctor.

What you must know about alcohol and other drugs
Avoid alcoholic beverages, sedatives (such as drugs that relax you and make you feel sleepy), antihistamines (such as diphenhydramine [Benadryl]), and other depressant drugs while taking meclizine because of the risk of additive sedative effects.

Special directions
• Don't take meclizine if you're allergic to it or to similar medications (such as buclizine [Bucladin-S Softabs], cyclizine [Marezine], or dimenhydrinate).
• Tell your doctor about other medical problems you have, especially narrow-angle glaucoma, asthma, an enlarged prostate, or a blockage of the genitourinary or GI tract. Meclizine may make these conditions worse.
• Take this medication 1 hour before starting your trip, and continue to take it regularly every travel day during the trip.
• Avoid hazardous activities, such as driving a car or using dangerous tools, until you know how the medication affects you. Meclizine may make you drowsy or less alert.
• If you've been vomiting a lot, be sure to drink plenty of fluids to prevent dehydration.
• If this medication makes your mouth dry, use sugarless gum or hard candy or ice chips. However, if dry mouth lasts for more than 2 weeks, see your doctor or dentist for further evaluation.

Important reminders
If you're pregnant or breast-feeding, check with your doctor before taking meclizine.

If you're an athlete, you should know that meclizine is banned by the U.S. Olympic Committee and can lead to disqualification in biathlon and pentathlon events.

Taking medroxyprogesterone

Dear Patient:

This medication is usually prescribed to treat abnormal bleeding of the uterus caused by hormonal imbalance, to treat amenorrhea (absence of menstruation), or to help treat cancer of the endometrium or kidney. Brand names include Amen and Provera.

How to take medroxyprogesterone
This medication is available in tablets. Carefully check the label, which tells you how much to take at each dose. Take only the prescribed amount.

What to do if you miss a dose
Take it as soon as you remember. However, if it's almost time for your next dose, skip the missed dose and resume your regular dosage schedule. Don't double dose.

What to do about side effects
Rarely, this medication may cause a blood clot—a life-threatening emergency. If you have any of the following symptoms, stop taking the medication and get medical help *immediately:* pain in the chest, groin, or leg; sudden shortness of breath or loss of coordination; sudden or severe headache; sudden slurring of speech; sudden vision loss or change in vision; or weakness, numbness, or pain in the arm or leg.

If this medication causes changes in your vaginal bleeding pattern, such as spotting, breakthrough bleeding, or prolonged bleeding, report these side effects to your doctor *promptly.*

What you must know about other drugs
Check with your doctor or pharmacist before taking rifampin (Rifadin), a tuberculosis drug, because it may make medroxyprogesterone less effective.

Special directions
• Don't take this medication if you're allergic to it or if you have a history of blood clots (thromboembolism), severe liver disease, breast or genital cancer, or undiagnosed abnormal vaginal bleeding. Medroxyprogesterone may make these disorders worse.
• Tell your doctor about other medical problems you have, especially heart or kidney disease, fluid retention, seizures, migraine headaches, depression, or breast or genital cancer.
• Contact your doctor if your menstrual period doesn't start within 45 days of your last period or if vaginal bleeding lasts an unusually long time.
• Brush and floss your teeth and massage your gums carefully and regularly to help prevent your gums from bleeding. See your dentist regularly.
• Have regular medical checkups so the doctor can check your progress, adjust your dosage if needed, and detect any side effects.

Important reminders
If you're pregnant, you shouldn't take this medication. If you become pregnant while taking it, stop taking it immediately because it may harm your fetus.

If you're breast-feeding, check with your doctor before taking this medication.

If you have diabetes, report symptoms of high blood glucose (such as increased thirst and urination) to the doctor.

Taking meperidine

Dear Patient:

This drug is usually prescribed to treat moderate to severe pain. The label may read Demerol.

How to take meperidine
This drug is available in tablets and a syrup. Take only the amount prescribed.

If you're using the *syrup* form, take it with a full glass (8 ounces) of water to reduce numbness of the mouth and throat.

What to do if you miss a dose
If you're taking this medication on a regular schedule, take the missed dose as soon as possible. But if it's almost time for your next regular dose, skip the missed dose and resume your regular schedule. Never take a double dose.

What to do about side effects
Get emergency help *immediately* if you think you may have taken an overdose of this medication. Symptoms include cold, clammy skin; confusion; seizures; severe dizziness or drowsiness; slow heartbeat; slow or troubled breathing; and severe weakness.

This drug may cause dizziness, drowsiness, light-headedness, faintness, urine retention, nausea, vomiting, or constipation. These side effects usually subside as your body adjusts to the drug. But check with your doctor if they persist or become bothersome.

What you must know about alcohol and other drugs
Don't drink alcoholic beverages or take sleeping pills, sedatives (such as drugs that relax you), or antihistamines (such as diphenhydramine [Benadryl]) while taking meperidine because of the risk of additive sedative effects.

Check with your doctor if you're taking other prescription or nonprescription medications. Other drugs may change the way meperidine works.

Special directions
• Don't take meperidine if you're allergic to it.
• Tell your doctor about other medical problems you have, especially heart rhythm problems, a head injury, liver or kidney problems, asthma, respiratory problems, glaucoma, seizures, or drug abuse or addiction.
• To reduce nausea or vomiting from the first few doses, lie down for a while after taking the dose. If these problems persist, call your doctor.
• This medication may make you feel faint, dizzy, or light-headed when rising from a lying or sitting position. To reduce this effect, get up slowly.
• Avoid hazardous activities, such as driving a car, because meperidine may make you drowsy or less alert.
• If you've been taking meperidine regularly for several weeks or more, don't stop taking it suddenly because this could cause withdrawal side effects. Check with your doctor for instructions on how to stop the drug gradually.

Important reminders
If you're pregnant or breast-feeding, check with your doctor before taking meperidine.

Children and older adults are especially sensitive to meperidine's effects.

If you're an athlete, you should know that meperidine is banned by the U.S. Olympic Committee.

Taking meprobamate

Dear Patient:

This medication is usually prescribed to treat anxiety or tension. Brand names include Equanil, Miltown, and Trancot.

How to take meprobamate
This medication is available in tablets and sustained-release capsules.

Carefully check the prescription label. Take only the prescribed amount.

What to do if you miss a dose
If you remember within an hour or so, take the missed dose as soon as possible. Otherwise, skip the missed dose and resume your regular dosage schedule. Never take a double dose.

What to do about side effects
If you think you've taken an overdose, get emergency help *immediately.* Symptoms of a meprobamate overdose include severe drowsiness, dizziness, light-headedness, shortness of breath, slow or troubled breathing, slow heartbeat, slurred speech, severe weakness, and staggering.

If you experience any of the following symptoms, contact your doctor *as soon as possible:* a fast, pounding, or irregular heartbeat; shortness of breath; troubled breathing; a rash, hives, or itching; confusion; or unusual bleeding or bruising.

What you must know about alcohol and other drugs
Avoid alcoholic beverages, sedatives (such as drugs that relax you and make you feel sleepy), antihistamines (such as diphenhydramine [Benadryl]), and other depressant drugs while taking this medication because of the risk of additive sedative effects.

Special directions
• Don't take this drug if you're allergic to it or to aspirin or if you have porphyria.
• Be sure your doctor knows your medical history, especially if you've had liver or kidney problems, seizures, depression, or drug abuse or addiction.
• Avoid hazardous activities, such as driving a car or using dangerous tools, because meprobamate may make you drowsy or less alert.
• Use sugarless gum or hard candy or suck on ice chips to relieve dry mouth.
• If you're taking meprobamate for a long time, be sure to have regular medical checkups so the doctor can check your progress and detect any unwanted side effects.
• If you've been taking meprobamate regularly for several weeks or more, don't stop taking it suddenly because this could cause withdrawal side effects. Check with your doctor for instructions on how to discontinue the drug gradually.

Important reminders
If you're pregnant, check with your doctor about taking meprobamate.

If you're breast-feeding, check with your doctor. This drug may make your baby drowsy.

If you're an athlete, you should know that meprobamate use is banned by the U.S. Olympic Committee and the National Collegiate Athletic Association.

Additional instructions

_____

_____

Taking mesalamine

Dear Patient:

This medication is usually prescribed to treat ulcerative colitis and other inflammatory diseases of the bowel. Another name of the medication is Rowasa.

How to take mesalamine

This medication is available in a rectal suspension and rectal suppositories. Carefully check the label, which tells you how much to take at each dose. Take only the amount prescribed.

If the doctor has prescribed the *suspension,* take it once a day as an enema, preferably at bedtime. You may need to take it for up to 6 weeks. Just before taking the enema, empty your bowel. Then shake the suspension well and administer the enema. Be sure to retain the medication for at least 8 hours.

What to do if you miss a dose

If you remember the same night, take the missed dose as soon as possible. If you don't remember until the next morning, skip the missed dose and resume your regular dosage schedule.

What to do about side effects

Stop taking the medication, and contact your doctor *immediately* if you develop a rash, wheezing, itching, hives, severe stomach or abdominal pain or cramps, fever, bloody diarrhea, or severe headache. These symptoms may mean that you have an intolerance to the medication or a sensitivity to sulfites.

Call your doctor as soon as possible if rectal irritation occurs.

You may experience a mild headache, mild stomach or abdominal pain or cramps, nausea, diarrhea, bloating, and flatulence or gas. These side effects usually go away as your body adjusts to the medication. But you should check with your doctor if they persist or become bothersome.

Special directions

• You shouldn't take this medication if you're allergic to it or to any of its contents (including sulfites).
• Tell your doctor about your medical history, especially if you've had kidney disease, because this drug may further harm your kidneys. Also inform your doctor if you're allergic to sulfasalazine (Azulfidine), olsalazine (Dipentum), or aspirin.
• Contact your doctor if you suddenly have rectal pain, bleeding, burning, itching, or other symptoms of irritation after you start using this medication.
• Continue to take this medication for the full time of treatment prescribed by your doctor, even if you feel better within several days. Don't miss any doses.
• Have regular medical checkups so the doctor can evaluate your progress.

Additional instructions

_____

_____

_____

_____

_____

_____

_____

Taking metaproterenol

Dear Patient:

This medication is usually prescribed to treat asthma. It's also used to treat bronchospasm (wheezing or difficulty breathing) associated with chronic bronchitis, emphysema, or other lung diseases or to prevent bronchospasm caused by exercise. Brand names include Alupent and Metaprel.

How to take metaproterenol

This medication is available as an inhalation aerosol, an inhalation solution, or an oral tablet or syrup. You may need to take it up to 12 times daily if you're using the inhalation aerosol, every 4 hours if you're using the inhalation solution in a nebulizer, or every 6 to 8 hours if you're taking it orally.

Carefully check the label, which tells you how much to take at each dose. Take only the amount prescribed.

To take the *aerosol,* shake the container. Then exhale through your nose completely. Inhale deeply through your mouth, then take the medication. Hold your breath for 10 seconds, then exhale slowly. Don't take more than two inhalations at a time unless prescribed. After the first inhalation, wait 1 to 2 minutes to see if you need a second inhalation.

If you're using this medication in a *nebulizer* or a *combination nebulizer and respirator,* make sure you understand how to use it. Ask your doctor or pharmacist if you have any questions.

What to do if you miss a dose

If you're using this medication regularly, take the missed dose as soon as you remember. If you have more doses left that day, take them at regularly spaced intervals. Never take a double dose.

What to do about side effects

If you think you may have taken an overdose, get emergency medical help *immediately.* Symptoms of an overdose include severe dizziness, light-headedness, headache, chills, fever, nausea, vomiting, severe muscle cramps, severe weakness, blurred vision, severe shortness of breath or troubled breathing, or unusual anxiety or restlessness.

Trembling, nervousness, and restlessness may occur. These side effects usually go away over time as your body adjusts to the medication. But you should check with your doctor if they persist or become bothersome.

If you're using an oral inhaler, you may notice an unusual or unpleasant taste. This symptom will go away when you stop using the medication.

What you must know about other drugs

Check with your doctor if you're taking a beta blocker because it may prevent metaproterenol from working properly. Beta blockers are drugs prescribed to treat high blood pressure or angina. Some examples are atenolol (Tenormin), labetalol (Normodyne), and propranolol (Inderal).

Notify your doctor or pharmacist if you're taking ergoloid mesylates (Hydergine), ergotamine (Ergomar), maprotiline (Ludiomil), or a tricyclic antidepressant (a drug for depression). These drugs may increase metaproterenol's effects on the heart and blood vessels.

Check with your doctor or pharmacist if you're taking a digitalis glycoside (a drug used to treat an abnormal heart rhythm) because this drug increases the chance for an irregular heartbeat when taken with metaproterenol.

(continued)

Taking metaproterenol *(continued)*

If you're taking a monoamine oxidase (MAO) inhibitor (a drug for depression), check with your doctor or pharmacist. Metaproterenol may increase the effects of the MAO inhibitor if the two drugs are taken within 2 weeks of each other.

Special directions
• You shouldn't take this medication if you're allergic to it. If you have tachycardia (a too-fast heart rhythm), you shouldn't take metaproterenol because it may worsen this condition.
• Be sure your doctor knows your medical history, especially if you have brain damage, seizures, diabetes, an underactive thyroid, heart disease, or blood vessel disease. Metaproterenol may make these conditions worse.
• Call your doctor *right away* if you still have trouble breathing or if your condition gets worse after you start using this medication.
• If you're using the *aerosol* form, keep the spray away from your eyes to avoid irritation.
• If you're using the *aerosol* form and are also using an adrenocorticoid aerosol or ipratropium (Atrovent) aerosol, take metaproterenol at least 5 minutes before the other aerosol, unless your doctor tells you otherwise. Adrenocorticoids available in aerosol form include beclomethasone (Beclovent), dexamethasone (Decadron Respihaler), and flunisolide (Aerobid).
• If your mouth and throat feel dry after taking this drug, try rinsing your mouth with water after each dose to help prevent this problem.
• Save the applicator because you may be able to get refills.

• Don't use more of the drug or use it more often than recommended (unless your doctor tells you to) because this could cause serious side effects.
• After using this medication for a long time, contact your doctor if you find that its effects don't last as long as they did when you first started using it.

Important reminders
If you're pregnant or breast-feeding, check with the doctor before taking metaproterenol.

If you're an older adult, you may be especially sensitive to the effects of this medication.

If you have diabetes, the doctor may need to adjust the dosage of your insulin or other diabetes medication.

Additional instructions

_____

_____

_____

_____

_____

_____

_____

_____

_____

_____

Taking methenamine

Dear Patient:

This medication is usually prescribed to prevent and treat infections of the urinary tract. Brand names of the medication include Hiprex, Mandelamine, and Urex.

How to take methenamine
This drug is available in regular and enteric-coated tablets, an oral suspension, and granules (for oral solution).

Carefully check the label on your prescription bottle, which tells you how much to take at each dose. Take only the amount prescribed by your doctor.

If you're taking the *enteric-coated tablets,* swallow them whole. Don't crush or break them.

If you're taking the *oral suspension,* use the proper device, such as a specially marked measuring spoon, to measure doses accurately. Don't use a household teaspoon.

If you're taking the *granules,* dissolve the packet contents in 2 to 4 ounces of cold water, stir well, then take the dose immediately.

What to do if you miss a dose
Take the missed dose right away. However, if it's almost time for your next regular dose, space the missed dose and the next dose 5 to 6 hours apart if the doctor has prescribed two daily doses. Space them 2 to 4 hours apart if the doctor has prescribed three or more daily doses. Then resume your regular dosage schedule.

What to do about side effects
Contact your doctor *right away* if you develop a rash or lower back pain, if you feel pain or burning when you urinate, or if you see blood in your urine.

What you must know about other drugs
If you're taking thiazide diuretics (water pills) or urinary alkalizers (drugs that make your urine less acidic), check with your doctor or pharmacist. These medications may prevent methenamine from working properly. Urinary alkalizers include acetazolamide (Diamox), methazolamide (Neptazane), sodium bicarbonate (baking soda), and antacids that contain calcium or magnesium.

Special directions
• You shouldn't take this medication if you're allergic to it or severely dehydrated or if you have severe liver or kidney disease.
• Before you start taking this medication, test your urine pH with Nitrazine paper because your urine must be acidic (pH 5.5 or below) for methenamine to work well. If you don't know how to test your urine, ask your doctor, nurse, or pharmacist.
• To help make your urine more acidic, eat more acidic foods, such as cranberries, cranberry juice with vitamin C added, prunes, and plums. Eat fewer alkaline foods, such as milk, other dairy products, and most fruits. Avoid taking antacids.
• Drink plenty of fluids during treatment.
• Continue to take this medication for the full time prescribed by the doctor, even if you feel better after a few days.

Additional instructions

_____

_____

Taking methimazole

Dear Patient:

This medication is usually prescribed to treat an overactive thyroid gland. Another name of the drug is Tapazole.

How to take methimazole
This medication is available in tablets.

Carefully check the prescription label. Take only the amount prescribed.

If the doctor has prescribed more than one daily dose, take the doses at evenly spaced intervals throughout the day and night. If you need help in planning the best times to take the doses, call your doctor or pharmacist.

Take this medication at a consistent time every day in relation to meals. Either take all doses with meals or take all doses on an empty stomach. If this drug upsets your stomach, you may want to take it with meals.

What to do if you miss a dose
Take the missed dose as soon as possible. However, if it's almost time for your next regular dose, take both doses together, then resume your regular dosage schedule. If you miss two or more doses, check with your doctor.

What to do about side effects
Call your doctor *immediately* if you experience nausea, vomiting, fever, chills, a sore throat, malaise, unusual bleeding, or yellowing of the eyes.

What you must know about other drugs
Check with your doctor or pharmacist if you're taking lithium (Lithane), potassium iodide (Pima), or iodinated glycerol (Iophen). These drugs may reduce your thyroid function too much and increase the chance for goiter (swollen thyroid gland) when taken with methimazole. Avoid nonprescription cough remedies because they may contain iodine, which may make methimazole less effective.

Special directions
• You shouldn't take this medication if you're allergic to it.
• Tell your doctor about other medical problems you have, especially an infection or liver disease.
• To maintain the proper amount of this medication in your blood, don't skip any doses.
• When your thyroid function becomes normal, the doctor may reduce your dosage.
• Ask your doctor whether you can eat shellfish or use iodized salt. The iodine in these substances may make methimazole less effective.
• If you're injured or get sick, you may need to stop taking this medication or you may need to take a different dosage for a while. Call your doctor for instructions.
• Contact your doctor if you have symptoms of an underactive thyroid, such as mental depression, intolerance to cold, or swelling. These symptoms may mean your dosage should be changed.
• This medication may take several weeks to work. Don't stop taking it without consulting your doctor.
• Tell the doctor or dentist before having surgery (including dental surgery).

Important reminders
If you're pregnant, make sure the doctor monitors you carefully during treatment.

If you're breast-feeding, check with your doctor before taking methimazole.

Taking methocarbamol

Dear Patient:

This medication is usually prescribed to relax muscles and to relieve pain and discomfort caused by muscle injury (such as sprains and strains). Brand names include Delaxin and Robaxin.

How to take methocarbamol
This medicaton is available in tablets. Carefully check the prescription label. Take only the amount prescribed. If you have trouble swallowing tablets, you may crush the tablets and mix them with food or liquid.

What to do if you miss a dose
Take it right away if you remember within an hour or so. Otherwise, skip the missed dose and resume your regular dosage schedule. Don't double dose.

What to do about side effects
Call your doctor *right away* if you develop a fever, a fast heartbeat, skin rash or redness, itching, hives, shortness of breath, troubled breathing, wheezing, tightness in the chest, stinging or burning of the eyes, red or bloodshot eyes, or a stuffy nose.

You may experience vision changes (including blurring or double vision), dizziness, light-headedness, or drowsiness. These effects usually go away as your body adjusts to the medication. But you should check with your doctor if they persist or become bothersome.

This medication may discolor your urine. This effect goes away once you stop taking the medication.

You may notice a metallic taste.

What you must know about alcohol and other drugs
Avoid alcoholic beverages, sedatives, antihistamines (such as diphenhydramine [Benadryl]), and other depressant drugs while taking methocarbamol because of the risk of oversedation.

Special directions
• You shouldn't take this medication if you're allergic to it.
• Tell your doctor about other medical problems you have, especially allergies, kidney disease, seizures, or a blood disease caused by an allergy to another medication. Also tell the doctor if you've ever abused or been dependent on drugs.
• To prevent stomach upset, take this drug with meals or milk.
• Avoid hazardous activities, such as driving a car or using dangerous tools. Methocarbamol may make you drowsy or less alert and may affect your vision.
• If you're taking this medication for more than a few weeks, have regular medical checkups so the doctor can evaluate your progress and detect any unwanted side effects.

Important reminders
If you're breast-feeding, check with your doctor before taking methocarbamol.

If you're an athlete, you should know that methocarbamol use is banned and tested for by the U.S. Olympic Committee and the National Collegiate Athletic Association.

Additional instructions

_____

_____

Taking methotrexate

Dear Patient:

This medication is often prescribed to treat psoriasis or rheumatoid arthritis. (It's also used to treat cancer. However, this instruction sheet doesn't apply to that use.) Brand names include Folex, Mexate, and Rheumatrex.

How to take methotrexate
This medication is available in tablets. Carefully check the prescription label. Take only the prescribed amount.

What to do if you miss a dose
Don't take the missed dose or double the next dose. Resume your regular schedule and call your doctor.

What to do about side effects
Call your doctor *immediately* if you have diarrhea; reddened skin; red spots on the skin; stomach pain; mouth or lip sores; black, tarry stools; bloody urine or stools; blurred vision; seizures; cough; hoarseness; fever; chills; lower back or side pain; painful urination; shortness of breath; or unusual bleeding or bruising.

Check with your doctor *promptly* if you have dark urine, dizziness, drowsiness, headache, unusual fatigue or weakness, or yellow eyes or skin.

Hair loss may occur. However, after you finish methotrexate treatment, your normal hair growth should return.

If nausea and vomiting occur, check with your doctor. If you vomit shortly after taking a dose, ask the doctor whether you should take the dose again or wait until the next scheduled dose.

What you must know about alcohol and other drugs
Avoid drinking alcoholic beverages, which may increase unwanted effects on the liver. Check with your doctor or pharmacist before taking other drugs, including nonprescription medications. Especially avoid taking aspirin and other drugs used for pain and inflammation because they may increase the risk of serious side effects.

Special directions
• Tell your doctor about other medical problems you have, especially a stomach ulcer, colitis, an immune system disease, liver or kidney disease, or a blood disorder.
• Don't get immunizations during treatment except with your doctor's approval. Also, avoid people who've recently taken oral polio vaccine.
• Practice birth control during and at least 3 months after treatment ends. Methotrexate may cause birth defects if either the mother or the father takes it at the time of conception or if the mother takes it during pregnancy.

Important reminders
If you're pregnant, don't take this medication because it may harm the fetus. If you think you've become pregnant while taking methotrexate, call your doctor right away.

If you're breast-feeding, check with your doctor before taking methotrexate because it may cause serious side effects in your baby.

If you're an older adult, you may be especially sensitive to the effects of methotrexate.

Taking methyldopa

Dear Patient:

This medication is usually prescribed to treat high blood pressure. It controls impulses along certain nerve pathways, which relaxes blood vessels. The prescription label may read Aldomet.

How to take methyldopa
This medication is available in tablets and an oral suspension. Carefully check the label. Take only the prescribed amount.

What to do if you miss a dose
Take it right away. However, if it's almost time for your next dose, skip the missed dose and resume your regular schedule. Don't double dose.

What to do about side effects
Call your doctor *immediately* if you develop a fever shortly after you start taking this medication.

Contact your doctor *as soon as possible* if you experience swelling of the feet or lower legs, depression, anxiety, nightmares, stomach pain or cramps, pale stools, diarrhea, nausea, vomiting, fever, chills, joint pain, troubled breathing, fast heartbeat, weakness, a rash, itching, dark or amber urine, or yellow eyes or skin.

Drowsiness, dry mouth, and headache may occur. Also, you may feel dizzy or light-headed when getting up from a lying or sitting position. Check with your doctor if these side effects persist or become bothersome.

What you must know about other drugs
Check with your doctor or pharmacist before taking levodopa. When combined with methyldopa, this drug may lower your blood pressure too much and cause other problems.

Contact your doctor or pharmacist before taking a tricyclic antidepressant or a monoamine oxidase (MAO) inhibitor (drugs for depression) or a phenothiazine (used for anxiety, nausea and vomiting, or psychosis). Combining one of these drugs with methyldopa may cause high blood pressure.

Don't take any nonprescription remedies (such as for colds, hay fever, or cough) without first checking with your doctor or pharmacist. These drugs may increase your blood pressure.

Special directions
• Be sure your doctor knows about your medical history, especially if you're taking diuretics (water pills) or other drugs to reduce your blood pressure. Also tell the doctor if you have Parkinson's disease, kidney or liver problems, or mental depression or if you've ever had liver problems when taking methyldopa in the past.
• Avoid hazardous activities, such as driving a car or using dangerous tools, until you know how the drug affects you. Methyldopa can make you drowsy or less alert.
• Follow any special diet the doctor prescribed, such as a low-salt diet.
• Don't suddenly stop taking this medication if you don't think it's working or if unpleasant side effects occur. Instead, contact your doctor.

Important reminder
If you're an older adult, you may be especially sensitive to methyldopa's side effects.

Taking methyldopa with hydrochlorothiazide

Dear Patient:

This medication is usually prescribed to treat high blood pressure. Methyldopa works by controlling nerve impulses along certain nerve pathways. This relaxes blood vessels so that blood passes through them more easily. Thiazide diuretics help reduce the amount of water in the body by increasing urine flow. Both of these actions help lower blood pressure. The label may read Aldoril.

How to take this drug
Take only the amount prescribed.

What to do if you miss a dose
Take the missed dose as soon as you remember. However, if it's almost time for your next regular dose, skip the missed dose and resume your regular dosage schedule. Never take a double dose.

What to do about side effects
Call your doctor *right away* if you develop a fever shortly after you start taking this medication.

Contact your doctor promptly if you have symptoms of too much potassium loss, such as an irregular heartbeat, muscle pain or cramps, nausea or vomiting, increased thirst, or unusual weakness or fatigue.

You may experience drowsiness, dry mouth, or a headache. Also, you may feel dizzy or light-headed when rising from a sitting or lying position. Check with your doctor if these effects persist.

What you must know about alcohol and other drugs
Limit alcoholic beverages. They increase the chance for dizziness and light-headedness.

Check with your doctor before taking other medications, especially nonprescription drugs (such as for colds, cough, hay fever, asthma, or appetite control), lithium (Lithane), methenamine (Urex), adrenocorticoids (cortisone-like drugs), digitalis (a heart medication), or a monoamine oxidase (MAO) inhibitor (for depression). These drugs affect the way this medication works.

Special directions
• Be sure your doctor knows your medical history, especially if you have or have had angina (chest pain), diabetes, gout, kidney or liver disease, lupus, depression, inflammation of the pancreas (pancreatitis), Parkinson's disease, or pheochromocytoma. Also tell him if you've ever had liver problems when taking methyldopa in the past.
• Avoid hazardous activities, such as driving a car, until you know how the drug affects you. This drug can make you drowsy or less alert.
• Keep taking this medication exactly as directed, even if you feel well.
• Follow any special diet the doctor prescribed, such as a low-salt diet.
• This medication may increase your sensitivity to sunlight. Stay out of direct sunlight, wear sunglasses and protective clothing, and apply a sun block.

Important reminders
If you're pregnant or breast-feeding, check with your doctor before taking this medication. If you're an older adult, you may be especially sensitive to the effects of this medication. If you have diabetes, this medication may increase your blood glucose level. Test your urine for glucose regularly.

Giving methylphenidate

Dear Caregiver:

This drug is usually given to treat attention-deficit disorder in children. It's sometimes used to treat narcolepsy (sudden episodes of sleeping) in adults. Brand names include Ritalin and Ritalin-SR.

How to give methylphenidate
This drug is available in regular and sustained-release tablets. Carefully check the prescription label. Administer only the amount prescribed.

If the doctor has prescribed the sustained-release tablets, make sure your child swallows them whole and doesn't break, crush, or chew them first.

To help the drug work better, you should give it to your child 30 to 45 minutes before meals. However, if the drug causes loss of appetite, give it after meals.

Give your child the last daily dose 6 hours before bedtime so it won't cause difficulty sleeping.

What to do if your child misses a dose
Give the missed dose as soon as possible, then give remaining doses for that day at regularly spaced intervals. Never give a double dose.

What to do about side effects
Call your doctor *right away* if your child has a fast heartbeat, bruising, chest pain, fever, joint pain, a rash, hives, uncontrolled body movements, vision changes, seizures, sore throat, or unusual weakness or fatigue.

Appetite loss, nervousness, or difficulty sleeping may occur at first. Check with the doctor if these symptoms persist or become bothersome.

Depression, unusual behavior, or unusual weakness or fatigue may occur after your child stops taking this drug. Report these side effects to the doctor.

What you must know about other drugs
Check with the doctor or pharmacist before giving your child amantadine (Symmetrel), amphetamines, asthma medications, or any nonprescription medications. Serious problems could occur when these drugs are combined with methylphenidate.

Don't give your child methylphenidate within 14 days of a monoamine oxidase (MAO) inhibitor (a drug for depression).

Special directions
• Be sure the doctor knows about your child's medical history. Methylphenidate increases the chance for seizures and may worsen Tourette's syndrome, glaucoma, high blood pressure, psychosis, severe anxiety, agitation, depression, or tics. Also, a child with a history of drug abuse or dependence is more likely to become dependent on methylphenidate.
• If your child has been taking this drug in large doses for a long time, the doctor may want to reduce the dosage gradually before stopping it completely.
• Don't let your child perform activities requiring alertness or good coordination until you know the effects of the drug.
• After long-term treatment, the doctor may recommend drug-free periods to reduce the risk of a slowed growth rate.

Important reminder
If your child has diabetes, the doctor may need to adjust the dosage of diabetes medication.

Taking methylprednisolone

Dear Patient:

This medication is usually given to treat severe inflammation caused by allergies, asthma, skin problems, or arthritis. Brand names for this medication include Depo-Medrol, Medrol, and Meprolone.

How to take methylprednisolone

This drug is available in tablets and as an enema. Carefully check the prescription label, and take only the prescribed amount. This drug can also be given as an injection by the nurse or the doctor.

If you're taking the *enema,* use the entire contents of the bottle unless your doctor tells you otherwise. Insert the rectal applicator tip gently. If the doctor has instructed you to take the enema slowly, shake the bottle every so often during administration.

What to do if you miss a dose

If you're taking one dose every other day, take the missed dose as soon as possible if you remember it the same morning. Then resume your regular schedule. If you don't remember until later, take the missed dose the next morning, then skip a day and start your regular schedule again.

If you're taking one dose a day, take the missed dose as soon as you remember, then resume your regular schedule. If you don't remember until the next day, skip the missed dose. Don't double the next one.

If you're taking several doses a day, take the missed dose as soon as possible, then resume your regular schedule. If you don't remember until it's time for your next regular dose, double the next dose.

What to do about side effects

Call your doctor *as soon as possible* if you have decreased or blurred vision, frequent urination, increased thirst, confusion, excitement, hallucinations, depression, mood swings, a false sense of well-being, unusual feelings of self-importance or of being mistreated, or restlessness.

If you've been taking this medication for a long time, report any of the following side effects to your doctor: nausea; vomiting; stomach pain or burning; skin problems; bloody or black, tarry stools; filling out of the face; irregular heartbeat; menstrual problems; muscle cramps, pain, or weakness; pain in the back, hips, arms, shoulders, ribs, or legs; pitting, scarring, or skin depression (at the place of injection); reddish purple lines on the arms, legs, face, trunk, or groin; swelling of the feet or lower legs; thin, shiny skin; unusual bruising; unusual weakness or fatigue; rapid weight gain; or wounds that won't heal.

This medication may cause an increased appetite, indigestion, nervousness, or trouble sleeping. Call your doctor if these side effects persist or become bothersome.

If you're taking the *enema,* call your doctor if you experience rectal pain, bleeding, burning, blistering, itching, or other irritation that wasn't present before you started using this medication.

If you take the medication for a long time, you may experience side effects when you stop taking it. For instance, you may have an upset stomach, loss of appetite, fatigue, weakness, joint pain, fever, dizziness, lethargy, depression, fainting, or dizziness or light-headedness

(continued)

Taking methylprednisolone *(continued)*

when rising from a sitting or lying position. Also, your inflammation may come back.

What you must know about alcohol and other drugs

Avoid drinking alcohol while taking this drug. Combining alcohol with this drug increases the chance for stomach problems. Check with your doctor or pharmacist if you're taking other drugs. They may change the way methylprednisolone works, methylprednisolone may change the way other drugs work, or serious problems could occur. For instance, barbiturates, phenytoin (Dilantin), and rifampin (Rifadin) may make methylprednisolone less effective. Aspirin and indomethacin (Indocin) may increase the risk of stomach upset and bleeding.

Special directions

• Tell your doctor about other medical problems you have, especially bone, heart, liver, or kidney disease; colitis; diverticulitis; a stomach or an intestinal disorder; diabetes; infection; glaucoma; high blood pressure; kidney stones; high cholesterol levels; an overactive or underactive thyroid; myasthenia gravis; or lupus. Also tell the doctor if you've ever had tuberculosis or if you've recently had surgery or a serious injury.
• Take this medication in the morning unless the doctor tells you otherwise.
• You may take the tablets with food if they cause stomach upset.
• Follow any special diet your doctor has prescribed, such as a low-salt, high-potassium diet. The doctor also may want you to add protein to your diet and take potassium supplements.
• Have regular medical examinations so the doctor can check your progress.

• Don't get immunizations when taking this medication unless your doctor approves them. Also, avoid people who've recently taken oral polio vaccine.
• If this medication is injected into one of your joints, don't put too much strain or stress on that joint at first. While the joint is healing, don't move it more than the doctor permits. Call the doctor if you have persistent redness or swelling at the place of injection.
• *Don't suddenly stop taking this medication after long-term use because this can be fatal.* Check with your doctor for instructions on reducing the dosage gradually before stopping treatment.

Important reminders

If you're pregnant or breast-feeding, tell your doctor before taking methylprednisolone.

Older adults are especially likely to develop high blood pressure or bone disease when taking this medication.

If you have diabetes, you may need to change the dosage of your diabetes medication. Call your doctor for instructions.

If you're an athlete, you should know that the U.S. Olympic Committee and the National Collegiate Athletic Association restrict athletes' use of this medication.

Additional instructions

_____

_____

_____

_____

_____

Taking metoclopramide

Dear Patient:

This medication may be prescribed to prevent nausea and vomiting after treatment with anticancer medications or to help diagnose stomach or intestinal problems. The doctor also may prescribe it to treat certain GI disorders or to help relieve nausea, vomiting, and bloating after meals. The medication label may read Reglan.

How to take metoclopramide
This drug is available in tablets and as a syrup. Carefully check the label. Take only the amount prescribed.

Take this medication 30 minutes before meals and at bedtime unless your doctor tells you otherwise.

What to do if you miss a dose
Take it as soon as you remember. However, if it's almost time for your next dose, skip the missed dose and resume your regular schedule. Don't double dose.

What to do about side effects
Call your doctor *promptly* if you experience a fever, chills, sore throat, loss of balance, odd tongue movements, arm or leg stiffness, shuffling walk, or difficulty swallowing or speaking.

If you're taking high doses, a panic-like sensation, lower leg discomfort, or unusual restlessness, nervousness, or irritability may occur within minutes. Report these effects to the doctor as soon as possible.

Drowsiness usually goes away over time. If it persists or becomes bothersome, check with your doctor.

What you must know about other drugs
Avoid sedatives (drugs that relax you and make you feel sleepy), antihistamines (such as diphenhydramine [Benadryl]), and other depressants while taking this drug because of the risk of oversedation.

Check with your doctor before taking a narcotic pain reliever or an anticholinergic drug (used to treat spastic disorders of the stomach or intestine). These drugs can prevent metoclopramide from working properly.

Special directions
• Don't take this medication if you're allergic to it or to a sulfonamide.
• Tell your doctor about other medical problems you have, especially stomach bleeding, breast cancer, intestinal blockage, Parkinson's disease, seizures, or severe kidney or liver disease.
• Avoid hazardous activities, such as driving a car or using dangerous tools, until you know how this medication affects you. Metoclopramide can make you drowsy or less alert.
• Don't take this medication for more than 12 weeks.

Important reminders
If you're an older adult, you may be especially sensitive to this medication if you take it for a long time. Children are more sensitive than adults to the effects of metoclopramide.

If you're an athlete, you should know that metoclopramide use is banned by the U.S. Olympic Committee and the National Collegiate Athletic Association.

Taking metolazone

Dear Patient:

This medication is usually prescribed to treat high blood pressure. The doctor also may prescribe it to treat heart failure or kidney disease. Brand names include Diulo, Mykrox, and Zaroxolyn.

How to take metolazone
This medication is available in tablets. Carefully check the prescription label. Take only the prescribed amount.

What to do if you miss a dose
Take it right away. However, if it's almost time for your next regular dose, skip the missed dose and resume your regular schedule. Don't double dose.

What to do about side effects
Call your doctor *right away* if you have fever; chills; lower back, side, or joint pain; severe stomach pain; a rash; hives; red spots on the skin; unusual bleeding or bruising; yellow skin or eyes; bloody urine or stools; or black, tarry stools.

Also call your doctor if you experience increased thirst, irregular heartbeat, muscle pain or cramps, nausea or vomiting, unusual fatigue or weakness, or mood or mental changes.

You may notice appetite loss, diarrhea, decreased sexual performance, stomach upset, and increased sensitivity to sunlight. Also, you may feel dizzy or light-headed when getting up from a sitting or lying position. Check with your doctor if these side effects persist or become bothersome.

What you must know about other drugs
Check with your doctor or pharmacist before taking another drug, especially nonprescription medications for colds, cough, hay fever, asthma, or appetite control.

Cholestyramine (Questran) and colestipol (Colestid), medications used to lower cholesterol levels, may prevent metolazone from working properly. Digitalis (a heart medication) may increase the chance for digitalis side effects. Nonsteroidal anti-inflammatory drugs (such as ibuprofen, indomethacin [Indocin], and naproxen [Naprosyn]) may decrease the effects of metolazone.

Special directions
• Don't take this medication if you're allergic to it.
• Tell your doctor about other medical problems you have, especially diabetes, gout, lupus, inflammation of the pancreas, or heart, blood vessel, liver, or kidney disease.
• Follow any special diet the doctor has prescribed, such as a low-salt, high-potassium diet.
• Keep taking this medication exactly as directed, even if you feel well.

Important reminders
If you're breast-feeding or you become pregnant while taking this medication, check with your doctor.

If you're an older adult, you may be especially likely to feel dizzy and light-headed and to lose too much potassium when taking this medication.

If you have diabetes, this medication may increase your blood glucose level. Be sure to test your blood or urine for glucose regularly.

If you're an athlete, you should know that metolazone use is banned by the U.S. Olympic Committee and the National Collegiate Athletic Association.

Taking metoprolol

Dear Patient:

This medication is usually prescribed to treat high blood pressure. The label may read Lopressor.

How to take metoprolol
This medication is available in regular and sustained-release tablets. Take only the amount prescribed. To help the drug work better, take the tablets with meals.

What to do if you miss a dose
Take the missed dose as soon as possible. However, if it's within 4 hours of your next regular dose, skip the missed dose and resume your regular dosage schedule. Never take a double dose.

What to do about side effects
Call your doctor *right away* if you experience wheezing or difficulty breathing, confusion, hallucinations, slow or irregular heartbeat, cold feet or hands, or swelling of the feet or ankles.

You may experience trouble sleeping, drowsiness, dizziness, light-headedness, reduced sexual ability, or unusual fatigue or weakness. Call your doctor if these effects persist.

What you must know about other drugs
Check with your doctor before taking other drugs, including nonprescription drugs. Some may prevent metoprolol from working properly.

Barbiturates and rifampin (Rifadin) may decrease the effects of metoprolol.

Chlorpromazine (Thorazine), cimetidine (Tagamet), and verapamil (Calan) may cause your blood pressure to drop too much when taken with metoprolol.

Monoamine oxidase (MAO) inhibitors (drugs for depression) may cause severe high blood pressure if taken within 14 days of metoprolol.

Special directions
• Be sure your doctor knows about your medical history, especially if you have heart or blood vessel disease, diabetes, kidney or liver disease, depression, asthma, hay fever, hives, bronchitis, emphysema, an unusually slow heartbeat, or an overactive thyroid.
• Ask your doctor about checking your pulse rate regularly while taking metoprolol. If it's slower than your usual rate (or less than 50 beats per minute), don't take the dose; call your doctor.
• If metoprolol makes you urinate frequently, take it early in the day to prevent sleep disruption.
• Avoid hazardous activities, such as driving a car. Metoprolol may make you drowsy or dizzy.
• Follow any diet the doctor prescribes.
• Don't stop taking this medication, even if you're feeling well or if side effects occur. Check with your doctor.

Important reminders
If you're pregnant or breast-feeding, check with your doctor before taking metoprolol. If you're an older adult, you may be especially sensitive to the effects of this medication.

If you have diabetes, check with your doctor. This drug may decrease your blood glucose level and may mask signs of low blood glucose (such as a change in your pulse rate). Also, the dosage of your diabetes medication may need to be changed.

If you're an athlete, you should know that metoprolol use is banned by the U.S. Olympic Committee and National Collegiate Athletic Association.

Taking metronidazole

Dear Patient:

This medication is usually prescribed to treat trichomoniasis (an infection of the sex organs) or amebiasis (an infection of the intestine). Brand names include Flagyl, Metizol, and Protostat.

How to take metronidazole
This medication is available in tablets and as an oral suspension. Carefully check the prescription label. Take only the amount prescribed.

To keep a constant amount of this medication in your blood, space doses evenly.

You may crush the tablets before swallowing, if necessary.

If this medication causes stomach upset, take it with meals.

What to do if you miss a dose
Take it as soon as you remember. However, if it's almost time for your next dose, skip the missed dose and resume your regular schedule. Don't double dose.

What to do about side effects
Call your doctor *immediately* if you have seizures or if you experience pain, tingling, numbness, or weakness in your hands or feet.

This medication may cause a metallic taste and may turn your urine reddish brown.

Headache, dizziness, light-headedness, diarrhea, nausea, vomiting, stomach pain, and appetite loss may occur. Call your doctor if these side effects persist or become bothersome.

What you must know about alcohol and other drugs
Avoid drinking alcoholic beverages or taking drugs that contain alcohol (such as cough syrup) during treatment and for at least 48 hours afterward.

Check with your doctor before taking an anticoagulant (blood thinner). Combining metronidazole with an anticoagulant may increase your chance for bleeding.

Special directions
• Be sure your doctor knows about your medical history, especially if you have heart or liver disease, blood problems, central nervous system problems (such as seizures), or edema (swelling).
• Avoid hazardous activities, such as driving a car or using dangerous tools, until you know how this medication affects you. Metronidazole may make you dizzy.
• If you're taking this medication to treat amebiasis, see your doctor for follow-up visits. You may need to provide stool specimens for 3 months after treatment ends to make sure your infection is gone. To prevent reinfection, wash your hands after bowel movements and before handling and eating food. Avoid eating raw foods.
• If you're taking this medication to treat trichomoniasis, avoid intercourse or use a condom. The doctor may want to treat your sexual partner while you're being treated.

Important reminder
If you're in the first 3 months of pregnancy or if you're breast-feeding, check with your doctor before taking this medication.

Using miconazole

Dear Patient:

This medication is usually prescribed to treat fungus infections, such as athlete's foot, jock itch, and vaginal yeast infections. Brand names include Micatin, Monistat-Derm, and Monistat.

How to use miconazole

This drug is available in cream, lotion, powder, spray, vaginal cream, and vaginal suppositories.

You can buy some preparations of this drug without a prescription. If you're treating yourself, carefully follow the instructions on the package.

If your doctor prescribed this medication or gave you special instructions on how to use a nonprescription preparation, follow those instructions carefully.

If you're using the *spray,* shake it well before applying. Spray it on the affected area from a distance of 4 to 6 inches. If you're using the spray on your feet, spray it between your toes, on your feet, and in your socks and shoes. Don't inhale the spray.

If you're using the *powder* on your feet, sprinkle it between your toes, on your feet, and in your socks and shoes.

If you're using the *vaginal cream* or *suppositories,* insert the applicator or suppository high into your vagina at bedtime for the number of days specified on the package or prescribed by your doctor.

What to do if you miss a dose

Administer it as soon as you remember. However, if it's almost time for your next dose, skip the missed dose and resume your regular schedule.

What to do about side effects

Call your doctor *as soon as possible* if you notice a rash, burning, redness, blistering, or another type of skin irritation that wasn't there before you started using miconazole.

Special directions

• Don't take this medication if you're allergic to it. If you have liver disease, check with your doctor before using this medication.
• Don't apply an airtight cover (such as plastic wrap) over the treated area unless the doctor tells you to because this may irritate your skin.
• If you plan to use a vaginal form and are using any other vaginal medication, check with your doctor or pharmacist before starting treatment.
• If you're using the vaginal cream or suppositories, wear a sanitary pad to prevent clothing stains. To help clear up your infection, wear only freshly washed, cotton underwear and avoid using tampons during treatment. If you have intercourse during treatment, don't stop using this medication. Avoid using a latex contraceptive diaphragm because this could cause an interaction with the medication. Also, your sexual partner may need to be treated.
• Take this medication for the full time of treatment, even if your condition improves. If your condition doesn't improve within 4 weeks or if it gets worse, call the doctor.

Important reminder

If you're pregnant, check with your doctor before using the vaginal form of this medication.

Applying minoxidil

Dear Patient:

This medication is prescribed to stimulate hair growth. The label may read Rogaine.

How to apply minoxidil
This medication is available as a topical solution.

Carefully check the label on your prescription applicator, which tells you how much to use at each dose. Use only the amount prescribed. Using more won't speed hair growth or cause more hair to grow. In fact, using too much might cause unwanted side effects.

Apply the medication once in the morning and again at bedtime, using the applicator provided. Before applying the morning dose, shampoo your hair and towel-dry it thoroughly. Then use the applicator to spread the medication. Start at the center of the bald area.

After applying your bedtime dose, let the medication dry for at least 30 minutes. This allows more to be absorbed by your scalp and less by your pillowcase.

What to do if you miss an application
Apply the missed dose as soon as possible, then resume your regular dosage schedule. However, if it's almost time for your next dose, skip the missed dose and go back to your regular schedule. Don't apply the medication twice or try to make up for a missed dose some other way.

What to do about side effects
Call your doctor *right away* if you have difficulty breathing, chest pain, a fast or irregular heartbeat, flushing, headache, dizziness, faintness, rapid weight gain, swelling of the feet or lower legs, or numbness or tingling in your hands, feet, or face.

Check with your doctor if your scalp starts burning or itching, if your face swells, or if you notice a rash.

Your skin may become reddened or dry and flake, and you may have increased hair growth on your face, arms, and back. These side effects usually go away over time as your body adjusts to the medication. But you should check with your doctor if they persist or become bothersome.

What you must know about other drugs
Don't apply other drugs to your scalp while using minoxidil. Other drugs may prevent minoxidil from working properly or cause unwanted side effects.

Special directions
• Be sure your doctor knows about your medical history, especially if you have heart disease or high blood pressure or if you've had other skin problems, irritation, or sunburn on your scalp.
• If you apply minoxidil by hand, wash your hands thoroughly when you're finished.
• Don't use a hair dryer during treatment because this might make the medication less effective.
• Stop using the medication temporarily if your scalp gets irritated or sunburned—but check with the doctor first.
• You may have to use minoxidil for 4 or more months before you see results, and you must use it every day. If you stop using it, hair growth stops and you can expect to lose any new hair within a few months.

Taking misoprostol

Dear Patient:

This medication is usually prescribed to prevent stomach ulcers in patients who are taking anti-inflammatory medications (such as aspirin). A brand name of this medication is Cytotec.

How to take misoprostol

This medication is available in tablets. You may need to take it four times a day.

Carefully check the prescription label. Take only the amount prescribed.

To make the medication work better, take it with or after meals and at bedtime.

What to do if you miss a dose

Take the missed dose as soon as possible. However, if it's almost time for your next regular dose, skip the missed dose and resume your regular dosage schedule. Never take a double dose.

What to do about side effects

Diarrhea and abdominal or stomach pain may occur. These side effects usually go away over time as your body adjusts to the medication. But you should check with your doctor if diarrhea lasts more than 1 week or if abdominal or stomach pain persists or becomes bothersome.

Special directions

• Be sure your doctor knows about your medical history, especially if you have blood vessel disease or have had uncontrolled seizures. Misoprostol may worsen blood vessel disease and may trigger seizures.

• Avoid smoking cigarettes because this may increase stomach acid secretion and make your ulcer worse.

• If the doctor has prescribed this medication to treat a duodenal ulcer, you may take an antacid to help relieve stomach pain (unless the doctor tells you not to). However, avoid antacids that contain magnesium because they may worsen diarrhea caused by misoprostol. Also, keep taking this medication for the full time of treatment, even if you start to feel better. However, don't take it for more than 4 weeks, unless the doctor wants you to continue treatment for another 4 weeks to make sure your ulcer heals completely.

Important reminders

If you're a woman of childbearing age, discuss the use of this medication with your doctor before starting treatment. You must have had a negative pregnancy test within 2 weeks before starting misoprostol. Also, you must begin taking this medication only on the second or third day of your next normal menstrual period, and you must use an effective birth control method during treatment.

If you become pregnant or even suspect you've become pregnant while taking this drug, stop taking it immediately and call the doctor. This drug may cause miscarriage, uterine contractions, and uterine bleeding.

If you're breast-feeding, check with your doctor before using misoprostol.

Additional instructions

_____

_____

Taking molindone

Dear Patient:

This medication is usually prescribed to treat emotional, nervous, or mental disorders. The label may read Moban.

How to take molindone
This medication is available in tablets and a solution. Take only the amount prescribed.

If you're taking the *solution,* drink it undiluted or mix it with water, milk, fruit juice, or a carbonated beverage. To reduce stomach irritation, take it with food or a full glass of water or milk.

What to do if you miss a dose
Take the missed dose as soon as you remember. However, if it's within 2 hours of your next regular dose, skip the missed dose and resume your regular schedule. Never take a double dose.

What to do about side effects
Before taking this medication, discuss the potential for permanent side effects with your doctor. This medication may cause a movement disorder that doesn't go away even after you stop taking it. Symptoms include lip smacking or puckering, cheek puffing, rapid or worm-like tongue movements, and other uncontrolled movements of the mouth, tongue, cheeks, jaw, arms, and legs.

Call your doctor *promptly* if you experience sedation, difficulty talking or swallowing, loss of balance, muscle spasms, restlessness or the need to keep moving, or trembling and shaking of the hands.

You may experience constipation, blurred vision, decreased sweating, difficult urination, drowsiness, dry mouth, headache, nausea, stuffy nose, and diz-ziness or light-headedness when getting up suddenly from a lying or sitting position. Check with your doctor if these side effects persist.

What you must know about alcohol and other drugs
Avoid alcoholic beverages, barbiturates, sedatives (such as drugs that relax you and make you feel sleepy), antihistamines (such as diphenhydramine [Benadryl]), and other depressant drugs while taking this medication because of the risk of additive sedative effects.

Don't take molindone within 1 to 2 hours of an antacid or a diarrhea medication because these drugs may make molindone less effective.

Special directions
• Be sure your doctor knows about your medical history, especially if you have or have had brain damage; a head injury; cerebrovascular, heart, respiratory, or liver disease; intestinal blockage; difficult urination; enlarged prostate; glaucoma; seizures; or Parkinson's disease.
• Avoid hazardous activities, such as driving a car, until you know how the drug affects you. Molindone can make you drowsy or less alert.
• Don't stop taking this medication without first checking with your doctor. The doctor may want to reduce your dosage gradually before stopping it.

Important reminders
If you're an older adult, you may be especially sensitive to molindone's effects. If you're an athlete, you should know that molindone use is banned by the U.S. Olympic Committee and the National Collegiate Athletic Association in some athletic events.

Taking morphine

Dear Patient:

Morphine is usually prescribed to relieve pain. Brand names include Astramorph, Duramorph, and MSIR.

How to take morphine

Take only the amount prescribed.

If you're taking the *extended-release tablets,* be sure to swallow them whole. Don't break, crush, or chew them.

If you're taking the *liquid* form, use a measuring spoon to measure your dose. Mix it with juice to improve its taste.

If you're using the *suppositories,* remove the foil wrapper and moisten the suppository with cold water. Lie on your side. Using your finger, push the suppository well up into your rectum.

If you're taking the *injection* form, your doctor or nurse will teach you how to administer it.

What to do if you miss a dose

If you're taking morphine on a regular schedule, take the missed dose as soon as you remember. But if it's almost time for your next regular dose, skip the missed dose and resume your regular schedule. Never take a double dose.

What to do about side effects

Get emergency help *immediately* if your heartbeat seems unusually fast, slow, or pounding; if you start wheezing or have trouble breathing; if your hands and face swell; or if you start sweating a lot.

Call your doctor *right away* if your breathing rate drops to 8 to 10 breaths a minute, if you have hallucinations, or if you feel confused, dizzy, or unusually weak or tired.

If itching or a rash develops, you may be having an allergic reaction. Stop the medication and contact your doctor.

Nausea, vomiting, or constipation may occur, especially at first. If these side effects continue, call your doctor.

What you must know about alcohol and other drugs

Don't take sleeping pills or antihistamines or drink alcoholic beverages during morphine treatment.

Check with your doctor or pharmacist if you're taking other prescription or nonprescription drugs. Other drugs may change the way morphine works.

Special directions

• Be sure your doctor knows about your medical history before you take morphine.
• Take morphine at regular times. Don't wait until your pain is severe.
• Get up slowly from a lying or sitting position to avoid feeling faint or dizzy.
• Avoid hazardous activities, such as driving a car, because morphine may make you drowsy.
• If morphine causes nausea, eat your meals after nausea subsides. If nausea is severe or if you vomit, ask the doctor for medication to prevent this.
• To help prevent constipation, eat a well-balanced, high-fiber diet, including bran, fruit, and raw, leafy vegetables.
• If you've been taking morphine regularly, don't stop taking it suddenly. Ask the doctor how to discontinue it gradually.

Important reminders

If you're pregnant or breast-feeding, check with your doctor before taking morphine. Children and older adults are especially sensitive to the effects of morphine. If you're an athlete, you should know that the use of morphine is banned by the U.S. Olympic Committee.

Applying mupirocin

Dear Patient:

This medication is usually prescribed to treat bacterial infections of the skin (such as impetigo). The label may read Bactroban.

How to apply mupirocin

This medication is available in an ointment.

In Canada, you can buy this medication without a prescription. If you're treating yourself, carefully follow the instructions on the package, which tell you how much to take at each dose.

If your doctor prescribed this medication or gave you special instructions on how to use it, follow those instructions carefully. Apply only the amount prescribed by the doctor.

The doctor will probably instruct you to apply mupirocin to affected skin areas two or three times daily. Before applying it, clean the affected area with soap and water and dry it thoroughly. Then apply a small amount of the ointment, rubbing it in gently.

What to do if you miss an application

Apply the missed dose as soon as possible. However, if it's almost time for your next regular dose, skip the missed dose and resume your regular dosage schedule.

What to do about side effects

This medication may cause a rash, redness, or dryness. Also, you may notice itching, burning, pain, tenderness, or swelling at the place where you apply it. These side effects usually go away over time as your body adjusts to the medication. But you should check with your doctor if they persist or become bothersome.

Call your doctor if you have other side effects.

Special directions

• You shouldn't use mupirocin if you're allergic to it.
• If desired, you may cover the treated area with a gauze dressing.
• Keep this medication out of your eyes.
• Don't apply mupirocin on burns.
• To make sure your infection heals completely, continue to use this medication for the full time of treatment prescribed by the doctor, even if your symptoms disappear. Don't skip any doses.
• Don't use this medication for a longer period than the doctor prescribes or the package instructions specify.
• Call you doctor or pharmacist if your condition doesn't improve within 3 to 5 days or if it gets worse.

Additional instructions

_____

_____

_____

_____

_____

_____

_____

_____

Taking nabumetone

Dear Patient:

This medication is usually prescribed to reduce joint pain, swelling, and stiffness caused by arthritis. The label may read Relafen.

How to take nabumetone
This medication is available in tablets.

Carefully check the prescription label. Take only the prescribed amount.

If nabumetone gives you heartburn, you may take it with food or an antacid. However, you should check with your doctor first.

What to do if you miss a dose
Take the missed dose as soon as you remember. However, if it's almost time for your next regular dose, skip the missed dose and resume your regular dosage schedule. Never take a double dose.

What to do about side effects
Call your doctor *right away* if you see blood in your urine, if you start urinating less often, or if you have diarrhea, black stools, sore throat, wheezing, dizziness, drowsiness, light-headedness, ringing in your ears, vision changes, swollen ankles, or a rash.

You may experience stomach or abdominal cramps or pain, headache, heartburn, indigestion, nausea, or vomiting. These side effects usually go away over time as your body adjusts to the medication. But you should check with your doctor if they persist or become bothersome.

What you must know about alcohol and other drugs
Don't drink alcoholic beverages while you're taking this drug. Alcohol may increase this drug's depressant effects.

Check with your doctor or pharmacist before taking other drugs. Many drugs increase the chance for serious side effects when taken with nabumetone. Especially avoid taking aspirin or steroids because these drugs increase the risk of GI side effects.

Special directions
• You shouldn't take this medication if you're allergic to it or to aspirin.
• Be sure your doctor knows about your medical history, especially if you have GI disease, stomach ulcers, kidney disease, or heart or blood vessel disease.
• Take all doses at the prescribed times. Don't postpone taking a dose to make the medication last longer than intended.
• Avoid hazardous activities, such as driving a car or using dangerous tools, because nabumetone may make you drowsy.
• Keep taking this drug even if your symptoms don't get better right away. Nabumetone may take about 1 month to achieve its full effect.
• If you're taking this medication for a long time, be sure to get regular medical checkups so the doctor can evaluate your progress.

Important reminders
If you're pregnant or breast-feeding, check with your doctor before taking this medication.

If you're an older adult, you may be especially sensitive to side effects of this medication.

Taking nadolol

Dear Patient:

This medication is usually prescribed to treat angina (chest pain) or high blood pressure. The label may read Corgard.

How to take nadolol
Carefully check the prescription label. Take only the amount prescribed.

What to do if you miss a dose
Take it right away if you remember within an hour or so. However, if it's within 8 hours of your next dose, skip the missed dose and resume your regular schedule. Don't double dose.

What to do about side effects
Call your doctor *right away* if you start wheezing, have difficulty breathing, or experience confusion, hallucinations, a slow or irregular heartbeat, cold feet or hands, or swelling of the feet or ankles.

You may have trouble sleeping, drowsiness, dizziness, light-headedness, reduced sexual ability, or unusual fatigue or weakness. These side effects usually go away over time as your body adjusts to the medication. But you should check with your doctor if they persist or become bothersome.

What you must know about other drugs
Check with your doctor before taking other drugs, including nonprescription drugs. Some drugs may prevent nadolol from working properly. Prescription drugs used to reduce blood pressure may increase the effects of nadolol on the heart.

Digitalis (a heart medication) may cause a too-slow heart rate when combined with nadolol.

Other drugs used to treat angina may cause increased effects on your blood pressure when taken with nadolol.

Epinephrine may constrict your blood vessels and slow your heart rate when taken with nadolol.

Special directions
• You shouldn't take nadolol if you're allergic to it.
• Be sure your doctor knows about your medical history, especially if you have heart or blood vessel disease, diabetes, kidney disease, liver disease, mental depression, asthma, hay fever, hives, bronchitis, emphysema, an unusually slow heartbeat, or an overactive thyroid.
• Ask your doctor about checking your pulse rate before each dose. Then while taking nadolol, check your pulse rate regularly. If it's slower than your usual rate, don't take the dose; call your doctor.
• Avoid hazardous activities, such as driving a car, because nadolol may make you drowsy or less alert.
• The doctor may need to increase your dosage gradually to find the amount that causes the best response.

Important reminders
If you have diabetes, check with your doctor. This drug may cause your blood glucose level to drop and may mask signs of low blood glucose (such as a change in your pulse rate). Also, the dosage of your diabetes medication may need to be changed.

If you're pregnant or breast-feeding, check with your doctor before taking nadolol. Also, be aware that older adults may be especially sensitive to the side effects of this medication. Athletes should be aware that nadolol is banned by the U.S. Olympic Committee and the National Collegiate Athletic Association.

Applying naftifine

Dear Patient:

This medication is usually prescribed to treat fungus infections, such as athlete's foot, jock itch, and ringworm of the body. The label may read Naftin.

How to apply naftifine
Apply naftifine twice a day unless your doctor tells you otherwise. Wash your hands first. Then apply enough cream to cover the affected skin and surrounding areas. Rub it in gently.

What to do if you miss an application
Apply the missed dose as soon as you remember. However, if it's almost time for your next regular dose, skip the missed dose and resume your regular dosage schedule.

What to do about side effects
You may notice burning or stinging on the treated area. These side effects usually go away over time as your body adjusts to the medication. But you should check with your doctor if they persist or become bothersome.

Special directions
• You shouldn't take this medication if you're allergic to it.
• Keep naftifine away from your eyes, nose, and mouth.
• Use naftifine for the full treatment time prescribed. If you stop using it too soon, your symptoms may return. Also, the doctor will probably instruct you to keep using the cream for 1 to 2 weeks after your symptoms go away. Don't skip doses.
• Call your doctor if your skin condition doesn't improve within 1 month or if it gets worse.

• If you're using this medication to treat *athlete's foot,* dry your feet carefully, especially between your toes, after bathing. Wear cotton socks and change them daily (more often if your feet sweat heavily). Avoid wearing wool socks or socks made of synthetic materials (such as nylon or rayon). After applying naftifine cream (but after it has disappeared into your skin), apply powder on the affected area. Make sure it's an antifungal powder, talcum powder, or another bland, absorbent powder. Sprinkle it on your feet, between your toes, and in your socks and shoes once or twice a day.
• If you're using naftifine to treat *jock itch,* dry your groin area carefully after bathing. Wear loose-fitting, cotton underwear. Avoid tight-fitting underwear made from rayon, nylon, or another synthetic material. After applying naftifine cream (but after it has disappeared into your skin), apply powder on your groin area once or twice a day. Make sure it's an antifungal powder, talcum powder, or another bland, absorbent powder.
• If you're using naftifine to treat *ringworm of the body,* dry yourself carefully after bathing. Try to prevent moisture buildup on the affected parts. Avoid excessive heat and humidity. Don't wear tight-fitting, poorly ventilated clothing. After applying naftifine cream (but after it has disappeared into your skin), sprinkle an antifungal powder, talcum powder, or another bland, absorbent powder on the affected areas.

Additional instructions

_____

_____

Taking nalidixic acid

Dear Patient:

This medication is usually prescribed to treat infections of the urinary tract. The label may read NegGram.

How to take nalidixic acid

This medicaton is available in tablets and an oral suspension. Carefully check the label. Take only the amount prescribed.

If you're taking the *oral suspension,* use a specially marked measuring spoon (not a household teaspoon).

For best results, take nalidixic acid with a full glass (8 ounces) of water on an empty stomach (1 hour before or 2 hours after meals). However, if this medication upsets your stomach, you may take it with food or milk.

What to do if you miss a dose

Take it as soon as you remember. But if it's almost time for your next dose and the doctor has prescribed three or more doses a day, space the missed dose and the next dose 2 to 4 hours apart, or double your next dose. Then resume your regular schedule.

What to do about side effects

Call the doctor *immediately* if you experience vision changes (including double vision, blurring, decreased vision, halos around lights, too-bright appearance of lights, or changes in color vision), seizures, hallucinations, mood changes, pale skin or stools, sore throat, fever, severe stomach pain, yellow skin or eyes, unusual bleeding or bruising, or unusual weakness or fatigue.

Abdominal pain, nausea, and vomiting may occur. These side effects usually go away over time as your body adjusts to the medication. But you should check with your doctor if they persist or become bothersome.

What you must know about other drugs

Check with your doctor or pharmacist before taking an anticoagulant (blood thinner). This drug may increase your chance for bleeding when taken with nalidixic acid.

Special directions

• You shouldn't take this medication if you're allergic to it.
• Be sure your doctor knows about your medical history, especially if you've had seizures, liver or kidney problems, or brain or spinal cord damage. Also tell him if you have glucose-6-phosphate dehydrogenase deficiency or hardening of the brain arteries.
• Avoid hazardous activities, such as driving a car or using dangerous tools, because nalidixic acid may make you dizzy or less alert and may impair your vision.
• If this medication makes you sensitive to sunlight, stay out of direct sunlight, wear protective clothing and sunglasses, and use a sun block.
• Take this medication for the full prescribed time, even if you feel better after a few days. Don't skip doses.
• Call your doctor if your symptoms don't improve within 2 days or if they get worse.

Important reminders

If you're pregnant or breast-feeding, check with your doctor before taking this medication. Also, be aware that this medication isn't recommended for use in infants or children.

Taking naproxen

Dear Patient:

This medication is usually prescribed to reduce joint pain, swelling, and stiffness caused by arthritis. The label may read Naprosyn.

How to take naproxen
This medication is available in regular and extended-release tablets and an oral suspension. Carefully check the label. Take only the prescribed amount.

Take each dose with a full glass (8 ounces) of water. Stay upright for about 30 minutes afterward.

If you're taking the *extended-release tablets,* be sure to swallow them whole. Don't crush or break them.

If you're taking the *regular tablets,* you may take them with food or an antacid if naproxen gives you heartburn. However, check with your doctor first.

If you're taking the *oral suspension,* don't mix it with an antacid.

What to do if you miss a dose
Take it as soon as you remember. However, if it's almost time for the next dose, skip the missed dose and resume your regular schedule. Don't double dose.

What to do about side effects
Call your doctor *right away* if you see blood in your urine, if you start urinating less often, or if you have diarrhea, black stools, sore throat, wheezing, dizziness, drowsiness, light-headedness, ringing in your ears, vision changes, swollen ankles, or a rash.

Headache, heartburn, indigestion, nausea, vomiting, or stomach or abdominal cramps or pain may occur. Call your doctor if these side effects persist or become bothersome.

What you must know about alcohol and other drugs
Avoid drinking alcoholic beverages while taking this drug. Alcohol may increase this drug's depressant effects.

Check with your doctor before taking other drugs. Many drugs increase the chance for serious side effects when taken with naproxen. Especially avoid aspirin and steroids because these drugs increase the risk of GI side effects.

Special directions
• You shouldn't take this medication if you're allergic to it or to aspirin.
• Be sure your doctor knows about your medical history, especially if you've had stomach or intestinal disease, ulcers, kidney disease, or heart or blood vessel disease.
• Avoid hazardous activities, such as driving a car or using dangerous tools, until you know how you react to naproxen because it may make you drowsy.
• Take all doses at the prescribed times. Don't postpone a dose to make the drug last longer than intended.
• Keep taking this medication even if your symptoms don't get better right away. Naproxen may take 1 month to achieve its effect.
• If you're taking this medication for a long time, get regular checkups so the doctor can evaluate your progress.

Important reminders
If you're pregnant, check with your doctor before taking this medication.

If you're an older adult, you may be especially likely to have GI side effects.

Applying neomycin

Dear Patient:

This medication is usually prescribed to treat skin infections, minor burns, or minor wounds. The label may read Myciguent.

How to apply neomycin

This drug is available in a cream and an ointment.

You can buy this medication without a prescription. If you're treating yourself, carefully follow the package instructions. If your doctor prescribed this medication or gave you special instructions on how to use it, follow those instructions carefully.

To apply neomycin, wash the affected area with soap and water, then dry it thoroughly. Apply a generous amount of medication to the affected area and rub it in gently. If you're using the *cream* form of neomycin, rub it in until it disappears. If you wish, you may cover the area with a gauze dressing.

What to do if you miss an application

Apply the missed dose to the affected area as soon as possible. However, if it's almost time for your next regular dose, skip the missed dose and resume your regular dosage schedule.

What to do about side effects

Call your doctor *immediately* if you have breathing problems, dizziness, fainting, or a fever or if you notice a rash, itching, redness, or other symptoms of skin irritation that weren't there before you started using this medication.

Report any hearing changes to the doctor.

What you must know about other drugs

Check with your doctor or pharmacist before applying another medication to the same skin area where you're using neomycin.

Special directions

• Check with your doctor before using this medication if you have a kidney problem or if you've ever had an allergic or unusual reaction to this medication or to another antibiotic, including the oral form of neomycin (Mycifradin), amikacin (Amikin), gentamicin (Garamycin), kanamycin (Kantrex), netilmicin (Netromycin), streptomycin, and tobramycin (Nebcin).
• If you're using this medication without a prescription, don't apply it on a puncture wound, deep wound, serious burn, or raw area unless your doctor approves this.
• Keep this medication away from your eyes.
• Continue to use this medication for the full time of treatment, even if your symptoms go away. This will help eliminate your infection completely.
• If your skin condition doesn't improve within 1 week or if it gets worse, call your doctor or pharmacist.
• Don't use this medication for a long time without your doctor's approval.

Additional instructions

_____

_____

_____

_____

Taking niacin

Dear Patient:

The doctor may prescribe this medication to treat niacin deficiency or to help lower blood cholesterol and fat levels. Brand names include Nia-Bid, Niacor, and Tega-Span.

How to take niacin
This drug is available in regular and extended-release tablets and capsules and an oral suspension.

Take niacin with milk or meals if it causes diarrhea or stomach upset.

If you're taking the *extended-release tablets,* swallow them whole. If they're scored, you may break them before swallowing, but don't crush or chew them.

If you're taking the *extended-release capsules,* swallow them whole. Don't chew, crush, or break them. If they're too large to swallow, mix the contents with jelly or jam and swallow without chewing.

What to do if you miss a dose
If you're taking niacin without a doctor's recommendation, missing 1 or 2 days is harmless. If the doctor prescribed niacin to treat high cholesterol levels, take the missed dose as soon as possible. However, if it's almost time for your next dose, skip the missed dose and resume your regular schedule. Never take a double dose.

What to do about side effects
If you're taking extended-release niacin, call your doctor *immediately* if you have darkened urine, light gray stools, appetite loss, severe stomach pain, or yellow skin or eyes.

You may feel dizzy or faint, especially when getting up quickly from a lying or sitting position. This effect should decrease after 1 or 2 weeks.

If you're taking high doses of niacin, you may have stomach pain, diarrhea, nausea, vomiting, dizziness, faintness, fever, frequent urination, itching, joint pain, muscle aches or cramps, lower back or side pain, unusual weakness or fatigue, or a fast, slow, or irregular heartbeat. Also, a feeling of warmth, skin flushing or redness, and headache may occur. Call your doctor if side effects persist or become bothersome.

Special directions
• Before using niacin, check with your doctor if your medical history includes diabetes, bleeding problems, glaucoma, gout, liver disease, low blood pressure, or a stomach ulcer.
• Avoid taking large doses of niacin except under your doctor's direction, after your need has been determined.
• If you're taking niacin to lower your cholesterol level, follow any special diet your doctor gave you (such as a low-fat, low-cholesterol diet). Take niacin only as directed. Check with your doctor before stopping treatment.
• If you're taking niacin as a vitamin supplement, keep in mind that such supplements aren't meant to replace a varied, well-balanced diet. Meat, eggs, and dairy foods contain niacin.

Important reminder
If you're pregnant or breast-feeding, check with your doctor before taking niacin.

Applying a nicotine patch

Dear Patient:

This drug is prescribed to help you stop smoking. You should use it only as part of a comprehensive stop-smoking program. Some brand names for this drug include Habitrol, Nicoderm, and Pro-step.

How to apply a patch
This drug is available by prescription only. It comes in a stick-on patch.

Carefully follow the instructions on the package, which tell you when and how often to apply a new patch and how long to leave it on. Typically, you should apply a new patch daily, preferably at the same time each day.

To apply the patch, choose a hairless part of your body, such as the outer part of your upper arm or your stomach or back above the waist. The chosen site should be free from cuts and irritation.

Press the patch firmly to your skin. Then wash your hands with water only.

What to do if you miss an application
Apply a new patch as soon as you remember. Then change the patch at the regular time.

What to do about side effects
Call your doctor *immediately* if you have symptoms of nicotine overdose: severe headache, vomiting, diarrhea, dizziness, weakness, or confusion.

The first patch you apply may cause mild itching, tingling, and burning. These problems should go away within 1 hour. If the skin under the patch becomes red or swollen or a rash ap-

pears, remove the patch and call your doctor; you could be allergic to it.

What you must know about other drugs
Check with your doctor or pharmacist to find out if the dosages of any drugs you're taking need to be changed.

Special directions
• Don't use this drug if you're allergic to nicotine or to any component in the patch.
• Be sure your doctor knows about your medical history, especially if you have high blood pressure, ulcers, kidney or liver disease, heart rhythm problems, or angina (chest pain) or if you've recently had a heart attack.
• Be sure to stop smoking completely before starting this drug to prevent nicotine overdose.
• To avoid skin irritation, apply each new patch to a different site. Wait at least 1 week before reusing a site.
• Discard patches properly—and always where children and animals can't reach them. Used patches contain enough nicotine to poison children and pets.
• If the patch falls off, apply a new one, then change it at your usual time.
• Continue to use this drug for the full time prescribed by your doctor. Don't stop using it suddenly.
• Follow the other parts of your stop-smoking program.

Important reminders
If you're pregnant, don't use this patch. If you become pregnant while using it, stop using the patch until you've talked to your doctor.

If you're breast-feeding, check with your doctor before using the patch.

Taking nifedipine

Dear Patient:

This medication is usually prescribed to treat angina (chest pain). It may also be used to treat Raynaud's disease (episodes of reduced blood supply to the fingers or toes). Brand names include Adalat and Procardia.

How to take nifedipine

This medication is available in capsules and sustained-release tablets. Carefully check the prescription label, and take only the prescribed amount.

Take nifedipine exactly as your doctor has ordered. Swallow capsules whole. Don't break, crush, or chew them.

What to do if you miss a dose

Take it as soon as you remember. But if it's almost time for your next dose, skip the missed dose and resume your regular schedule. Don't double dose.

What to do about side effects

Call your doctor if you have ankle swelling, a very fast or very slow heartbeat, shortness of breath, severe headache, or fainting.

Chest pain may occur when you first start taking nifedipine. Although such pain is usually temporary, report it to the doctor *immediately.*

Constipation, dizziness, flushing, headache, and nausea may occur. These side effects usually go away over time as your body adjusts to the medication. Check with your doctor if they persist or become bothersome.

What you must know about other drugs

Check with your doctor before taking other drugs, including nonprescription medications. Heart failure or very low blood pressure may occur if you take nifedipine with other angina medication or with drugs used to treat blood pressure or heart rhythm problems.

Special directions

• You shouldn't take this medication if you're allergic to it.
• Be sure your doctor knows about your medical history, especially if you've had heart failure or constriction of the aorta.
• Call your doctor if this medication doesn't relieve your chest pain.
• Avoid hazardous activities, such as driving a car, because nifedipine may make you dizzy or light-headed.
• Avoid eating excessive amounts of calcium-rich foods, such as cheese.
• Be sure to check with your doctor before taking calcium supplements.
• If swelling occurs, the doctor may want you to drink less fluid and limit your salt intake.
• Schedule your activities so you can get enough rest.
• Get up slowly from a sitting or lying position to help prevent dizziness.
• If constipation occurs, drink more fluids and add more bulk to your diet. Consult your doctor about taking a bulk laxative if needed.
• Keep taking this medication as prescribed, even if you feel better.
• Don't stop taking this medication suddenly. The doctor may need to reduce your dosage gradually.

Important reminders

If you're pregnant, check with your doctor before taking nifedipine. If you're an older adult, you may be especially sensitive to the effects of nifedipine.

Taking nitrofurantoin

Dear Patient:

This medication is usually prescribed to treat urinary tract infections. Brand names include Furadantin, Macrodantin, and Nitrofuracot.

How to take nitrofurantoin
This medication is available in tablets, capsules, and an oral suspension.

Carefully check the prescription label, and take only the prescribed amount.

If you're taking the *oral suspension,* shake it forcefully before each dose. Use a specially marked measuring spoon (not a household teaspoon) to measure doses accurately.

What to do if you miss a dose
Take the missed dose as soon as you remember. However, if it's almost time for your next regular dose and the doctor has prescribed three or more daily doses, space the missed dose and the next dose 2 to 4 hours apart. Then resume your regular dosage schedule.

What to do about side effects
Contact your doctor *immediately* if you have chest pain, fever, chills, sore throat, cough, troubled breathing, dizziness, drowsiness, headache, numbness or tingling of the face or mouth, joint pain, itching, a rash, yellow skin or eyes, or unusual tiredness or weakness.

This drug may cause stomach or abdominal pain or upset, diarrhea, nausea, vomiting, and appetite loss. These side effects usually go away over time as your body adjusts to the drug. Check with your doctor if they persist or become bothersome.

This drug may turn your urine brown or darker.

What you must know about other drugs
Check with your doctor or pharmacist before taking other drugs. Taken at the same time, many drugs can worsen the side effects of nitrofurantoin.

Antacids that contain magnesium may make nitrofurantoin less effective. If you must take such an antacid, take it at least 1 hour before or after nitrofurantoin.

Special directions
• Don't take this medication if you're allergic to it.
• Be sure your doctor knows about your medical history, especially if you have glucose-6-phosphate dehydrogenase deficiency, kidney or lung disease, diabetes, asthma, anemia, vitamin B deficiency, electrolyte imbalance, or nerve damage.
• To reduce stomach upset, take this drug with milk or meals.
• Store this medication in its original container, and keep it away from all metals except aluminum and stainless steel.

Important reminders
If you're pregnant or breast-feeding, check with your doctor before using nitrofurantoin.

If you have diabetes, don't use the copper sulfate test (Clinitest) to test your urine glucose because nitrofurantoin may cause a false-positive result. Check with your doctor about which test to use.

Additional instructions

_____

_____

Taking nitroglycerin tablets

Dear Patient:

This medication is prescribed to prevent or relieve angina (chest pain) attacks. It's also called by the brand names Nitrogard and Nitrostat.

How to take nitroglycerin tablets

Place one tablet under your tongue, between your lip and gum, or between your cheek and gum. Let it dissolve there. Don't chew, crush, or swallow the tablet.

To *prevent* an angina attack, take a tablet 5 to 10 minutes before expected physical exertion or emotional distress that has caused an attack in the past.

To *relieve* an angina attack, place one tablet in your mouth when you start to feel an attack coming on. If your pain doesn't go away within 5 minutes, take a second tablet. If you still have pain after another 5 minutes, take a third tablet. If three tablets don't provide relief, call your doctor and have someone take you to the nearest hospital. Never take more than three tablets.

What to do about side effects

Call your doctor *right away* if you get a severe or prolonged headache, dry mouth, or blurred vision.

This medication may cause a fast pulse rate, flushing of your face and neck, headache, nausea, vomiting, and restlessness. Also, it may make you feel dizzy or light-headed when you get up from a sitting or lying position. These side effects usually go away over time as your body gets used to the medication. Check with your doctor if these effects persist or become bothersome.

What you must know about alcohol and other drugs

Drink alcoholic beverages in moderation, if at all. Alcohol will increase the chance for feeling dizzy or light-headed when you get up quickly from a lying or sitting position.

Check with your doctor or pharmacist before taking other heart or blood pressure medications. When taken with nitroglycerin, these drugs may decrease your blood pressure too much.

Special directions

• Be sure your doctor knows about your medical history, especially if you have kidney or liver disease or an overactive thyroid or if you've recently had a heart attack.
• This drug works best when you're sitting or standing. Sitting is safer than standing because you may become dizzy or light-headed soon after taking a tablet. If you get dizzy or light-headed while sitting, take a few deep breaths and bend forward with your head between your knees.
• Don't eat, drink, smoke, or use chewing tobacco while the nitroglycerin tablet is dissolving in your mouth.
• Get new tablets after 3 months, even if you have some left in the container.
• If you've been taking this medication regularly for several weeks or more, don't suddenly stop using it because this may bring on angina attacks. Your doctor may instruct you to gradually reduce your dosage before stopping completely.

Important reminder

If you're an older adult, you may be especially sensitive to the effects of nitroglycerin.

Applying nitroglycerin ointment

Dear Patient:

This ointment is prescribed to prevent or reduce the number of angina (chest pain) attacks. It's also called by the brand names Nitro-Bid, Nitrol, and Nitrostat.

How to apply nitroglycerin ointment

Carefully check the label on your prescription tube, and apply only the amount prescribed at each dose.

Measure the prescribed amount of ointment onto the special paper. Spread it lightly over the area specified by the doctor—usually your upper arm or chest. *Don't rub it into your skin.* For best results, spread the ointment to cover an area about the size of the application paper (roughly 3½ inches by 2¼ inches). Cover the ointment with paper and tape it in place.

You may want to cover the paper (including the side edges) with plastic wrap to protect your clothes from stains. However, check with your doctor first. This covering will make your skin absorb more medication and may increase the chance for side effects.

What to do if you miss an application

Apply the missed application as soon as you remember. However, if your next scheduled application is within 2 hours, skip the missed one and resume your regular schedule. Don't increase the amount you apply.

What to do about side effects

Call your doctor *right away* if you get a severe or prolonged headache, dry mouth, or blurred vision.

This ointment may cause a headache, fast pulse rate, flushing of the face and neck, nausea, vomiting, and restlessness. Also, you may feel dizzy or lightheaded when rising from a sitting or lying position. These side effects usually go away over time as your body gets used to the medication. Check with your doctor if these side effects persist or become bothersome.

What you must know about alcohol and other drugs

Drink alcoholic beverages in moderation, if at all, because they will increase the chance for feeling dizzy or lightheaded when you get up quickly from a lying or sitting position.

Check with your doctor before taking other heart or blood pressure medications. When taken with your ointment, these medications may lower your blood pressure too much.

Special directions

• Be sure your doctor knows about your medical history, especially if you have glaucoma, kidney or liver disease, an overactive thyroid, or severe anemia or if you've recently had a heart attack, stroke, or head injury.
• To prevent skin irritation and other problems, apply each dose to a different skin site.
• If you're using this medication for several weeks or more, don't suddenly stop using it because this may bring on angina attacks. Your doctor may tell you to gradually reduce your dosage before stopping completely.

Important reminder

If you're an older adult, you may be especially sensitive to the effects of nitroglycerin.

Applying a nitroglycerin patch

Dear Patient:

This medication is prescribed to treat attacks of angina (chest pain). It's also called by the brand names Deponit, Nitro-Dur, and Transderm-Nitro.

How to apply a patch
This medication comes in a stick-on patch.

Carefully check the label on the prescription package, which tells you how often to apply a new patch. Apply a patch only as often as prescribed by your doctor.

To apply the patch, choose a clean, dry skin area with little or no hair. The area should be free from cuts, scars, or irritation. Don't choose the lower part of your arm or leg because the drug won't work as well at these sites.

What to do if you miss an application
Apply a new patch as soon as you remember. Then resume your regular schedule.

What to do about side effects
Call your doctor *right away* if you get a severe or prolonged headache, dry mouth, or blurred vision.

This medication may cause a fast pulse rate, flushing of your face and neck, headache, nausea, vomiting, and restlessness. Also, it may make you feel dizzy or light-headed when you get up from a sitting or lying position. These side effects usually subside as your body gets used to the medication. Check with your doctor if these effects persist or become bothersome.

What you must know about alcohol and other drugs
Drink alcoholic beverages in moderation, if at all. Alcohol will increase the chance for feeling dizzy or light-headed when you get up quickly from a lying or sitting position.

Check with your doctor or pharmacist before taking other heart or blood pressure medications. Taken with nitroglycerin, these medications may lower your blood pressure too much.

Special directions
• Be sure your doctor knows about your medical history, especially if you have glaucoma, kidney or liver disease, an overactive thyroid, or severe anemia or if you've recently had a heart attack, stroke, or head injury.
• Always remove the previous patch before applying a new one.
• To prevent skin irritation or other problems, apply each new patch to a different skin area.
• If you think this medication isn't working properly, don't trim or cut the patch to adjust the dosage. Instead, check with your doctor.
• If you've been using this medication for several weeks or more, don't suddenly stop using it because this may bring on angina attacks. Your doctor may instruct you to gradually reduce your dosage before stopping treatment completely.

Important reminder
If you're an older adult, you may be especially sensitive to the effects of nitroglycerin.

Taking nizatidine

Dear Patient:

Your doctor has prescribed nizatidine to treat your duodenal ulcers or prevent their return. The label may read Axid.

How to take nizatidine
Nizatidine comes in capsules. Follow the directions on the prescription label exactly. If you're taking one capsule daily, take it at bedtime unless your doctor gives you other instructions. If you're taking two capsules, take one in the morning and one at bedtime.

Continue to take this medication even after you begin to feel better. Stopping too soon may prevent your ulcer from healing completely.

What to do if you miss a dose
Take it as soon as possible. However, if it's almost time for your next dose, skip the missed capsule and take your next dose as scheduled. Don't double dose.

What to do about side effects
Call your doctor *at once* if you start to bleed or bruise easily or you become unusually tired. Also tell him right away if you develop rashes or other skin problems.

This medication may make you sleepy or sweaty or, rarely, may cause an irregular heartbeat. Check with your doctor if these symptoms persist or are troublesome.

What you must know about other drugs
Tell your doctor if you're taking other medications and check with him before taking new medications. In particular, reveal if you regularly take aspirin in high doses because nizatidine may increase aspirin's side effects.

If you take antacids to relieve stomach pain, wait 30 minutes to 1 hour between taking the antacid and nizatidine.

Special directions
• Nizatidine may aggravate certain medical conditions. For this reason, tell your doctor if you have other medical problems, especially kidney or liver disease.
• Before you have skin tests for allergies or tests to measure how much acid is in your stomach, tell your doctor you're taking nizatidine. This medication may affect the test results.
• Avoid foods and other substances that irritate your stomach, such as alcohol, carbonated soft drinks, and citrus products.
• Don't smoke while taking this medication because cigarette smoking reduces nizatidine's effectiveness. If you can't stop smoking completely, at least wait until after you've taken your last dose for the day.
• Keep appointments for follow-up examinations, so your doctor can check your progress.

Important reminders
If you're pregnant or breast-feeding, check with your doctor about using nizatidine.

If you're an older adult, you may be especially prone to nizatidine's side effects, particularly dizziness and confusion.

Additional instructions

_____

_____

_____

Taking norfloxacin

Dear Patient:

Your doctor has prescribed norfloxacin to treat your bacterial infection. This medication usually is prescribed to treat urinary tract infections. The label may read Noroxin.

How to take norfloxacin
Norfloxacin comes in tablets. Follow your doctor's instructions exactly. Take your tablet with a full glass (8 ounces) of water on an empty stomach, either 1 hour before or 2 hours after meals. Also, try to drink several extra glasses of water every day.

For best results, take your tablets at evenly spaced times during the day and night. For example, if you take two doses daily, you might take one dose at 8 a.m. and the other at 8 p.m.

Continue to take your medication, even after you begin to feel better. Stopping too soon might allow your infection to return.

What to do if you miss a dose
Take it as soon as possible. But if it's almost time for your next dose, skip the missed tablet and go back to your regular dosing schedule. Don't double dose.

Try not to forget a dose because norfloxacin works best with a constant amount in your blood or urine.

What to do about side effects
Call your doctor *right away* if you start to wheeze, have difficulty breathing, or break out in hives or a rash.

Check with your doctor if you become dizzy, drowsy, or unusually tired. Also tell him if you develop constipation, heartburn, nausea, a dry mouth, headache, or trouble sleeping.

What you must know about other drugs
Tell your doctor about other medications you're taking. If you use antacids or sucralfate (Carafate), an ulcer medication, don't take these drugs with norfloxacin. Instead, take antacids or sucralfate at least 2 hours after you take norfloxacin.

Your doctor also needs to know if you're taking nitrofurantoin (Macrodantin), another medication for urinary tract infections, or probenicid (Benemid), a gout medication.

Special directions
• Tell your doctor if you have other medical problems, especially kidney disease or a history of seizures.
• Because norfloxacin may increase your sensitivity to light, wear sunglasses and use a sunscreen while outdoors on bright days. Call your doctor if you have a severe reaction from the sun.
• Norfloxacin can make you drowsy, so make sure you know how you react to it before you drive or perform other activities that might be dangerous if you're not fully alert.

Important reminders
If you're pregnant or breast-feeding, don't use norfloxacin unless your doctor instructs you to do so.

Don't give this medication to infants, children, or adolescents because it may cause bone problems.

Additional instructions

_____

_____

Taking nortriptyline

Dear Patient:

Your doctor has prescribed nortriptyline to treat your depression. Brand names include Aventyl and Pamelor.

How to take nortriptyline

This medication comes in capsules and an oral solution. Follow the directions for using nortriptyline exactly.

To lessen stomach upset, take nortriptyline with food unless your doctor has told you to take it on an empty stomach.

If you're taking the *oral solution,* use the dropper provided to measure each dose. Dilute each dose with about one-half cup (4 ounces) of water, milk, or orange juice. Then drink the liquid.

Check with your doctor before you stop taking this medication.

What to do if you miss a dose

Adjust your dosage schedule as follows.

If you take one dose a day at bedtime, don't take the missed dose the next morning because it may cause side effects during the waking hours. Check with your doctor instead.

If you take more than one dose a day, take the missed dose as soon as possible. If it's almost time for your next dose, skip the missed dose and take your next dose as scheduled. Don't double dose.

What to do about side effects

Check with your doctor if you have blurred vision, a dry mouth, increased sweating, constipation, dizziness, drowsiness, rapid or irregular heartbeat, or difficulty urinating.

What you must know about alcohol and other drugs

Don't drink alcoholic beverages while taking nortriptyline because the combination may cause oversedation. For the same reason, don't use other medications that slow the nervous system, such as sleeping pills, sedatives, tranquilizers, and cold, flu, and allergy medications.

Be sure to tell your doctor about other medications you're taking. In particular, he needs to know if you take barbiturates (for seizures or sedation); cimetidine, or Tagamet (for ulcers); epinephrine, or Sus-Phrine (for asthma or severe allergic reactions); or medications for depression or other emotional problems.

Special directions

• Tell your doctor if you have other medical problems. They may affect the use of this medication.
• Because this medication may make you drowsy, avoid driving or performing other activities requiring alertness until you know how it affects you.
• If nortriptyline makes your mouth feel dry, use sugarless gum or hard candy, ice chips, or a saliva substitute.

Important reminders

If you're pregnant or breast-feeding, don't use nortriptyline, unless you've discussed the risks and benefits with your doctor.

Children and older adults are especially prone to nortriptyline's side effects.

Additional instructions

Taking oral nystatin

Dear Patient:

Your doctor has prescribed nystatin by mouth to treat your fungal infection. Brand names include Mycostatin, Nilstat, and Nystex.

How to take nystatin
This medication comes in tablets, lozenges, an oral solution, and a dry powder that's mixed with water. Follow your doctor's directions for taking nystatin exactly.

If you're taking the *lozenges,* hold the lozenge in your mouth to allow it to dissolve slowly. Don't chew or swallow lozenges whole.

If you're taking the *oral solution,* place half of the dose in each side of your mouth. Then swish the dose in your mouth, gargle, and swallow.

If you're using the *dry powder,* follow these steps:
• Read the prescription label to find out what proportions of water and powder to use for each dose.
• Thoroughly mix the powder and water. Then take the medication by dividing the whole amount into several portions.
• Swish each portion in your mouth for as long as possible, gargle, then swallow.

Continue to take nystatin, as directed, even if your symptoms disappear. Stopping too soon might allow your infection to return.

What to do about side effects
Check with your doctor if you have digestive upset, such as diarrhea, nausea, vomiting, or stomach pain.

Special directions
• To prevent fungal infections of your mouth, take good care of your teeth and mouth. Don't overuse mouthwash or wear poorly fitting dentures because doing so may lead to a mouth infection.
• Check with your doctor or pharmacist about how to store the form of nystatin you're using. Keep nystatin lozenges in the refrigerator. Don't allow the oral solution to freeze.

Important reminder
If you're giving nystatin to a child under age 5, avoid the lozenge form to prevent choking.

Additional instructions

_____

_____

_____

_____

_____

_____

_____

_____

_____

_____

_____

Applying topical nystatin

Dear Patient:

Topical nystatin is prescribed to treat a fungal infection of the skin or vagina. Brand names include Nystex, Nilstat, and Mycostatin.

How to apply nystatin

For a skin infection, this medication comes in cream, ointment, and powder forms. For a vaginal infection, it's available as vaginal tablets. Follow your doctor's directions for applying nystatin.

If you have a *skin infection,* apply just enough cream or ointment to cover the affected area. If you're using the powder on your feet, sprinkle it between your toes, on your feet, and in socks and shoes.

Don't cover the treated skin with a bandage, wrap, or other tight dressing unless directed to do so by your doctor.

If you have a *vaginal infection,* you'll probably insert the tablets with an applicator. Check with your doctor about how to use the applicator. Keep using this medication even if you begin to menstruate during the time of treatment.

Continue to use nystatin for as long as your doctor directs, even if your symptoms disappear. Stopping too soon might allow your infection to return.

What to do about side effects

Check with your doctor if you have skin or vaginal irritation that wasn't present before you began using nystatin.

If you're using vaginal tablets, expect some vaginal drainage. Wear a sanitary napkin to protect your clothing.

Special directions

• Let your doctor know if you're allergic to nystatin. Also reveal if you have other allergies, especially to foods, other medications, or preservatives.

• If you have a vaginal infection, practice good health habits to prevent reinfection. Wear cotton panties (or panties or pantyhose with cotton crotches) instead of synthetic underclothes. Also wear only freshly washed underwear.

Important reminder

If you're pregnant and have a vaginal infection, check with your doctor before using the applicator to insert the vaginal tablets.

Additional instructions

_____

_____

_____

_____

_____

_____

_____

_____

_____

_____

Applying nystatin with triamcinolone

Dear Patient:

Your doctor has prescribed nystatin with triamcinolone to treat your fungal infection and relieve the discomfort it's causing. Brand names include Derma-comb, Myco II, or Tristatin II.

How to apply this drug
This combination medication comes in cream and ointment forms. Follow your doctor's directions for using this medication exactly. Don't use it more often or for a longer time than your doctor prescribes.

To apply the cream or ointment, rub a small amount into the affected area gently and thoroughly. Take care to keep it away from your eyes.

Don't put a bandage, wrap, or other tight dressing over the treated skin unless your doctor directs you to do so. Wear loose-fitting clothing when using this medication on your groin area.

Use the medication for the full time of treatment, even if your symptoms go away. Stopping too soon might allow your infection to return.

What to do if you miss a dose
Apply the medication as soon as possible. But if it's almost time for your next dose, skip the missed dose and take your next dose on schedule.

What to do about side effects
Call your doctor *right away* if you start to have skin irritation, such as blistering, burning, dryness, itching, or peeling.

If you use this medication for a long time, you may experience other side effects. Let your doctor know if you start to have:

• acne or oily skin
• increased growth or loss of hair
• reddish purple lines on your arms, face, legs, trunk, or groin
• thin skin with easy bruising.

Special directions
• Because certain medical conditions may prevent your using this medication, tell your doctor if you have (or have had in the past) other medical problems, especially herpes, chicken pox, tuberculosis, or viral infections of the skin.
• Don't use this medication for other skin problems without checking first with your doctor.
• If your skin problem isn't better within 2 to 3 weeks, check with your doctor.
• If you're using this medication to treat a child's diaper rash, avoid tight-fitting diapers and plastic pants.

Important reminders
If you're pregnant or breast-feeding, check with your doctor before using this medication.

If you have severe diabetes, also talk to your doctor before using this medication. In rare instances, it can raise blood and urine glucose levels.

Additional instructions

_____

_____

_____

_____

_____

Taking ofloxacin

Dear Patient:

Your doctor has prescribed ofloxacin to treat your bacterial infection. This antibiotic is used to kill the bacteria that cause gonorrhea, urinary tract infections, and other infections. The label may read Floxin.

How to take ofloxacin
This medication comes in tablets. Take them exactly as ordered. For best results, take each dose with a full glass (8 ounces) of water. Drink several extra glasses of water daily unless your doctor tells you otherwise.

Continue to take ofloxacin, even after you begin to feel better. Stopping too soon may allow your infection to return.

What to do if you miss a dose
Take it as soon as possible. However, if it's almost time for your next dose, skip the missed dose and take your next dose as scheduled. Don't double dose.

What to do about side effects
Call your doctor *right away* if you start to wheeze, feel short of breath, have difficulty breathing, or break out in a rash or hives.

Check with your doctor if you have abdominal pain, diarrhea, dizziness, drowsiness, headache, light-headedness, nausea, vomiting, nervousness, or trouble sleeping.

What you must know about other drugs
Tell your doctor about other medications you're taking because many drugs can interfere with absorption of ofloxacin. These include aluminum- or magnesium-containing antacids; iron supplements; sucralfate (Carafate), an ulcer drug; and products that contain zinc.

If you take blood thinners, you should know that combined use with ofloxacin may increase the risk of bleeding. If you take theophylline (Theo-Dur), a drug for asthma or bronchitis, ofloxacin may worsen the side effects from this medication.

Special directions
• Be sure your doctor knows about your medical history, especially if you have brain or spinal cord disease or a kidney problem.
• Because ofloxacin may make you drowsy, make sure you know how you react to it before you drive or perform other activities that might be dangerous if you're not fully alert.
• This medication may make you unusually sensitive to sunlight, so limit your exposure to direct sun.

Important reminder
If you're pregnant or breast-feeding, don't use ofloxacin unless you and your doctor have discussed the possible risks.

Additional instructions

_____

_____

_____

_____

_____

_____

Taking omeprazole

Dear Patient:

This medication is used to treat duodenal ulcers, severe or chronic heartburn, and other problems in which the stomach has too much acid. The label may read Prilosec.

How to take omeprazole

Omeprazole comes in delayed-release capsules. Carefully check the label, and follow the directions exactly as ordered. Don't break, chew, or crush the capsule—swallow it whole.

Keep taking omeprazole for the full treatment period even after you feel better.

What to do if you miss a dose

Take it as soon as possible. However, if it's almost time for your next dose, skip the missed dose and take your next scheduled dose. Don't double dose.

What to do about side effects

Call your doctor *immediately* if you have:
• bloody or cloudy urine
• difficult, frequent, or painful urination
• easy bruising or bleeding
• fever
• persistent sores or ulcers in the mouth
• sore throat
• unusual tiredness.

Check with your doctor if you get a cough, a headache, back or chest pain, or a rash. Also let him know if you have digestive troubles, such as abdominal or stomach pain, constipation, diarrhea, gas, heartburn, nausea, or vomiting.

What you must know about other drugs

Tell the doctor about other medications you're taking. Some medicatons are more likely to cause side effects if taken with omeprazole. These drugs include blood thinners, the muscle relaxant diazepam (Valium), and the seizure medication phenytoin (Dilantin).

Special directions

• Tell your doctor about other medical problems you have, especially liver disease. Also mention if you're allergic to omeprazole or to other substances, such as foods or dyes.
• Keep appointments for follow-up examinations, so your doctor knows when you can stop taking this medication.
• After you start therapy, several days may pass before you experience pain relief. Until then, you may take antacids with omeprazole unless your doctor gives you other instructions.

Important reminder

If you're pregnant or breast-feeding, check with your doctor before taking this medication.

Additional instructions

_____

_____

_____

_____

_____

_____

_____

Taking oxacillin

Dear Patient:

Your doctor has prescribed oxacillin to treat your bacterial infection. The label may read Bactocill or Prostaphlin.

How to take oxacillin

This antibiotic, a form of penicillin, comes in capsules and an oral solution. Follow the medication instructions exactly. For best results, take your medication 1 hour before or 2 hours after meals.

Try to take the doses at evenly spaced times to keep a constant amount of oxacillin in your blood or urine.

Keep taking this medication for the full treatment period even after you feel better. Stopping too soon may allow your infection to return.

What to do if you miss a dose

Take it as soon as possible. However, if it's almost time for your next dose, adjust your dose as follows.

If you take two doses daily, space the missed dose and the next dose about 5 hours apart.

If you take three or more doses daily, space the missed dose and the next dose 2 to 4 hours apart.

Then resume your regular dosing schedule.

What to do about side effects

Stop taking oxacillin *at once* and call for emergency medical help if you have symptoms of an allergic reaction. These symptoms include difficulty breathing, light-headedness, fever, chills, a rash, hives, itching, and wheezing.

Check with your doctor if you have diarrhea or other digestive troubles, especially if these side effects persist or become bothersome.

Rarely, this medication may cause seizures. If you experience a seizure, a friend or family member must call for medical help *at once.*

What you must know about other drugs

Tell your doctor if you're taking probenecid (Benemid), a medication for gout, because this medication can increase blood levels of oxacillin.

Special directions

• Tell the doctor about your medical history, especially if you have allergies, bleeding problems, kidney disease, mononucleosis, or stomach or intestinal disease.
• If you're allergic to oxacillin or another form of penicillin, don't use this medication. If you're allergic to penicillin, carry a medical identification card or wear a medical identification bracelet stating this.
• Before you have medical tests, tell the doctor that you're taking oxacillin because it may affect the results.

Important reminder

If you're breast-feeding, check with your doctor before using this medication.

Additional instructions

_____

_____

_____

_____

Taking oxycodone

Dear Patient:

Your doctor has prescribed oxycodone to help relieve your pain. The label may read Roxicodone.

How to take oxycodone
This narcotic medication is available in tablets and an oral solution. Follow the directions exactly as ordered. Don't take more oxycodone than directed because it may become habit-forming or cause an overdose.

Check with your doctor before you stop taking this medication.

What to do if you miss a dose
Take it as soon as possible. However, if it's almost time for your next dose, skip the missed dose and take your next dose on schedule. Don't double dose.

What to do about side effects
Confusion, seizures, difficulty breathing, severe dizziness or drowsiness, slow heartbeat, and weakness are possible signs of overdose. If you have any of these side effects, call for emergency medical help *right away.*

This medication can make you sleepy or drowsy or can create a false sense of well-being. And it can cause nausea, vomiting, constipation, or difficult urination. Check with your doctor if you develop any of these symptoms, especially if they continue or become severe.

What you must know about alcohol and other drugs
Don't drink alcoholic beverages while taking oxycodone because the combination can lead to oversedation.

For the same reason, avoid taking medications that slow the nervous system unless your doctor gives you other directions. These depressant medications include many allergy and cold medications, sleeping pills, and muscle relaxants.

If you regularly take blood thinners, aspirin, or products containing aspirin, check with your doctor before using oxycodone. Combined use may lead to easy bleeding.

Special directions
• Tell your doctor if you have other medical problems. They may affect the use of this medication.
• Because oxycodone may make you drowsy, make sure you know how it affects you before you perform hazardous activities, such as driving or operating machinery.
• Oxycodone may make you feel faint, dizzy, or light-headed, especially when you get up suddenly from a lying or sitting position. To prevent falls, get up slowly from these positions.
• Tell your doctor or dentist that you're taking this medication before you have surgery.

Important reminders
If you're pregnant or breast-feeding, check with your doctor before using this medication.

If you're an athlete, you should know that oxycodone is banned and tested for by the U.S. Olympic Committee.

Additional instructions

_____

_____

Taking oxycodone with acetaminophen

Dear Patient:

This medication contains two kinds of pain relievers: a narcotic analgesic (oxycodone) and acetaminophen. Brand names include Percocet, Roxicet, and Tylox.

How to take this drug
This medication is available in capsules, tablets, and an oral solution. Follow the instructions exactly. Don't take more than the prescribed amount of this medication because it may become habit-forming or lead to overdose. If you think this medication isn't helping you, check with your doctor.

What to do if you miss a dose
Take it as soon as you remember it. However, if it's almost time for your next dose, skip the missed dose and take your next dose on schedule. Don't double dose.

What to do about side effects
Call for emergency help *immediately* if you think you may have taken an overdose. Symptoms include cold, clammy skin; confusion; seizures; difficulty breathing; severe dizziness or drowsiness; increased sweating; slow heartbeat; stomach cramps; and weakness.

Call your doctor *at once* if you have:
• black, tarry stools
• bloody or dark urine
• easy bruising or bleeding
• facial swelling
• irregular heartbeat or breathing
• mental depression
• skin problems
• sore throat or fever.

Also check with your doctor if this medication makes you feel dizzy or faint or causes nausea or vomiting.

What you must know about alcohol and other drugs
Don't drink alcoholic beverages while taking this medication because the combination may lead to oversedation. For the same reason, avoid other medications that depress the nervous system, including many cold and flu remedies, muscle relaxants, sleeping pills, and seizure medications.

Check with your doctor before you take aspirin, aspirin-containing products, or nonsteroidal anti-inflammatory drugs, such as Motrin and Naprosyn.

Special directions
• Tell your doctor if you have other medical problems, especially alcohol or drug abuse, emotional problems, brain disease or head injury, or diseases of any of the major organs.
• Because this medication can make you dizzy or drowsy, make sure you know how it affects you before you perform hazardous activities, such as driving or operating machinery.
• Tell your doctor or dentist that you're taking this medication before you have surgery.

Important reminders
If you're pregnant or breast-feeding, check with your doctor before using this medication.

Children and older adults may be especially sensitive to the effects of this medication.

If you're an athlete, you should know that the oxycodone in this medication is banned and tested for by the U.S. Olympic Committee.

Taking oxycodone with aspirin

Dear Patient:

This medication contains two kinds of pain relievers: a narcotic analgesic (oxycodone) and aspirin. Brand names include Percodan, Percodan-Demi, and Roxiprin.

How to take oxycodone with aspirin

This medication comes in tablets. Take it exactly as directed. Don't take more than the prescribed amount because it may become habit-forming or lead to overdose. If this medication isn't relieving your pain, check with your doctor.

What to do if you miss a dose

Take it as soon as you remember it. However, if it's almost time for your next dose, skip the missed dose and take your next dose on schedule. Don't double dose.

What to do about side effects

Call for emergency help *immediately* if you think you may have taken an overdose. Symptoms include cold, clammy skin; confusion; seizures; severe dizziness or drowsiness; increased sweating or thirst; slow heartbeat; severe stomach pain; vision problems; and weakness.

Call your doctor *right away* if you have:
• black, tarry stools
• confusion
• dark urine
• facial swelling
• irregular heartbeat or breathing
• mental depression
• rashes or other skin problems
• unusual tiredness or weakness
• vomiting that looks like coffee grounds.

Check with your doctor if you feel faint or dizzy or have stomach upset.

What you must know about alcohol and other drugs

Don't drink alcoholic beverages while taking this medication because the combination may cause oversedation. For the same reason, avoid taking other drugs that depress the nervous system, including many cold and flu remedies, muscle relaxants, and sleeping pills.

Check with your doctor before you take other medications, especially blood thinners, acetaminophen (Tylenol), aspirin or aspirin-containing products, diabetes medications, probenecid (Benemid) for gout, and zidovudine (AZT).

Special directions

• Tell your doctor if you have other medical problems. They may affect the use of this medication. Also mention if you're allergic to any medication.
• Because this medication may make you drowsy, make sure you know how it affects you before you drive or perform other activities that require full alertness.

Important reminders

If you're pregnant or breast-feeding, check with your doctor before using this medication.

If you're an older adult, you may be especially prone to this drug's side effects.

If you're an athlete, you should know that the oxycodone in this medication is banned and tested for by the U.S. Olympic Committee.

Additional instructions

_____

_____

Taking penbutolol

Dear Patient:

Your doctor has prescribed penbutolol to treat your high blood pressure. The label may read Levatol.

How to take penbutolol
Penbutolol comes in tablets. Follow your doctor's instructions exactly. Try not to miss any doses because your condition may worsen if you don't take this medication regularly.

Don't stop taking penbutolol suddenly. Check with your doctor first.

What to do if you miss a dose
Take it as soon as possible. However, if it's within 8 hours of your next dose, skip the missed dose and resume your regular schedule. Don't double dose.

What to do about side effects
Call your doctor *right away* if you start to have difficulty breathing, cold hands and feet, confusion, hallucinations, irregular heartbeat, depression, nightmares, a rash, or swelling of your feet or ankles.

Check with your doctor if you feel dizzy, drowsy, or unusually tired or weak. Also tell him if you have trouble sleeping or with your sexual function.

What you must know about other drugs
Tell the doctor about other prescription or nonprescription medications you're taking. In particular, your doctor needs to know if you take other medications for high blood pressure, such as clonidine (Catapres). Also tell him if you use nonsteroidal anti-inflammatory drugs, such as aspirin or ibuprofen (Motrin), or if you're taking drugs for diabetes or asthma.

Special directions
• Tell the doctor if you have other medical problems, especially asthma, bronchitis, emphysema, a slow heart rate, depression, diabetes, or diseases of the heart, kidneys, liver, or thyroid.
• Because penbutolol may make you dizzy, make sure you know how it affects you before you drive or perform other activities that require full alertness.
• Tell your doctor or dentist that you're taking this medication before you have surgery.

Important reminders
If you're pregnant or breast-feeding, check with your doctor before using penbutolol.

If you're an older adult, you may be especially prone to penbutolol's side effects.

If you have diabetes, this medication may cause your blood glucose level to fall or may mask signs of low blood glucose.

If you're an athlete, be aware that penbutolol is banned and tested for by the U.S. Olympic Committee and the National Collegiate Athletic Association.

Additional instructions

_____

_____

_____

_____

_____

_____

Taking penicillin G

Dear Patient:

Your doctor has prescribed penicillin G to treat your bacterial infection.

How to take penicillin G

Penicillin G comes in tablet and oral liquid forms. Take this medication exactly as your doctor directs.

If you're taking the *oral liquid,* use a specially marked measuring spoon (not a household teaspoon) or dropper to measure each dose.

If you're taking the *tablets,* don't drink acidic beverages, such as fruit juices, within 1 hour of taking penicillin G.

Try to take your medication at evenly spaced times day and night. Continue to take penicillin G as directed, even if you start to feel better. Stopping too soon may allow your infection to return.

What to do if you miss a dose

Take it as soon as possible. But if it's almost time for your next dose, follow these guidelines.

If you take two doses a day, space the missed dose and the next dose 5 to 6 hours apart.

If you take three or more doses a day, space the missed dose and the next dose 2 to 4 hours apart.

Then resume your regular schedule.

What to do about side effects

Call for emergency help *at once* if you have an allergic reaction to penicillin G. Symptoms include difficulty breathing, light-headedness, a rash, hives, itching, or wheezing.

Call your doctor *right away* if you have severe abdominal or stomach cramps, bloody or decreased urine, seizures, severe diarrhea, fever, joint pain, sore throat, or unusual bleeding or bruising.

Check with your doctor if this medication causes mild diarrhea, nausea, vomiting, or sore mouth or tongue.

What you must know about other drugs

Tell the doctor about other medications you're taking. Probenicid (Benemid), a gout medication, may increase blood levels of penicillin G.

Don't take diarrhea medication without first checking with your doctor. Severe diarrhea may be a sign of a serious side effect.

Special directions

• Tell your doctor if you have other medical problems, especially asthma, bleeding disorders, mononucleosis, or kidney, stomach, or intestinal disease. Also mention if you're allergic to any penicillin or another medication.
• Before you have medical tests, tell the doctor you're taking penicillin G because it may affect the test results.
• If you're allergic to penicillin, your doctor may want you to carry a medical identification card or wear a medical identification bracelet stating this.

Important reminders

If you're breast-feeding, check with your doctor before using this medication.

Additional instructions

_____

_____

_____

_____

Taking pentamidine

Dear Patient:

Pentamidine is prescribed to prevent or treat pneumocystis pneumonia. If you're receiving the *injection* form of this medication, the label may read Pentam 300. If you're using the *inhalant* form, the label may read NebuPent.

How to take pentamidine
Take pentamidine exactly as directed by your doctor.

If you're using the *inhalant* form, use the aerosal device until the chamber is empty. This may take as long as 45 minutes.

If you're receiving the *injection* form, lie down during the injection. That's because the medication may cause your blood pressure to drop suddenly, making you feel light-headed or dizzy.

Continue to take pentamidine as directed, even after you begin to feel better. Stopping too soon may allow your infection to return.

What to do if you miss a dose
If you're using the *inhalant* device and you miss a dose, use your medication as soon as possible. If you miss an *injection,* check with your doctor about when to receive the next dose.

What to do about side effects
Call your doctor *right away* if you have:
• decreased urination
• sore throat and fever
• easy bleeding or bruising
• symptoms of low blood glucose: anxiety; chills; cold sweats; cool, pale skin; headache; increased hunger; nervousness; shakiness
• symptoms of low blood pressure: blurred vision, confusion, dizziness, fainting or light-headedness, and unusual tiredness or weakness.

Also check with your doctor if you develop diarrhea, loss of appetite, nausea, or vomiting.

If you're receiving the injections, tell your doctor if you have pain, redness, or swelling at the injection site.

What you must know about other drugs
Tell the doctor about other medications you're taking. In particular, you may be at risk for kidney damage if you take pentamidine with certain antibiotics; amphotericin B (Fungizone), a drug for fungal infections; cisplatin (Platinol), a cancer medication; or zidovudine (AZT), an AIDS medication.

Special directions
• Tell your doctor if you have other medical problems, especially anemia, asthma, diabetes, bleeding disorders, low blood pressure, and kidney, heart, or liver disease. Also mention if you're allergic to pentamidine.
• If you're receiving the injections, apply warm compresses to the injection site if the area hurts.
• If you're using the inhalant, don't smoke because it can cause coughing and difficulty breathing.

Important reminder
If you're pregnant or breast-feeding, check with your doctor before using this medication.

Additional instructions

_____

_____

Taking pentazocine

Dear Patient:

Your doctor has prescribed pentazocine to relieve your pain. If you're taking the *tablet* form of this narcotic pain reliever, the label may read Talwin-Nx. If you're using the *injection* form, the label may read Talwin.

How to take pentazocine
If you're taking the *tablets,* carefully follow the prescription directions. If you're *injecting* yourself with pentazocine at home, make sure you understand and follow your doctor's instructions exactly.

Don't take more pentazocine or use it for a longer time than directed because it may become habit-forming. If you think this medication isn't helping your pain, check with your doctor.

What to do if you miss a dose
Take it as soon as you remember. However, if it's almost time for your next dose, skip the missed dose and take your next dose at the scheduled time. Don't double dose.

What to do about side effects
Get emergency help *at once* if you think you may have taken an overdose. Symptoms include seizures; confusion; severe nervousness, restlessness, dizziness, weakness, or drowsiness; and slow or troubled breathing.

Let your doctor know if you feel dizzy, light-headed, faint, or drowsy. Also tell him if you have difficulty urinating or nausea and vomiting.

What you must know about alcohol and other drugs
Don't drink alcoholic beverages while taking pentazocine. Combined use in-creases the depressant effects of the medication. For the same reason, don't take other depressant medications, such as sleeping pills, tranquilizers, and cold and flu medications unless your doctor tells you otherwise. Likewise, avoid other narcotic pain relievers, such as Darvon.

Special directions
• Tell your doctor if you have other medical problems, especially lung disease, colitis, or a history of seizures, emotional problems, or alcohol or drug abuse. Also reveal if you have any disease that affects a major organ, such as the heart, kidneys, and liver.
• Because this medication may make you drowsy or light-headed, don't drive or perform activities requiring alertness until you know how you respond.
• Don't stop taking pentazocine suddenly without checking first with your doctor. Your doctor may want you to reduce your dosage gradually to lessen the chance of withdrawal effects.

Important reminders
If you're pregnant or breast-feeding, check with your doctor before using this medication. If you're an older adult, you may be especially prone to pentazocine's side effects.

If you're an athlete, you should know that pentazocine is banned and tested for by the U.S. Olympic Committee.

Additional instructions

_____

_____

_____

Taking pentobarbital

Dear Patient:

Pentobarbital is prescribed to relax you. It belongs to a group of medications called barbiturates, which act by slowing down the nervous system. Brand names may include Nembutal and Nembutal Sodium.

How to take pentobarbital
This medication comes in capsule, elixir, and suppository forms. Take it exactly as your doctor directs. Because it can become habit-forming, don't take it for a longer time than your doctor recommends.

To use the suppository, first remove the foil wrapper. Then moisten the suppository with cold water. Next, lie down on your side and use your finger to push the suppository well up into your rectum. Wash your hands afterward.

What to do if you miss a dose
If you're taking this medication regularly, take a missed dose as soon as possible. However, if it's almost time for your next dose, skip the missed dose and go back to your regular schedule. Don't double dose.

What to do about side effects
Get emergency help *immediately* if you think you may have taken an overdose. Symptoms include:
• severe drowsiness, confusion, or weakness
• shortness of breath
• slow heartbeat
• slow or troubled breathing
• slurred speech
• staggering.

Check with your doctor if you become drowsy or lethargic or feel as if you have a hangover.

What you must know about alcohol and other drugs
Don't drink alcoholic beverages while you're taking pentobarbital because the combination may cause oversedation. Likewise, don't take other depressant medications, such as many allergy and cold medications, narcotic pain relievers, and sleeping pills, without checking first with your doctor.

Tell your doctor about other medications you're taking. In particular, he needs to know if you're using adrenocorticoids (cortisone-like medications); blood thinners; griseofulvin (Grisactin), an antifungal medication; or birth control pills.

Special directions
• Tell your doctor if you have other medical problems. They may affect the use of this medication.
• Because pentobarbital may make you drowsy or light-headed, don't drive or perform activities requiring alertness until you know how it affects you.
• After prolonged use, don't suddenly stop taking this medication.

Important reminders
If you're pregnant or breast-feeding, check with your doctor before using this medication.

If you're an older adult, you may be especially prone to pentobarbital's side effects.

If you're an athlete, you should know that pentobarbital is banned and, in some cases, tested for by the U.S. Olympic Committee and the National Collegiate Athletic Association.

Taking pentoxifylline

Dear Patient:

Your doctor has prescribed pentoxifylline to improve your blood circulation. This medication is used to relieve leg pain and cramps caused by poor circulation. The label may read Trental.

How to take pentoxifylline
Pentoxifylline comes in extended-release tablets. Take your medication with meals to lessen the chance of stomach upset. You may also take the tablets with an antacid unless your doctor tells you otherwise.

Swallow the tablet whole—don't chew, crush, or break it.

Don't stop taking this medication suddenly without first checking with your doctor. Also, realize that it may take several weeks before you feel that pentoxifylline is working.

What to do if you miss a dose
Take it as soon as possible. But if it's almost time for your next dose, skip the missed dose and take your next dose on schedule. Don't double dose.

What to do about side effects
Pentoxifylline can cause headache, dizziness, heartburn, nausea, or vomiting. Check with your doctor if these symptoms continue or bother you.

Rarely, this medication causes chest pain or an irregular heartbeat. If you have these symptoms, call your doctor as soon as possible.

What you must know about other drugs
Tell your doctor about other medications you're taking. Taking pentoxifylline with blood thinners may increase your risk of bleeding. If you take medications for high blood pressure, your doctor may need to adjust your dosage of these medications because pentoxifylline can increase their effect.

Special directions
• Tell your doctor if you have other medical problems, especially stomach ulcers and kidney or liver disease. Also mention if you've ever had an unusual or allergic reaction to caffeine or any foods or medications.
• Because nicotine can narrow your blood vessels, cigarette smoking may worsen your condition. Therefore, if you smoke, make an effort to quit, such as by joining a smoking-cessation program.

Important reminders
If you're pregnant or breast-feeding, check with your doctor before you take pentoxifylline.

If you're an older adult, you may be especially prone to side effects from pentoxifylline.

Additional instructions

_____

_____

_____

_____

_____

_____

_____

Taking perphenazine

Dear Patient:

This medication is used to treat psychological disorders and to relieve severe nausea, vomiting, or hiccups. The label may read Trilafon.

How to take perphenazine
Perphenazine comes in tablets and an oral solution. Take your medication exactly as your doctor directs. Take your dose with food, water, or milk to prevent stomach irritation.

To use the concentrated oral solution, dilute your dose in fruit juice, ginger ale, or semisolid food, such as applesauce. Don't mix your medication with colas, black coffee, grape or apple juice, or tea.

Don't stop taking perphenazine without first checking with your doctor.

What to do if you miss a dose
If you take one dose daily, take the missed dose as soon as possible. If you don't remember until the next day, skip it and go back to your regular schedule.

If you take more than one dose a day, take the missed dose within 1 hour if you remember it. If not, skip the missed dose and go back to your regular dosing schedule. Don't double dose.

What to do about side effects
Call your doctor *right away* if you develop a fever, fast heartbeat, difficulty breathing, and increased sweating. Also call *immediately* if you start to feel extremely tired or unwell.

Tell your doctor if this medication causes uncontrolled movements of your mouth, tongue, or other body parts. Also tell him if you have blurred vision, a dry mouth, difficulty urinating, or constipation. Let your doctor know if perphenazine makes you feel dizzy or faint, especially when you get up from a sitting or lying position.

What you must know about alcohol and other drugs
Don't drink alcoholic beverages while taking this medication because it could cause oversedation. For the same reason, avoid other medications that depress the nervous system, including tranquilizers and sleeping pills.

To avoid harmful drug interactions, check with your doctor before you use other medications. If you take antacids, take them at least 2 hours before or after taking perphenazine.

Special directions
• Tell your doctor if you have other medical problems because perphenazine can aggravate many medical conditions.
• Before you have medical tests, tell the doctor that you're taking perphenazine because it may affect the test results.
• Because perphenazine may make you dizzy, make sure you know how you react to it before you drive or perform other activities that require alertness.

Important reminders
If you're pregnant or breast-feeding, check with your doctor before taking perphenazine.

Children and older adults are especially prone to perphenazine's side effects.

If you're an athlete, be aware that perphenazine is banned and sometimes tested for in shooting events by the U.S. Olympic Committee and the National Collegiate Athletic Association.

Taking phenazopyridine

Dear Patient:

This medication will help to ease the pain of your infected or irritated urinary tract. Brand names include Azo-Standard, Baridium, or Di-Azo.

How to take phenazopyridine

Phenazopyridine comes in tablets. Follow your doctor's directions exactly about how and when to take this medication. If you bought it without a prescription, carefully read the package instructions first.

To prevent stomach upset, take the tablets with meals or a snack.

You may stop using this medication after 3 days if your pain is relieved unless your doctor gives you other instructions.

What to do if you miss a dose

Take it as soon as possible. However, if it's almost time for your next dose, skip the missed dose and take your next dose on schedule. Don't double dose.

What to do about side effects

Check with your doctor *right away* if you have any of these symptoms:
• bluish skin
• shortness of breath or difficulty breathing
• a rash
• unusual tiredness or weakness
• yellow eyes or skin.

Let your doctor know if this medication makes you dizzy or nauseous or gives you a headache.

Don't be surprised if phenazopyridine turns your urine reddish orange. This is to be expected and won't harm you.

Special directions

• If you have kidney or liver disease, tell your doctor because these medical problems may affect the use of phenazopyridine.
• Before you have medical tests, tell the doctor that you're taking this medication because it may affect the test results.
• Because phenazopyridine may make you dizzy, make sure you know how you react to it before you drive or perform other activities requiring alertness.
• If you have another urinary tract problem in the future, don't use any left-over phenazopyridine without first checking with your doctor.

Important reminder

If you have diabetes, this medication may cause false test results with urine glucose or urine ketone tests. Check with your doctor for more information about this, especially if your diabetes isn't well controlled.

Additional instructions

_____

_____

_____

_____

_____

_____

_____

Taking phenobarbital

Dear Patient:

Phenobarbital is used to prevent seizures caused by epilepsy and other disorders. It's also used as a sedative to produce relaxation, such as before surgery. The label may read Barbita or Solfoton.

How to take phenobarbital
Phenobarbital comes in these forms: tablet, capsule, oral solution, and elixir. Follow your doctor's directions exactly. Don't increase your dose because phenobarbital can become habit-forming.

If you're taking the capsule or tablet form, swallow it whole—don't chew or crush it. If you're taking this medication for epilepsy, take it every day in regularly spaced doses, as prescribed.

What to do if you miss a dose
Take it as soon as possible. However, if it's almost time for your next dose, skip the missed dose and take your next dose on schedule. Don't double dose.

What to do about side effects
Call for emergency medical help *at once* if you think you may have taken an overdose. Symptoms of overdose include severe drowsiness, weakness, and confusion; slurred speech; and difficulty breathing.

Check with your doctor *right away* if you have any skin problems. Also let him know if this medication makes you feel drowsy, lethargic, or like you're "hung over."

What you must know about alcohol and other drugs
Avoid drinking alcoholic beverages while taking phenobarbital because the combination can lead to oversedation. For the same reason, don't use other medications that depress the nervous system, including tranquilizers, sleeping pills, and many cold and flu remedies.

To prevent harmful drug interactions, tell your doctor about other medications you're taking. If you take blood thinners, birth control pills, or estrogen, be aware that phenobarbital may not work well.

Special directions
• Tell your doctor if you have other medical problems, especially asthma, lung disease, or porphyria. Also reveal if you're depressed or in chronic pain.
• Before you have medical tests, tell the doctor that you're taking this medication because it may affect the test results.
• Because phenobarbital may make you drowsy, make sure you know how you react to it before you drive or perform other activities requiring alertness.

Important reminders
If you're pregnant or breast-feeding, don't take phenobarbital without specific instructions from your doctor.

If you're an older adult, you may be especially sensitive to phenobarbital's side effects.

If you're an athlete, you should know that phenobarbital is banned and sometimes tested for by the U.S. Olympic Committee and the National Collegiate Athletic Association.

Additional instructions

_____

_____

Using nasal phenylephrine

Dear Patient:

This medication will help to relieve your stuffy nose. Phenylephrine is used to relieve nasal congestion caused by hay fever or other allergies, colds, or sinus trouble. The label may read Alconefrin, Neo-Synephrine, or Sinex.

How to use phenylephrine

This medication comes in a nose jelly, nose drops, and a nose spray. Follow your doctor's directions exactly. If you bought your medication without a prescription, carefully read the package directions before using. Also, before you use this medication, blow your nose gently.

To use the *nose drops,* tilt your head back and squeeze the drops into each nostril. Keep your head tilted back for a few minutes. Rinse the dropper with hot water, dry it with a clean tissue, and recap.

To use the *nose spray,* hold your head upright and spray the medication into each nostril. Sniff briskly while squeezing the bottle. Spray once or twice, then wait a few minutes for the medication to work. Blow your nose and repeat until the complete dose is used.

To use the *nose jelly,* place a pea-size amount of the jelly up each nostril. Sniff it well back into the nose.

Don't use phenylephrine longer than directed because doing so may worsen your runny or stuffy nose.

What to do if you miss a dose

Use it right away if you remember within 1 hour or so of the missed dose. However, if you don't remember until later, skip the missed dose and take your next dose on schedule. Don't double dose.

What to do about side effects

Check with your doctor if your heart starts to pound irregularly or too rapidly. These symptoms suggest that you've used too much phenylephrine. When you use this medication, your nose may burn, sting, or feel dry. Let your doctor know if these symptoms continue or become bothersome.

Special directions

• Tell your doctor if you have other medical problems, especially heart or blood vessel disease, high blood pressure, glaucoma, diabetes, an overactive thyroid, or diseases of the liver or pancreas.
• Before you have a hearing test, tell the doctor that you're taking phenylephrine because it may affect the test results.

Important reminders

If you're giving this medication to a child, check with the doctor first because children are especially prone to side effects from phenylephrine.

If you're an athlete, you should know that phenylephrine is banned and tested for by the U.S. Olympic Committee. Use of nasal phenylephrine can lead to disqualification in most athletic events.

Additional instructions

_____

_____

_____

_____

_____

Using ophthalmic phenylephrine

Dear Patient:

This medication will relieve the redness of your eyes. Phenylephrine eyedrops also are used to treat some other eye problems and to enlarge the pupils before eye examinations. The label may read AK-Dilate, Neo-Synephrine, and Prefrin Liquifilm.

How to use phenylephrine eyedrops
Follow your doctor's directions exactly. If you bought this medication without a prescription, carefully read the package directions before using. Don't use more of the eyedrops or use them more often than your doctor ordered. To instill the eyedrops, follow these steps:
• First, wash your hands.
• Tilt your head back and pull the lower eyelid away from the eye to form a pouch.
• Squeeze the drops into the pouch and gently close your eye.
• Wash your hands again.

What to do if you miss a dose
Instill it as soon as possible, However, if it's almost time for your next dose, skip the missed dose and instill your next dose on schedule. Don't double dose.

What to do about side effects
Check with your doctor if you're told your blood pressure is elevated. When you instill the eyedrops, your eyes may burn, sting, water, or become more sensitive to light. Check with your doctor if these symptoms continue or become bothersome.

What you must know about other drugs
Tell your doctor about other medications you're taking. Your doctor may want you to avoid certain medications to prevent harmful interactions. In particular, medications to avoid or use with your doctor's supervision are those for high blood pressure, Parkinson's disease, and depression or other psychiatric problems.

Special directions
• Tell your doctor if you have other medical problems, especially heart or blood vessel disease, high blood pressure, glaucoma, diabetes, an overactive thyroid, or diseases of the liver or pancreas.
• Before you have a hearing test, tell the doctor that you're taking phenylephrine because it may affect the test results.
• Because your eyes may be more sensitive to light while you use this medication, wear sunglasses that block ultraviolet light when you're in a bright room or outside on sunny days.

Important reminders
If you're giving this medication to a child, check with the doctor first because children are especially prone to side effects from phenylephrine. Older adults are also especially prone to its side effects.

If you're an athlete, you should know that phenylephrine eyedrops are banned by the U.S. Olympic Committee.

Additional instructions

_____

_____

_____

_____

Taking phenytoin

Dear Patient:

This medication is used to control seizures and treat several other medical problems. The label may read Dilantin or Diphenylan.

How to take phenytoin
Phenytoin comes in capsules, chewable tablets, and an oral liquid. Don't take more or less than your doctor orders. Take phenytoin with meals to reduce stomach upset. If you're taking the *liquid* form, use a specially marked measuring spoon (not a household teaspoon) to measure your dose. If you're taking the *capsules,* be sure to swallow them whole.

What to do if you miss a dose
Adjust your dosing schedule as follows.

If you take one dose a day, take the missed dose as soon as possible. But if you don't remember until the next day, skip it and take your next dose on schedule.

If you take more than one dose a day, take the missed dose as soon as possible. However, if it's within 4 hours of your next dose, skip the missed dose and take your next dose on schedule. Don't double dose.

What to do about side effects
Call your doctor *right away* if you have skin problems, palpitations, or difficulty breathing. Also call if you have a fever, become extremely weak or tired, or feel very unwell.

Check with your doctor if you experience confusion, dizziness, vision changes, sleeplessness, or slurred speech. Also report uncontrolled movements, nausea, vomiting, and bleeding gums.

What you must know about alcohol and other drugs
Check with your doctor before drinking alcoholic beverages because alcohol may prevent phenytoin from working well.

Tell your doctor about other medications you're taking. Some of the many medications you need to avoid or use only with your doctor's supervision are blood thinners, antihistamines (found in cold and allergy medications), the ulcer drug cimetidine (Tagamet), and aspirin.

Special directions
• Tell your doctor if you have other medical problems, especially a heart condition, porphyria, and liver or kidney disease.
• Make sure you know how you react to phenytoin before you drive or perform other activities requiring alertness.
• See your dentist regularly, and inform him you're taking phenytoin.

Important reminders
If you're pregnant or breast-feeding, check with your doctor before taking this medication.

If you have diabetes, be aware that phenytoin may affect the results of blood and urine glucose tests.

If you're an athlete, you should know that phenytoin is banned and sometimes tested for in biathlon and modern pentathlon events by the U.S. Olympic Committee.

Using pilocarpine

Dear Patient:

Your doctor has ordered pilocarpine to treat your glaucoma or another eye condition. This medication comes in the form of eyedrops, eye gel, and an eye system. Brand names include Adsorbocarpine, Pilocar, and Pilopine HS.

How to use pilocarpine
Follow your doctor's instructions exactly. Don't use more pilocarpine or use it more often than your doctor orders. Also, before you use pilocarpine, wash your hands. Then follow these steps.

If you're using *eyedrops,* first tilt your head back. Use your index finger to pull the lower eyelid away from the eye, forming a pouch. Squeeze the drops into the pouch and gently close your eyes for 1 to 2 minutes. Don't blink.

If you're using *eye gel,* first pull the lower eyelid away to form a pouch. Squeeze a thin strip of gel into the pouch. Gently close your eyes for 1 to 2 minutes.

Right after using the eyedrops or eye gel, wash your hands to remove any pilocarpine that might be on them. Also, take care to keep your medication bottle germfree. Don't let the applicator tip touch any surface, including your eye.

Before you use the *eye system,* read the patient instructions that come with this medication. If you have any questions, check with your doctor.

What to do if you miss a dose
If you forget to use the eyedrops or eye gel, do so as soon as possible. But if it's almost time for your next dose, skip the missed dose and take your next dose on schedule. Don't double dose.

What to do about side effects
When you use this medication, it may make your brow or head hurt or cause eye pain. For a short time after you use pilocarpine, your vision may be blurred or you may notice a change in your near or distant vision, especially at night.

If these symptoms persist or become bothersome, check with your doctor.

What you must know about other drugs
Tell your doctor about other medications you're taking. To prevent harmful interactions, you need to avoid certain other drugs, especially some eye medications, such as phenylephrine (used to treat eye redness) and carbachol (Carbacel), another medication for glaucoma.

Special directions
• Tell your doctor if you have other medical problems, especially asthma, other eye problems, heart disease, urinary difficulty, stomach ulcers, an overactive thyroid, or Parkinson's disease.
• If you're using the eyedrops or eye gel, make sure your vision is clear before you drive or perform other activities that might be dangerous if you can't see well.

Additional instructions

_____

_____

_____

_____

_____

Taking pimozide

Dear Patient:

Pimozide is prescribed to treat the symptoms of Tourette's syndrome. Pimozide works in the central nervous system to help reduce vocal outbursts and uncontrolled, repeated body movements (tics) that can disrupt everyday living. The label may read Orap.

How to take pimozide

Pimozide comes in tablets. Follow your doctor's instructions for taking this medication exactly. Don't use more of it or take it more often or longer than your doctor orders.

Don't stop taking this medication suddenly without first checking with your doctor. Your doctor may want you to reduce your dosage gradually to give your body time to adjust.

What to do if you miss a dose

Take it as soon as possible. Then take any remaining doses for the day at regularly spaced times. Don't double dose.

What to do about side effects

Get emergency help *at once* if you start to experience seizures, difficulty breathing, fast heartbeat, high fever, heavy sweating, severe muscle stiffness, loss of bladder control, or extreme fatigue.

Call your doctor *right away* if you have difficulty speaking or swallowing, loss of balance, mood changes, muscle spasms, or unusual changes in your body movements.

Check with your doctor if pimozide makes you feel faint, dizzy, or drowsy. Also tell him if you have blurred vision, constipation, dryness of your mouth, a rash, or breast swelling or soreness.

What you must know about alcohol and other drugs

Avoid drinking alcoholic beverages while taking pimozide because the combination may make you overly drowsy. For the same reason, don't use other medications that depress the nervous system, including tranquilizers, sleeping pills, and many cold and flu medications.

Tell your doctor about prescription and nonprescription medications you're taking. To prevent harmful interactions, you need to avoid a variety of other medications, including certain drugs for depression, mental illness, and stomach or abdominal cramps.

Special directions

• Tell your doctor if you have other medical problems, especially breast cancer or diseases of the heart, kidneys, or liver. Also reveal if you've ever had tics other than those caused by Tourette's syndrome. Other medical problems may affect the use of this medication.
• Make sure you know how you react to pimozide before you drive or perform other activities that might be dangerous if you're not fully alert.
• Before you have surgery, dental work, or emergency care, tell the doctor that you're taking pimozide.

Important reminders

If you're pregnant, check with your doctor before using this medication.

If you're an older adult, you may be especially prone to side effects from pimozide.

Taking pirbuterol

Dear Patient:

Your doctor has prescribed pirbuterol to open the air passages in your lungs and help you breathe easier. This medication is used to treat the symptoms of asthma, chronic bronchitis, emphysema, and other lung diseases. The label may read Maxair.

How to take pirbuterol
Pirbuterol comes in an aerosol inhaler. Follow your doctor's instructions for taking pirbuterol. Don't use more of it or take it more often than your doctor directs.

Shake the aerosol canister well before each use. Keep the spray away from the eyes because it may cause irritation. Also, don't take more than two inhalations at any one time unless your doctor gives you other instructions. Wait 1 to 2 minutes after the first inhalation to be sure that a second inhalation is necessary.

What to do if you miss a dose
If you're using the inhaler on a regular schedule, take a missed dose as soon as possible. Then take any remaining doses for that day at regularly spaced times. Don't double dose.

What to do about side effects
Let your doctor know if pirbuterol makes you feel nervous or dizzy or if you have headaches or trouble sleeping. Also tell him if you develop palpitations or a fast heartbeat and if your throat feels dry or sore.

Occasionally, pirbuterol causes changes in smell or taste. Don't worry. These effects are temporary and will go away when you stop using this medication.

What you must know about other drugs
Tell your doctor if you're taking beta blockers, such as propranolol (Inderal), to treat high blood pressure or a heart condition. Taking these medications with pirbuterol may reduce its helpful effects on your lungs.

Before you begin taking any new medication, check first with your doctor.

Special directions
• Tell your doctor if you have other medical problems, especially heart disease or a seizure disorder. Other medical problems may affect the use of this medication.
• If pirbuterol makes your throat and mouth feel dry, rinsing your mouth with water after each dose may help.
• If the dosage of pirbuterol you've been using no longer seems to work, check with your doctor. This may mean your condition is getting worse.

Important reminder
If you're pregnant, check with your doctor before using this medication.

Additional instructions

_____

_____

_____

_____

_____

_____

Taking piroxicam

Dear Patient:

Your doctor has prescribed piroxicam to treat your arthritis. This medication is used to relieve joint swelling, pain, and stiffness. The label may read Feldene.

How to take piroxicam

Piroxicam comes in capsules. Follow your doctor's instructions for taking this medication. To lessen stomach upset, take your dose with food or an antacid. Also, avoid lying down for 15 to 30 minutes after taking your dose to prevent irritation of your esophagus (food tube).

Take your medication faithfully every day, as directed. Realize that it may take several weeks before you start to feel better.

What to do if you miss a dose

If you remember the missed dose within 1 to 2 hours, take it as soon as possible. Otherwise, skip the missed dose and take your next dose on schedule. Don't double dose.

What to do about side effects

Occasionally, piroxicam can cause serious bleeding from the digestive tract. Call your doctor *at once* if you have warning signs of internal bleeding, such as black, tarry stools; severe abdominal or stomach pain; severe, continuing nausea or heartburn; or vomiting of blood or material that looks like coffee grounds.

Piroxicam also can cause nausea, heartburn, drowsiness, dizziness, and increased light sensitivity. Let your doctor know if these symptoms continue or become bothersome.

What you must know about other drugs

Tell your doctor if you're taking other medications. Don't use aspirin without your doctor's okay because piroxicam may not work as well. If you take lithium (Lithane), a drug for manic-depressive disorder, your doctor may need to adjust your lithium dosage.

Tell your doctor if you take blood thinners or diabetes medications because these drugs may cause harmful effects when used with piroxicam.

Special directions

• Tell your doctor if you have other medical problems, especially stomach ulcers or other digestive disorders, diabetes, and heart or liver disease. Also reveal if you've ever had an unusual or allergic reaction to aspirin or another medication.
• Because piroxicam may make you more sensitive to sunlight, limit your exposure to bright sun.
• If this medication makes you drowsy or dizzy, don't drive or perform other activities that require alertness.

Important reminders

If you're pregnant or breast-feeding, check with your doctor before using this medication.

If you're an older adult, you may be especially prone to side effects from piroxicam.

If you have diabetes, check carefully for infection because piroxicam may mask signs.

Additional instructions

Taking potassium chloride

Dear Patient:

Because your body needs additional potassium for good health, your doctor has prescribed supplements of potassium chloride. These supplements will help to restore potassium that your body may have lost after illness or treatment with certain medications. Brand names include K+ 10, Kaochlor 10%, and Kaon-Cl.

How to take potassium chloride
Potassium chloride comes in tablets, extended-release tablets and capsules, an oral liquid, and a soluble powder. If you're taking the *liquid* or *soluble powder,* dilute your dose in at least 4 ounces of cold water or juice to prevent stomach irritation. With the soluble powder, wait for any fizzing to stop before you drink the dissolved medication.

If you're taking the *extended-release capsules or tablets,* swallow them whole—don't chew, crush, or break them. If you have trouble swallowing, check with your doctor or pharmacist.

Take your medication with food or right after meals to prevent stomach upset.

What to do if you miss a dose
If you remember the missed dose within 2 hours, take it with food or liquids as soon as possible. Then go back to your regular dosing schedule. But if you don't remember until later, skip the missed dose and take your next dose on schedule. Don't double dose.

What to do about side effects
Stop taking this medication and call your doctor *right away* if you have:

- confusion
- irregular or slow heartbeat
- "pins and needles" feeling in your hands, feet, or lips
- shortness of breath or difficulty breathing
- unusual tiredness or weakness
- unexplained anxiety
- weakness or heaviness of your legs.

This medication may also cause nausea, vomiting, abdominal pain, or diarrhea. Call your doctor if these effects persist or become bothersome.

What you must know about other drugs
Tell your doctor if you're taking other medications. He may want you to avoid certain medications that slow intestinal movements (including anticholinergic drugs, such as atropine) because their use with potassium chloride may increase the risk of side effects.

Make sure your doctor knows if you're taking angiotensin-converting enzyme inhibitors (Vasotec) or potassium-sparing diuretics (Dyrenium) because their combined use may cause potassium levels to rise dangerously high.

Special directions
- Tell your doctor if you have other medical problems, especially Addison's disease, stomach ulcers, severe diarrhea, and kidney or heart disease. Other medical problems may affect the use of this medication.
- Don't use salt substitutes or drink low-salt milk unless your doctor tells you to do so. These products may contain potassium and might cause you to have too much potassium. Also, check for added potassium in the ingredients lists of processed foods.

Taking prazosin

Dear Patient:

Your doctor has prescribed prazosin to treat your high blood pressure. This medication works by relaxing blood vessels, allowing blood to pass through them more easily. This helps to lower blood pressure. The label may read Minipress.

How to take prazosin

Prazosin comes in capsules. Your doctor may direct you to take your first dose at bedtime because the first dose of prazosin sometimes causes dizziness and irregular heartbeat. If so, take care not to fall if you get up during the night.

Take your doses at the same times every day to help you remember to take your medication.

What to do if you miss a dose

Take it as soon as possible. However, if it's almost time for your next dose, skip the missed dose and take your next dose on schedule. Don't double dose.

What to do about side effects

Prazosin may make you feel dizzy, faint, or light-headed, especially when you get up suddenly from a lying or sitting position. Getting up slowly may help.

If this medication makes you feel drowsy, nauseous, or tired or gives you a headache, tell your doctor.

What you must know about other drugs

Tell your doctor if you're taking other medications. If you're taking beta blockers (for high blood pressure or a heart condition), you should know that combining these medications with prazosin may lower your blood pressure too much.

Special directions

• Tell your doctor if you have other medical problems, especially chest pain, kidney disease, or a heart condition. Other medical problems may affect the use of this medication.
• Remember, prazosin won't cure your high blood pressure, but it will help to control it. Therefore, you may have to take high blood pressure medication for the rest of your life.
• Along with prazosin, your doctor may prescribe a special low-salt diet for you because a diet too high in salt can increase blood pressure. If so, you need to limit salty foods, such as canned soup, pickles, ketchup, olives, hot dogs, soy sauce, and carbonated beverages.
• Keep all appointments for follow-up visits, even if you feel well, so your doctor can check your progress and adjust your medication, if necessary.

Important reminder

If you're an older adult, you may be especially prone to side effects from prazosin, especially dizziness and light-headedness. Therefore, take care to prevent falls.

Additional instructions

_____

_____

_____

_____

_____

Taking prednisone

Dear Patient:

Prednisone is used to relieve severe inflammation and to treat a number of diseases. Brand names include Deltasone, Orasone, and Sterapred.

How to take prednisone
Prednisone comes in tablet, oral solution, and syrup forms. Take your medication exactly as your doctor directs. Don't take more or less or use it more often or longer than prescribed. To prevent stomach upset, take your dose with food. Never stop taking prednisone suddenly without first checking with your doctor; doing so could be fatal.

What to do if you miss a dose
Adjust your dosing schedule as follows.

If you take one dose every other day, take the missed dose as soon as possible if you remember it the same morning. If not, wait and take it the next morning. Then skip a day and start your regular dosing schedule again.

If you take one dose daily, take the missed dose as soon as possible. If you don't remember until the next day, skip the missed dose and take your next dose on schedule. Don't double dose.

If you take several doses a day, take the missed dose as soon as possible, then go back to your regular dosing schedule. If you don't remember until your next dose is due, double the next dose.

What to do about side effects
Prednisone can act on your metabolism to make your potassium levels too low or your blood glucose level too high. Call your doctor *at once* if you have symptoms of low potassium: dizziness, tiredness, weakness, leg cramps, nau-

sea, or digestive upset. Also call him if you have symptoms of high blood glucose: frequent urination and thirst.

Also tell your doctor *right away* if you have bloody or black, tarry stools or difficulty sleeping. Predisone may also affect your mood and cause euphoria.

What you must know about other drugs
Tell your doctor if you're taking other medications. Check with him before you take aspirin or indomethacin (Indocin) because these pain relievers increase the risk of stomach distress when taken with prednisone. Also check with your doctor before you have vaccinations.

If you take barbiturates (sedatives) or medications for seizures or tuberculosis, your doctor may need to adjust your prednisone dosage.

Special directions
• Tell your doctor if you have other medical problems, especially ulcers, high blood pressure, diabetes, and kidney, liver, or bone disease. Other medical problems may affect the use of this medication.
• Before you have medical tests, tell the doctor you're taking prednisone because it may affect the test results.

Important reminders
If you're pregnant or breast-feeding, check with your doctor before taking prednisone.

If you're an athlete, be aware that the U.S. Olympic Committee and the National Collegiate Athletic Association have restrictions on prednisone use.

Taking primidone

Dear Patient:

Your doctor has prescribed primidone to treat your seizure disorder. Brand names include Myidone and Mysoline.

How to take primidone
Primidone comes in tablet and oral suspension forms. Take this medication exactly as your doctor directs. For best results, take it in regularly spaced doses, as ordered by your doctor.

Don't stop taking primidone suddenly without first checking with your doctor. He may want you to reduce your dosage gradually.

What to do if you miss a dose
Take it as soon as possible. But if it's within 1 hour of your next dose, skip the missed dose and take your next dose on schedule. Don't double dose.

What to do about side effects
Occasionally, primidone can make you feel drowsy or cause nausea, vomiting, double vision, or loss of coordination. Check with your doctor if you have any of these side effects, especially if they continue or become bothersome.

What you must know about alcohol and other drugs
Check with your doctor about drinking alcoholic beverages. Drinking alcoholic beverages while taking primidone may lead to oversedation. For the same reason, check with your doctor before you take other medications that slow down your nervous system, such as muscle relaxants, anesthetics, sleeping pills, and cold and flu remedies.

Tell your doctor if you're taking other medications. In particular, your doctor may need to watch your progress closely if you're taking phenytoin (Dilantin) or carbamazepine (Tegretol), two other medications used to prevent seizures.

Special directions
• Tell your doctor if you have other medical problems, especially asthma or other lung diseases, porphyria, and liver disease. Other medical problems may affect the use of this medication.
• Before you have diagnostic tests on your liver, tell the doctor you're taking primidone because it may affect the test results.
• Because primidone can make you drowsy, make sure you know how it affects you before you drive or perform other activities that might be dangerous if you're not fully alert.
• Keep all appointments for follow-up visits, so your doctor can check your progress.

Important reminders
If you're pregnant or breast-feeding, don't use primidone unless instructed by your doctor.

If you're an older adult, you may be especially prone to primidone's side effects.

If you're an athlete, you should know that primidone is banned and sometimes tested for by the U.S. Olympic Committee and the National Collegiate Athletic Association.

Additional instructions

_____

_____

_____

Taking probucol

Dear Patient:

Your doctor has prescribed probucol to lower your blood cholesterol. This medication may help to prevent medical problems caused by cholesterol clogging your blood vessels. The label may read Lorelco.

How to take probucol

Probucol comes in tablets. Follow your doctor's directions exactly. Take your medication with meals for best results.

Continue to take your medication, as directed, even if you feel well. Don't stop taking probucol without checking first with your doctor.

What to do if you miss a dose

Take it as soon as possible. But if it's almost time for your next dose, skip the missed dose and take your next dose on schedule. Don't double dose.

What to do about side effects

Let your doctor know if probucol causes any digestive distress, such as diarrhea, gas, abdominal pain, bloating, nausea, or vomiting. Also tell him if you begin to sweat heavily for no apparent reason.

What you must know about other drugs

Tell your doctor about other medications you're taking. In particular, your doctor should know if you're taking medications for depression or a heart condition. Use of such medications with probucol may cause serious irregularities in your heartbeat.

Also tell your doctor if you're taking another cholesterol-lowering drug called clofibrate (Atromid-S) because combined use with probucol may cause harmful effects.

Special directions

• Tell your doctor if you have other medical problems, especially gallbladder disease or gallstones, liver disease, or a heart condition. Other medical problems may affect the use of this medication.
• Carefully follow the special diet your doctor gave you because eating properly is necessary for probucol to work well.
• Because probucol is less effective if you're very overweight, your doctor may want you to go on a reducing diet. However, check with your doctor first before you start a weight-loss diet.
• Before you have medical tests, tell the doctor that you're taking probucol because it may affect the test results.
• Keep all appointments for follow-up visits so your doctor can check your progress and make sure your medication is working to lower your cholesterol levels.

Important reminders

If you're planning to become pregnant, don't use probucol. Use birth control for 6 months after stopping the medication so that your body can be entirely rid of probucol before you conceive. Likewise, if you're breast-feeding, don't use this medication.

Additional instructions

_____

_____

_____

Taking procarbazine

Dear Patient:

Procarbazine is prescribed to treat cancer. This medication stops the growth of cancer cells by destroying them. The label may read Matulane.

How to take procarbazine

Procarbazine comes in capsules. Follow your doctor's directions exactly. Don't use more or less or take procarbazine more often than prescribed. Don't stop taking this medication, even if it makes you feel ill, without first checking with your doctor.

If you vomit soon after taking a dose, check with your doctor to find out whether you should take another dose or wait until the next scheduled dose.

What to do if you miss a dose

If you remember the missed dose in a few hours, take it as soon as you remember. But if several hours have passed or if it's almost time for your next dose, skip the missed dose and take your next dose on schedule. Don't double dose.

What to do about side effects

Stop taking procarbazine and call your doctor *at once* if you have chest pain, rapid or irregular heartbeat, severe headache, or a stiff neck. Also call your doctor *right away* if you become extremely tired or weak or if you start to bruise or bleed easily.

This medication may cause nausea, vomiting, or loss of appetite. Ask your doctor, nurse, or pharmacist how to lessen these side effects. Watch for signs of infection, such as fever and sore throat, and report them to your doctor. Also report hallucinations.

What you must know about alcohol and other drugs

Don't drink alcoholic beverages while taking procarbazine because the combination can cause harmful side effects.

Also, tell your doctor about other medications you're taking. In general, you need to avoid medications that slow down the nervous system, such as tranquilizers, sleeping pills, anesthetics, and cold and flu remedies.

Don't use the pain reliever meperidine (Demerol) with procarbazine because this combination can cause life-threatening low blood pressure.

Also check with your doctor before you have vaccinations or take new medications—even aspirin.

Special directions

• Tell your doctor if you have other medical problems, especially an infection or liver or kidney disease.
• Don't eat foods that have a high tyramine content, such as cheeses and Chianti wine. Ask your doctor for a complete list of foods to avoid.
• Because procarbazine may make you drowsy, make sure you know how you react to it before you drive or perform other activities that might be dangerous if you're not fully alert.

Important reminders

Tell your doctor if you're pregnant or intending to have children in the future. If you're breast-feeding or plan to do so during treatment, also check with your doctor.

Older adults may be especially sensitive to side effects from procarbazine.

Taking prochlorperazine

Dear Patient:

Prochlorperazine is used to relieve or prevent nausea and vomiting. It's also used to manage some psychiatric problems. The label may read Compazine.

How to take prochlorperazine
This medication comes in several forms. Follow your doctor's directions exactly. If you're taking prochlorperazine by mouth, take it with food, water, or milk. If you're taking the extended-release capsules, swallow them whole—don't crush, break, or chew them.

What to do if you miss a dose
If you take one dose a day, take the missed dose as soon as possible. But if you don't remember the missed dose until the next day, skip it and go back to your regular dosing schedule.

If you take more than one dose a day, take the missed dose right away if you remember within 1 hour or so. But if you don't remember until later, skip it and take your next dose on schedule. Don't double dose.

What to do about side effects
Call your doctor *right away* if you have fever, chills, headache, extreme tiredness, or skin problems.

Check with your doctor if you feel dizzy or have blurred vision, a fast heartbeat, dry mouth, constipation, or difficulty urinating. This medication also can cause a movement disorder called tardive dyskinesia, so be sure to report any uncontrolled movements of your mouth, tongue, or other body parts.

What you must know about alcohol and other drugs
Don't drink alcoholic beverages while taking prochlorperazine because the combination can cause oversedation. For the same reason, avoid medications that slow down the nervous system, including tranquilizers, sleeping pills, and cold and flu remedies.

Tell your doctor about other medications you're taking. In particular, your doctor may want to watch your progress closely if you're taking medications for Parkinson's disease or depression.

If you take antacids, take them at least 2 hours before or after you take prochlorperazine.

Special directions
• Tell your doctor if you have other medical conditions, especially heart or blood disease, glaucoma, seizure disorder, Parkinson's disease, or kidney or liver problems. Other medical problems may affect the use of this medication.
• Because prochlorperazine may make you dizzy, make sure you know how you react to it before you drive or perform other activities requiring alertness.
• This medication may make you more sensitive to light, so cover up outdoors and limit your sun exposure.

Important reminders
If you're pregnant or breast-feeding, check with your doctor before taking this medication.

Children and older adults are especially prone to prochlorperazine's side effects.

Be aware that this medication is banned and may be tested for by the U.S. Olympic Committee and the National Collegiate Athletic Association.

Taking promazine

Dear Patient:

Promazine is used to treat nervous, mental, and emotional disorders. The label may read Sparine.

How to take promazine
This medication comes in tablets and a syrup. Follow your doctor's directions exactly. Take your medication with food or a full glass (8 ounces) of water or milk.

What to do if you miss a dose
If you take more than one dose a day, take the missed dose right away if you remember within 1 hour or so. But if you don't remember until later, skip it and take your next dose on schedule. Don't double dose.

What to do about side effects
Call your doctor *right away* if you have fever, chills, headache, or extreme tiredness. Also call *at once* if you start sweating heavily or have a fast heartbeat or difficulty breathing.

Check with your doctor if you feel dizzy, your skin turns yellow, or you start to have blurred vision, dry mouth, constipation, or difficulty urinating.

Promazine can cause a movement disorder called tardive dyskinesia, so be sure to report any uncontrolled movements of your mouth, tongue, or other body parts.

What you must know about alcohol and other drugs
Don't drink alcoholic beverages while taking promazine because the combination can cause oversedation. For the same reason, avoid medications that slow down the nervous system, including tranquilizers, sleeping pills, and cold and flu remedies.

Tell your doctor about other medications you're taking. In particular, your doctor needs to know if you're taking blood thinners or medications for Parkinson's disease, depression, manic-depressive disorder, or high blood pressure.

If you take antacids, take them at least 2 hours before or after you take promazine.

Special directions
• Tell your doctor if you have other medical conditions, especially heart or blood disease, glaucoma, a seizure disorder, Parkinson's disease, or kidney, lung, or liver problems. Other medical problems may affect the use of this medication.
• Because promazine may make you dizzy, make sure you know how you react to it before you drive or perform other activities requiring alertness.
• This medication may make you more sensitive to light, so cover up outdoors and limit your sun exposure.

Important reminders
If you're pregnant or breast-feeding, check with your doctor before taking this medication.

Children and older adults are especially prone to promazine's side effects.

If you're an athlete, you should know that this medication is banned by the U.S. Olympic Committee and the National Collegiate Athletic Association.

Additional instructions

_____

_____

Taking propafenone

Dear Patient:

Your doctor has prescribed propafenone to correct your irregular heartbeat to a normal rhythm. The label may read Rythmol.

How to take propafenone
Propafenone comes in tablets. Take this medication exactly as your doctor directs even if you feel well. Don't take more or less of it than prescribed.

For best results, take propafenone at evenly spaced times day and night. To prevent stomach upset, take your medication with food.

What to do if you miss a dose
If you remember the missed dose within 4 hours, take it as soon as possible. But if you don't remember until later, skip it and take your next dose on schedule. Don't double dose.

What to do about side effects
Call your doctor *right away* if you have chest pain, palpitations, a fast or irregular heartbeat, difficulty breathing, or unusual weakness and fatigue.

This medication also may make you dizzy or cause taste changes; let your doctor know if these side effects continue or become bothersome.

What you must know about other drugs
Tell your doctor if you're taking other medications. Other medications can interact with propafenone and possibly cause problems. In particular, your doctor needs to know if you're taking blood thinners, other heart medications (such as digoxin), the ulcer drug cimetidine (Tagamet), or high blood pressure medications.

Special directions
• Tell your doctor if you have other medical conditions, especially asthma, bronchitis, emphysema, and kidney or liver disease. Also reveal if you've had other heart problems, such as a recent heart attack, or if you have a pacemaker. Other medical problems may affect the use of this medication.
• Because propafenone may make you dizzy, make sure you know how you react to it before you drive or perform other activities that might be dangerous if you're not fully alert.
• This medication may make you more sensitive to light, so cover up outdoors and limit your sun exposure.
• Before you have surgery (including dental surgery) or emergency treatment, tell the doctor or dentist that you're taking propafenone.
• Your doctor may want you to carry a medical identification card or wear a medical identification bracelet stating that you're taking propafenone.

Important reminder
If you're pregnant, check with your doctor before taking this medication.

Additional instructions

_____

_____

_____

_____

_____

_____

Taking propantheline

Dear Patient:

Your doctor has prescribed propantheline to help relieve stomach cramps, spasms, and acid stomach. Brand names include Norpanth and Pro-Banthine.

How to take propantheline

Take this medication exactly as the label directs. Take it 30 to 60 minutes before meals. And take your bedtime dose at least 2 hours after your last meal of the day. Swallow the tablets whole; don't chew or crush them.

What to do if you miss a dose

If you forget to take a dose, don't make it up. Just start your schedule all over again with the next dose. Never take a double dose.

What to do about side effects

Call your doctor *right away* if you develop difficulty with urinating or swallowing, dizziness, drowsiness, eye pain, headaches, nervousness, rapid heartbeat or palpitations, or a rash.

Also call him if you have constipation, decreased sweating, heartburn, nausea, or vomiting or if your eyes are unusually sensitive to bright light.

What you must know about alcohol and other drugs

Avoid alcoholic beverages because they may worsen your condition. Make sure your doctor knows all the medications you're taking. Before you take other medications, consult your doctor or pharmacist. Other medications can interact with propantheline and possibly cause problems.

Special directions

• Tell your doctor if you have other medical problems, especially glaucoma, difficult urination, myasthenia gravis, or diseases of the digestive tract, heart, liver, or kidneys. Other medical problems may affect the use of this medication.
• Because propantheline may make you drowsy, make sure you know how you react to it before you drive or perform other activities that might be dangerous if you're not fully alert.
• Your body sweats less while you're taking this medication. To avoid heatstroke, don't exercise too strenuously or stay outside too long in hot weather.
• If your eyes seem unusually sensitive to sunlight, protect them by wearing sunglasses or a wide-brimmed hat.
• While you're taking this medication, avoid eating spicy or acidic foods because they can upset your stomach.
• To prevent constipation, be sure to drink lots of extra water or other fluids.

Important reminders

If you're pregnant or breast-feeding, check with your doctor before taking this medication.

Older adults may be especially prone to side effects from propantheline.

Additional instructions

_____

_____

_____

_____

_____

Taking propoxyphene

Dear Patient:

Your doctor has prescribed propoxyphene to help relieve your pain. The label may read Darvocet-N, Darvon, or Dolene.

How to take propoxyphene

A narcotic analgesic, propoxyphene comes in three forms: tablets, capsules, and an oral suspension. Take propoxyphene exactly as the label directs. If you feel your medication isn't working well, don't take more than the prescribed dose. Check with your doctor instead. If you take too much of this medication or take it for too long, it could become habit-forming.

Also, don't stop taking propoxyphene suddenly. Your doctor may want to reduce your dosage gradually to lessen the chance of withdrawal side effects.

What to do if you miss a dose

Take it as soon as you remember. However, if it's almost time for your next dose, skip the missed dose and go back to your regular dosing schedule. Don't double the dose.

What to do about side effects

The most common side effect from propoxyphene is dizziness. This medication may also make you feel drowsy or cause nausea or vomiting. Let your doctor know if these symptoms continue or become bothersome.

What you must know about alcohol and other drugs

Avoid drinking alcoholic beverages while taking propoxyphene because the combination can cause oversedation. For the same reason, check with your doctor before using medications that slow down the central nervous system, such as sleeping pills, tranquilizers, sedatives, and many cold, flu, and allergy remedies.

Special directions

• Tell your doctor if you have other medical problems, especially heart, liver, lung, or kidney disease. Also tell him if you have asthma, a seizure disorder, or a history of drug or alcohol abuse. Other medical problems may affect the use of this medication.
• Because propoxyphene may make you dizzy, make sure you know how you react to it before you drive or perform other activities that might be dangerous if you're not fully alert.
• If this medication makes your mouth feel dry, you may use sugarless hard candy or gum, ice chips, or a saliva substitute. If your dry mouth continues for more than 2 weeks, see your dentist.

Important reminders

If you're pregnant or breast-feeding, check with your doctor before taking this medication.

If you're an older adult, you may be especially prone to propoxyphene's side effects.

If you're an athlete, you should know that propoxyphene is banned and tested for by the U.S. Olympic Committee.

Additional instructions

_____

_____

_____

Taking propranolol

Dear Patient:

Propranolol is prescribed to relieve angina (chest pain) and treat certain heart conditions. It may also be used to prevent some kinds of severe headaches. The label may read Inderal, Inderal LA, or Ipran.

How to take propranolol

Propranolol comes in these forms: tablets, extended-release capsules, and an oral solution. Take propranolol exactly as the doctor orders. Take it at the same time each day, so you're less likely to forget. Take propranolol with meals.

Once a day, preferably before the first dose, take your pulse (if instructed by your doctor). If your pulse rate is less than 50 beats a minute, don't take the next dose. Instead, call your doctor as soon as possible.

Don't stop taking propranolol suddenly—doing so may increase your angina.

What to do if you miss a dose

Take the missed dose right away if you remember within 1 hour or so. However, if it's within 8 hours of your next regular dose, skip the missed dose and resume your regular dosage schedule. Never take a double dose.

What to do about side effects

Call your doctor *right away* if you have a persistent cough, shortness of breath, difficulty breathing, unusual tiredness, lethargy, restlessness, and anxiety.

Check with your doctor if you feel depressed or dizzy or can't sleep at night. Also call him if you start wheezing, develop a rash, or have a very slow heart rate.

What you must know about other drugs

To avoid harmful interactions, tell your doctor if you're taking other medications. Also, check with him before you take new medications.

In particular, your doctor needs to know if you're taking insulin or other drugs for diabetes; the ulcer drug cimetidine (Tagamet); asthma medications; and medications for heart conditions.

Special directions

• Tell your doctor if you have other medical problems, especially other heart problems, asthma, lung disease, diabetes, low blood glucose, an overactive thyroid, and liver disease. Other medical problems may affect the use of this medication.
• Because propranolol may make you dizzy, make sure you know how you react to it before you drive or perform other activities that might be dangerous if you're not fully alert.
• To minimize dizziness, rise slowly from a sitting or lying position and avoid sudden position changes.
• To avoid insomnia, take your last dose no later than 2 hours before bedtime.
• Before you have surgery, tell the doctor that you're taking propranolol.

Important reminders

If you're pregnant or breast-feeding, check with your doctor before taking this medication.

If you're an athlete, you should know that propranolol is banned and tested for by the U.S. Olympic Committee and the National Collegiate Athletic Association.

Taking propylthiouracil

Dear Patient:

Because your thyroid gland makes too much thyroid hormone, your doctor has prescribed propylthiouracil. This medication works by making it harder for the body to use iodine to make thyroid hormone.

How to take propylthiouracil

Propylthiouracil comes in tablets. Take your medication exactly as the label directs. Don't take more or less or use it longer or more often than your doctor prescribed.

Take your tablets with meals to prevent stomach upset unless your doctor gives you other instructions. Also, if you're taking more than one dose a day, try to take your medication at evenly spaced times day and night.

Don't stop taking propylthiouracil without first checking with your doctor.

What to do if you miss a dose

Take it as soon as you remember. However, if it's almost time for your next dose, take both doses together. Then go back to your regular dosing schedule. If you miss more than one dose, check with your doctor.

What to do about side effects

Call your doctor *right away* if your skin starts to turn yellow, you gain unexpected weight, or your feet and ankles start to swell. Also call your doctor *at once* if you have fever, chills, a sore throat, or mouth sores.

This medication may cause nausea, vomiting, or easy bruising or bleeding. If these side effects occur, check with your doctor; your dosage may need to be adjusted.

What you must know about other drugs

Check with your doctor before you use other prescription or nonprescription medications. In particular, your doctor may want you to avoid iodine-containing medications, such as some cough medicines and potassium iodide (Pima). Using these medications with propylthiouracil may lead to a goiter or decrease thyroid activity too much.

Special directions

• Tell your doctor if you have other medical problems, especially an infection or liver disease. Other medical problems may affect the use of this medication.
• Check with your doctor *right away* if you're injured or get an infection or illness of any kind. Your doctor may want you to stop taking propylthiouracil or change your dosage.
• Before you have medical tests, tell the doctor that you're taking propylthiouracil because it may affect the test results.
• Ask your doctor if it's okay for you to eat iodine-containing foods, such as iodized salt and shellfish.

Important reminder

If you're pregnant or breast-feeding, check with your doctor before using this medication.

Additional instructions

_____

_____

_____

_____

Taking pseudoephedrine

Dear Patient:

Pseudoephedrine is used to relieve stuffiness of your nose or sinuses. It's also used to relieve ear congestion caused by ear infection or inflammation. Brand names include Cenafed, Sudafed, and Sufedrin.

How to take pseudoephedrine
This medication comes in tablets, extended-release tablets and capsules, a syrup, and an oral solution. If your doctor prescribed this medication, follow his directions exactly. If you bought the medication without a prescription, carefully read the package instructions before using.

If you're taking the extended-release tablets or capsules, swallow them whole; don't chew, crush, or break them.

To prevent trouble with sleeping, take your last dose for the day a few hours before bedtime.

What to do if you miss a dose
If you remember the missed dose within 1 hour or so, take it right away. If you don't remember until later, skip the missed dose and take your next dose on schedule. Don't take a double dose.

What to do about side effects
Check with your doctor if this medication makes you feel anxious, nervous, or restless or causes palpitations or trouble sleeping.

What you must know about other drugs
Check with your doctor before you use new prescription or nonprescription medications. Also, tell your doctor about other medications you're taking, especially medications for high blood pressure.

If you're taking a monoamine oxidase (MAO) inhibitor (a drug used to treat depression and other emotional problems), don't use pseudoephedrine because the combination can cause a life-threatening rise in blood pressure.

Special directions
• Tell your doctor if you have other medical problems, especially high blood pressure, heart disease, an overactive thyroid, diabetes, or difficult urination. Other medical problems may affect the use of this medication.
• If pseudoephedrine makes your mouth feel dry, use sugarless gum or hard candy, melt bits of ice in your mouth, or use a saliva substitute.
• If you don't feel better within 5 days or if you also have a high fever, check with your doctor. These signs may mean you have some other medical problem.

Important reminders
If you're pregnant or breast-feeding, check with your doctor before using pseudoephedrine.

If you're an athlete, you should know that pseudoephedrine is banned and tested for by the U.S. Olympic Committee.

Additional instructions

_____

_____

_____

_____

Taking pseudoephedrine with triprolidine

Dear Patient:

This medication contains a decongestant (pseudoephedrine) and an antihistamine (triprolidine). It's used to relieve a stuffy nose caused by colds or hay fever. Brand names may include Actifed, AllerAct Decongestant, and Tripodrine.

How to take this drug

This medication comes in tablets, capsules, extended-release capsules, and a syrup. Follow your doctor's directions exactly. If you bought the medication without a prescription, carefully read the package instructions before using it. If this medication irritates your stomach, take it with food or a full glass (8 ounces) of milk or water.

If you're taking the extended-release capsules, swallow them whole. If the capsule is too big to swallow easily, mix its contents with applesauce and swallow without chewing.

If this medication causes trouble with sleeping, take your last dose a few hours before bedtime.

What to do if you miss a dose

Take it as soon as possible. But if it's almost time for your next dose, skip the missed dose and take your next dose on schedule. Don't take a double dose.

What to do about side effects

Check with your doctor if this medication makes you feel anxious, nervous, or restless or causes palpitations or trouble sleeping.

The antihistamine in this medication may make you feel drowsy, dizzy, or less alert than normal. Tell your doctor if these symptoms continue or become bothersome.

What you must know about alcohol and other drugs

Avoid alcoholic beverages while taking this medication because the combination may cause oversedation. For the same reason, don't use medications that slow down the central nervous system, such as sleeping pills, tranquilizers, and other medications for colds, flu, and allergies.

Check with your doctor or pharmacist before you take other medications, especially those for appetite control, high blood pressure, stomach cramps, and depression.

Special directions

• Tell your doctor if you have other medical problems, especially asthma, diabetes, an enlarged prostate, glaucoma, high blood pressure, an overactive thyroid, or heart or blood vessel disease. Other medical problems may affect the use of this medication.
• Because this medication may make you drowsy, make sure you know how you react to it before you drive or perform other activities that require alertness.

Important reminders

If you're pregnant, check with your doctor before using this medication. Don't use it if you're breast-feeding.

Children and older adults may be especially sensitive to side effects.

If you're an athlete, you should know that the U.S. Olympic Committee tests for pseudoephedrine. Athletes may be disqualified if amounts in the urine exceed certain limits.

Taking psyllium

Dear Patient:

This medication is used to encourage bowel movements to relieve constipation. Brand names include Cillium, Metamucil, and Perdiem Plain.

How to take psyllium

Psyllium comes in the form of chewable pieces, wafers, and mixable granules and powders. If your doctor prescribed this medication, follow his directions exactly. If you bought psyllium without a prescription, carefully read the package instructions before using it.

If you're using the dry powder or granule forms, always mix your dose with liquid first. Never swallow the dry powder or granules. After mixing, drink your medication immediately—or it may congeal.

Drink lots of fluids while taking psyllium. Drink a full glass (8 ounces) of cold water or fruit juice with each dose. Then drink a second glass of water or juice. Throughout the day, try to drink at least 6 to 8 full glasses of liquid. Don't take this medication before meals because you may no longer be hungry.

What to do about side effects

If you take too much psyllium or swallow the dry powder or granules without liquid, this medication may block the digestive tract. Call your doctor *right away* if you have severe constipation or difficulty swallowing.

Psyllium also may cause some digestive distress, such as nausea, vomiting, abdominal cramps, or diarrhea. Check with your doctor if these symptoms continue or become bothersome. Also tell him if you develop a rash while taking psyllium.

Special directions

• Tell your doctor if you have other medical problems, especially ulcers or other digestive disease. Also mention if you're on a low-sodium diet because this medication is high in sodium. And tell your doctor if you must limit foods that contain phenylalanine.

• Don't get into the "laxative habit." If you overuse laxatives, you may become dependent on these medications to have a bowel movement. In severe cases, laxative overuse may damage the nerves, muscles, and other tissues of the digestive tract.

• You may have to wait 2 to 3 days for this medication to work. However, many people have bowel movements within 12 hours after taking psyllium.

• To prevent constipation, eat plenty of whole-grain foods, such as bran and other cereals, as well as vegetables and fresh fruits. Getting regular exercise and drinking lots of fluids also will help to keep you regular.

Important reminder

If you have diabetes, choose a sugar-free brand of psyllium.

Additional instructions

_____

_____

_____

_____

_____

_____

Applying pyrethrins with piperonyl butoxide

Dear Patient:

This medication is used to treat head, body, and pubic lice infections. The lice absorb this medication, which kills them.

If you're using the *shampoo,* the label may read Tisit Shampoo or A-200 Shampoo Concentrate. If you're using the *topical gel or solution,* the label may read Tisit or A-200 Gel Concentrate.

How to apply this drug
If your doctor prescribed this medication, follow his directions exactly. If you bought it without a prescription, carefully read the package instructions before using it.

If you're using the *gel* or *solution,* follow these steps: Apply enough medication to thoroughly wet the skin or dry hair and scalp. Let the medication remain on the treated area for exactly 10 minutes. Wash the treated area with warm water and soap or regular shampoo. Rinse thoroughly and dry with a clean towel.

If you're using the *shampoo,* follow these steps: Apply enough medication to thoroughly wet the dry hair and scalp. Let the medication remain on the treated scalp for exactly 10 minutes. Work the shampoo into a lather, using a small amount of water. Rinse well and dry with a clean towel. After rinsing and drying, use a nit-removal comb to remove dead lice and eggs (nits) from your hair.

Wash your hands right after using this medication. Repeat the treatment 1 week to 10 days after the first treatment, as directed.

Keep this medication away from your eyes, mouth, and nose. Also, apply it in a well-ventilated room, so you don't inhale the vapors.

What to do about side effects
With repeated use, this medication may irritate your skin. Call your doctor if you develop a rash or an infection.

Special directions
• If you have hay fever or are allergic to ragweed, check with your doctor before you use this medication. Also, if you have a skin problem, such as severe inflammation or rawness, see your doctor before applying the drug.
• To prevent the spread of lice, machine wash all clothing, bedding, towels, and washcloths in very hot water. Then dry them using the hot cycle of a dryer for at least 20 minutes. Clothing or bedding that can't be washed should be dry-cleaned and sealed in a plastic bag for 2 weeks.
• Wash all hairbrushes and combs in very hot soapy water for 5 to 10 minutes.
• Clean the house or room by thoroughly vacuuming upholstered furniture, rugs, and floors.
• If more than one person lives in your household, all members should be checked for lice and, if they're infected, treated.

Additional instructions

_____

_____

_____

Taking quinidine

Dear Patient:

This medication is used to correct an irregular heartbeat to a normal rhythm or to slow an overactive heart. Brand names include Duraquin, Cardioquin, and Quinora.

How to take quinidine

Quinidine comes in the form of capsules, tablets, and extended-release tablets. Follow your doctor's directions for taking this medication exactly, even if you feel well.

To make sure your medication is well absorbed, take your dose with a full glass (8 ounces) of water on an empty stomach 1 hour before or 2 hours after meals. However, if you have stomach upset, your doctor may want you to take your dose with food or milk.

If you're taking the extended-release tablets, swallow them whole—don't chew, crush, or break them.

Don't stop taking quinidine without first checking with your doctor.

What to do if you miss a dose

If you remember the missed dose within 2 hours, take it as soon as possible. However, if you don't remember until later, skip the missed dose and take your next dose on schedule. Don't take a double dose.

What to do about side effects

Call your doctor *at once* if you have blurred vision or other vision changes; dizziness, light-headedness, or fainting; fever; severe headache; hearing changes, such as buzzing in the ears; or wheezing, shortness of breath, or trouble breathing.

Check with your doctor if this medication causes nausea, vomiting, or diarrhea.

What you must know about other drugs

Tell your doctor if you're taking other medications. Also check with him before you take new medications. In particular, your doctor needs to know if you use blood thinners, other heart medications, sedatives, seizure medications (for example, barbiturates), antacids, the ulcer drug cimetidine (Tagamet), and medications that make the urine less acidic, such as acetazolamide (Diamox).

Special directions

• Tell your doctor if you have other medical problems, especially asthma, emphysema, blood diseases, myasthenia gravis, an overactive thyroid, psoriasis, and kidney or liver disease. Other medical problems may affect the use of this medication.
• Keep all appointments for follow-up visits so your doctor can check your progress.
• Before having surgery (including dental surgery), tell the doctor or dentist that you're taking this medication.

Important reminder

If you're pregnant, check with your doctor before using quinidine.

Additional instructions

_____

_____

_____

Taking ranitidine

Dear Patient:

Ranitidine is prescribed to treat duodenal and gastric ulcers and to prevent their return. It's also used to treat some conditions in which the stomach makes too much acid. The label may read Zantac.

How to take ranitidine
Ranitidine comes in syrup and tablet forms. Follow your doctor's directions for taking this medication exactly. If you're taking one dose daily, take it at bedtime, unless otherwise directed. If you're taking two doses daily, take one in the morning and one at bedtime. If you're taking several doses a day, take them with meals and at bedtime for best results.

Take this medication for the full time of treatment, even after you start to feel better.

What to do if you miss a dose
Take it as soon as possible. However, if it's almost time for your next dose, skip the missed dose and take your next dose on schedule. Don't double dose.

What to do about side effects
Check with your doctor if this medication makes you feel dizzy, confused, nauseous, or constipated. Also let your doctor know if you get a rash or headache or if your heart starts to beat very slowly.

What you must know about other drugs
Tell your doctor if you're taking other medications. Also check with him before you take new medications. If you're using antacids to relieve stomach pain, wait 30 minutes to 1 hour between taking the antacid and ranitidine.

To prevent harmful drug interactions, your doctor also needs to know if you use blood thinners, muscle relaxants, or medications for diabetes or an irregular heartbeat.

Special directions
• Tell your doctor if you have other medical problems, especially kidney or liver disease. Other medical problems may affect the use of this medication.
• Before you have skin tests or tests to determine how much acid your stomach produces, tell the doctor you're taking ranitidine. This medication may affect the test results.
• Because ranitidine may make you drowsy or dizzy, make sure you know how you react to it before you drive or perform other activities that might be dangerous if you're not fully alert.
• Don't smoke while taking ranitidine because cigarette smoking reduces its effectiveness.
• Stay away from foods and other substances that can irritate your stomach, such as aspirin, citrus products, and carbonated drinks.

Important reminders
If you're pregnant, check with your doctor before using ranitidine. If you're breast-feeding, don't use this medication unless instructed to do so by your doctor.

Older adults may be especially prone to ranitidine's side effects, particularly confusion and dizziness.

Additional instructions

_____

_____

Taking reserpine

Dear Patient:

Your doctor has prescribed reserpine to lower your high blood pressure. Brand names include Serpalan and Serpasil.

How to take reserpine
This medication comes in tablets. Follow your doctor's directions for taking reserpine exactly, even if you feel well. If this medication upsets your stomach, take your tablets with meals or milk.

Don't stop taking reserpine suddenly without checking first with your doctor.

What to do if you miss a dose
Skip it. Don't take the missed dose and don't double the next one. Instead, take your next dose on schedule.

What to do about side effects
Call your doctor *right away* if you start having nightmares. Also call if you feel drowsy, dizzy, depressed, faint, or unusually nervous. Tell him if you start to gain weight unexpectedly or if you have a dry mouth, stuffy nose, slow heartbeat, or stomach upset.

If you're male, let your doctor know if you become impotent while taking this medication.

What you must know about alcohol and other drugs
Don't drink alcoholic beverages except with your doctor's okay because combined use with reserpine may cause oversedation. For the same reason, check with your doctor before you take medications that slow down the nervous system, such as cold, flu, and allergy remedies; sleeping pills; and tranquilizers.

Tell your doctor if you're taking other medications. Also check with him before you take new prescription or nonprescription medications.

To prevent harmful drug interactions, tell your doctor if you take monoamine oxidase (MAO) inhibitors (such as Marplan) for depression or other emotional problems.

Special directions
• Tell your doctor if you have other medical problems, especially asthma, allergies, seizure disorder, stomach ulcers, depression, Parkinson's disease, pheochromocytoma, or heart or kidney disease. Other medical problems may affect the use of this medication.
• Because reserpine may make you drowsy or dizzy, make sure you know how you react to it before you drive or perform other activities that might be dangerous if you're not fully alert.
• If reserpine makes your mouth dry, use sugarless gum or hard candy, ice chips, or a saliva substitute.
• To prevent dizziness, get up slowly when you rise from a sitting or lying position.

Important reminders
If you're pregnant or breast-feeding, don't use reserpine without discussing the risks and benefits with your doctor.

If you're an older adult, you may be especially prone to reserpine's side effects, especially drowsiness and dizziness.

Additional instructions

_____

_____

Taking reserpine and hydralazine with hydrochlorothiazide

Dear Patient:

Your doctor has prescribed this combination medication to lower your high blood pressure. Brand names include Ser-Ap-Es, Cam-Ap-Es, and Unipres.

How to take this drug

Follow your doctor's directions exactly for taking this medication. If the tablets upset your stomach, take them with meals or milk.

This medication may make you urinate more frequently. Adjusting your dose may help to prevent this increase in urine from affecting your sleep. If you take one dose daily, take it in the morning after breakfast. If you take more than one dose daily, take the last dose no later than 6 p.m., unless your doctor gives you other instructions.

What to do if you miss a dose

Take it as soon as possible. But if it's almost time for your next dose, skip the missed dose and take your next dose on schedule. Don't double dose.

What to do about side effects

Call your doctor *right away* if you start having nightmares. Also call if you feel drowsy, dizzy, depressed, faint, unusually nervous, or weak. And tell him if you start to gain weight unexpectedly or if you have a dry mouth, stuffy nose, slow heartbeat, or stomach upset.

If you're male, let your doctor know if you become impotent while taking this medication.

What you must know about alcohol and other drugs

Don't drink alcoholic beverages except with your doctor's okay because combined use with this medication may cause oversedation. For the same reason, check with your doctor before you take medications that slow down the nervous system, such as cold, flu, and allergy remedies; sleeping pills; and tranquilizers.

Tell your doctor if you're taking other medications. Also check him with before you take new prescription or nonprescription medications.

To prevent harmful drug interactions, tell your doctor if you take lithium (Lithane), heart medication, or adrenocorticoids (cortisone-like medications). Also reveal if you take monoamine oxidase (MAO) inhibitors (such as Marplan) for depression or other emotional problems.

Special directions

• Tell your doctor if you have other medical problems, especially asthma, allergies, diabetes, seizure disorder, stomach ulcers, gallstones, gout, depression, Parkinson's disease, pheochromocytoma, or heart, kidney, or liver disease. Other medical problems may affect the use of this medication.
• Because this medication may make you drowsy or dizzy, make sure you know how you react to it before you drive or perform other activities that might be dangerous if you're not fully alert.

Important reminders

If you're pregnant or breast-feeding, don't use this medication without discussing the risks and benefits with your doctor.

If you're an older adult, you may be especially prone to this medication's side effects.

Taking rifampin

Dear Patient:

Your doctor has prescribed rifampin to treat your tuberculosis. Brand names include Rifadin and Rimactane.

How to take rifampin
Take this medication exactly as directed for as long as the doctor prescribes. Take it 1 hour before or 2 hours after meals. However, if rifampin upsets your stomach, your doctor may tell you to take it with food.

What to do if you miss a dose
Take it as soon as possible. But if it's almost time for your next dose, skip the missed dose and take your next dose on schedule. Don't double dose.

What to do about side effects
Call your doctor *immediately* if you have any of the following: appetite loss, bloody or cloudy urine, bone and muscle pain, breathing problems, chills, dizziness, headache, nausea, or vomiting.

Also call him promptly if you experience shivering, sore throat, unusual bleeding or bruising, fever, joint pain and inflammation (especially in the feet), abdominal pain, yellowish skin or eyes (jaundice), dark urine, or light-colored stools.

Some side effects may subside as your body adjusts to the medication. These include diarrhea, itching, reddened skin or a rash, sore mouth or tongue, and stomach cramps.

What you must know about alcohol and other drugs
Avoid drinking alcoholic beverages while taking rifampin because the combination may damage your liver.

Tell your doctor if you're taking other prescription or nonprescription medications because rifampin decreases the effectiveness of many other medications. For instance, if you're taking an oral contraceptive, you may need to use another method of birth control. If you're taking a heart medication, a blood thinner, or diabetes medication, the doctor may need to change the dosage.

Special directions
• Tell your doctor if you have other medical problems, especially liver disease or alcoholism. Other medical problems may affect the use of this medication.
• Remember, rifampin will turn your body fluids and secretions reddish orange or reddish brown. It can permanently discolor soft contact lenses, but it doesn't affect hard lenses.
• Call your doctor if your symptoms seem worse or don't subside after 2 to 3 weeks of therapy.
• Because rifampin may make you drowsy, make sure you know how you react to it before you drive or perform other activities that might be dangerous if you're not fully alert.
• Take precautions to avoid injuries or accidental bleeding because rifampin affects the blood's clotting ability.

Important reminders
If you're female, use contraception while taking rifampin because it can cause birth defects.

If you're pregnant or breast-feeding, don't use this medication without careful discussion with your doctor.

Using ophthalmic scopolamine

Dear Patient:

Your doctor has prescribed scopolamine eyedrops to dilate your pupils. This medication is used before eye examinations, before and after eye surgery, and to treat certain eye conditions. The label on your eyedrop container may read Isopto Hyoscine.

How to use scopolamine eyedrops

First, wash your hands. Then follow these steps: Tilt your head back. With your middle finger, apply pressure to the inside corner of the eye. (And continue to apply pressure for 2 to 3 minutes after you've instilled the drops in your eye.) Using your index finger, pull the lower eyelid away from the eye to form a pouch. Squeeze the drops into the pouch. Gently close your eyes. Don't blink. To help the eyedrops become absorbed, keep your eyes closed for 1 to 2 minutes. Wash your hands again.

To keep your eyedrop bottle as germ-free as possible, take care not to touch the applicator tip to any surface, including your eye. Close the bottle tightly between uses.

What to do if you miss a dose

Instill the drops as soon as possible. However, if it's almost time for your next dose, adjust your dosing schedule as follows.

If you instill one dose daily, skip the missed dose. Instill the next day's dose on schedule.

If you instill more than one dose daily, skip the missed dose and instill the next dose on schedule. Don't double dose.

What to do about side effects

If you begin to have blurred vision or irritated eyes, check with your doctor, especially if these symptoms continue or become bothersome. You may also notice that your eyes are unusually sensitive to bright lights.

Special directions

• Tell your doctor if you have other medical problems, especially glaucoma, other eye problems, Down's syndrome, or spastic paralysis. Other medical problems may affect the use of this medication.
• Because scopolamine eyedrops may blur your vision, make sure you can see clearly before you drive or perform other activities that might be dangerous if you're not seeing well.
• Expect your eyes to be more sensitive than usual to light while using this medication. Wear sunglasses to protect your eyes when you're outdoors or in a brightly lighted room.

Important reminders

If you're an older adult, you may be especially prone to side effects from scopolamine eyedrops. If your vision becomes blurred, take extra care to prevent slips and falls.

Additional instructions

_____

_____

_____

_____

_____

Applying the scopolamine patch

Dear Patient:

Your doctor has prescribed scopolamine to prevent nausea and vomiting caused by your motion sickness. The label may read Transderm-Scōp.

How to apply the scopolamine patch

This medication comes in the form of a small patch—a transdermal disk—that you wear behind your ear. First, carefully read the patient directions that come with the transdermal disk. Wash and dry your hands well before and after handling the disk. Apply the disk to a hairless skin area behind the ear.

Apply the disk the night before or several hours before your trip. Don't place it over any cuts or irritations on your skin.

If the disk loosens, remove it and replace it with a new disk on another clean area of skin behind the ear.

When you no longer need the medication, remove and discard it. Wash your hands and the skin that was beneath the disk. The disks are designed to deliver medication for up to 3 days.

What to do about side effects

Check with your doctor if this medication makes you drowsy or dries your mouth, especially if these symptoms continue or bother you.

Also, while using the disk or even after removing it, your eyes may be more sensitive than usual to light. You may also notice the pupil in one eye is larger than the pupil in the other eye. Call your doctor if this side effect persists or troubles you.

Special directions

• Tell your doctor if you have other medical problems, especially glaucoma, asthma, lung disease, myasthenia gravis, or intestinal disease. Other medical problems may affect the use of this medication.

• Because scopolamine may make you drowsy, make sure you know how you react to it before you drive or perform other activities that might be dangerous if you're not fully alert.

• This product comes with a patient brochure containing helpful information. You may want to request it from your pharmacist.

• If scopolamine makes your mouth feel dry, use sugarless gum or hard candy, ice chips, or a saliva substitute. If your mouth still feels dry after 2 weeks, see your dentist.

Important reminders

If you're breast-feeding, check with your doctor before using scopolamine.

If you're an athlete, you should know that scopolamine is banned and sometimes tested for in biathlon and modern pentathlon events by the U.S. Olympic Committee.

Don't use the transdermal disk on children.

Additional instructions

_____

_____

_____

_____

_____

_____

Taking spironolactone

Dear Patient:

Spironolactone is used to treat high blood pressure and a condition called hyperaldosteronism. This diuretic (water pill) makes you urinate more, while also increasing the amount of potassium in your body. The label may read Aldactone.

How to take spironolactone
Spironolactone comes in tablets. Take this medication exactly as directed. For better absorption, take the tablets with meals.

What to do if you miss a dose
Take it as soon as possible. However, if it's almost time for your next dose, skip the missed dose and take your next dose on schedule. Don't double dose.

What to do about side effects
Call your doctor if you experience abdominal cramps, diarrhea, loss of appetite, or nausea; confusion, drowsiness, fatigue, headache, loss of coordination, or weakness; a rash; or excessive thirst. Also call him if you have breast enlargement (in men) or, in women, breast soreness, deepening voice, increased facial hair, or menstrual irregularities.

What you must know about other drugs
Tell your doctor about other medications you're taking. Also, check with him before you take new medications.

Don't take aspirin or aspirin-containing drugs because spironolactone may not work well. Your doctor also needs to know if you take the heart medication digoxin (Lanoxin), potassium pills, or other water pills.

Special directions
• Tell your doctor if you have other medical problems, especially diabetes, urinary problems, and kidney or liver disease. Other medical problems may affect the use of this medication.
• Don't use salt substitutes (which contain a lot of potassium) or eat potassium-rich foods (for example, bananas, carrots, and nonfat dry milk) without first checking with your doctor. Spironolactone can cause you to retain too much potassium.
• Because spironolactone may make you drowsy, make sure you know how it affects you before you drive or perform other activities that might be dangerous if you're not fully alert.
• Keep all appointments for follow-up examinations so your doctor can check your progress. Your doctor may order a higher dose of spironolactone at first and then reduce the amount as your body adjusts.

Important reminders
If you're pregnant, don't use spironolactone unless your doctor instructs you to do so.

If you're an athlete, you should know that diuretics are banned and tested for by the U.S. Olympic Committee and the National Collegiate Athletic Association.

Additional instructions

_____

_____

_____

_____

Taking sucralfate

Dear Patient:

Your doctor has prescribed sucralfate to treat your stomach ulcer. This medication works by forming a barrier over your ulcer. This protects the ulcer from stomach acid and allows it to heal. Another name for this drug is Carafate.

How to take sucralfate
Take sucralfate 1 hour before meals and at bedtime. Why? Because sucralfate works best on an empty stomach. For this reason, take the medication only with water.

If you have difficulty swallowing, try placing the sucralfate tablet in an ounce of water. Let the tablet sit in the water at room temperature until it dissolves. Then drink the fluid.

Make sure that you continue taking the medication for as long as your doctor has prescribed, even after you've begun to feel better.

What to do if you miss a dose
Take the dose as soon as possible. But if it's almost time for your next dose, skip the missed dose and take the next one at the regular time. Don't take two doses at once.

What to do about side effects
You may become constipated while you're taking this drug. If you do, call your doctor. He may prescribe a laxative to relieve the problem.

What you must know about other drugs
Antacids can keep sucralfate from working properly. So don't take an antacid for a half hour before a scheduled dose of sucralfate. Then, after taking a dose of sucralfate, wait another half hour before you take an antacid.

Also, because sucralfate can interfere with the way some other drugs work, check with your doctor or pharmacist if you're taking any other drugs while taking sucralfate. In particular, be sure to tell your doctor if you're taking an antibiotic.

Special directions
• If you have a history of kidney failure or an intestinal obstruction, let your doctor know. He may want to change your medication.
• While you're taking sucralfate, avoid activities that could worsen your condition. For example, don't smoke because smoking increases the production of acid in your stomach and could worsen your stomach ulcer. Also, don't drink alcoholic beverages, take aspirin, or eat foods that irritate your stomach.
• Store your medication in a cool, dry place—not in your bathroom medicine cabinet or near the kitchen sink. Protect the medication from direct light, and don't put it in the refrigerator.
• Don't take this medication for more than 8 weeks.

Important reminder
If you're pregnant or breast-feeding, check with your doctor before taking this medication.

Additional instructions

_____

_____

_____

Using sulfacetamide

Dear Patient:

Your doctor has prescribed sulfacetamide to treat your eye infection. This medication has several brand names, including Bleph-10, Cetamide, and Sodium Sulamyd.

How to use sulfacetamide

If you're using sulfacetamide *eyedrops,* follow these steps. First wash your hands. Then tilt your head back and pull your lower eyelid away from your eye to form a pouch. Without touching your eye with the applicator, instill the prescribed amount of drops into the pouch. Then gently close your eye and don't blink. Keep your eye closed for 1 to 2 minutes to give the medication time to saturate the area. If you think you didn't get the drop of medication into your eye properly, use another drop.

If you're using sulfacetamide *eye ointment,* follow these steps. Wash your hands. Pull your lower eyelid away from your eye to form a pouch. Without touching your eye with the applicator tip, squeeze a thin strip of ointment, about ½ inch to 1 inch long, into the pouch. Gently close your eye. Keep your eye closed for 1 to 2 minutes to give the medication time to saturate the area.

After you finish using the medication, wash your hands again.

Use all of the medication as prescribed by your doctor, even if your symptoms subside after a few days.

What to do if you miss a dose

Take the medication as soon as possible. However, if it's almost time for your next dose, skip the missed dose and take the next dose on schedule.

What to do about side effects

You may notice that your eyes sting or burn for a few minutes after you use the drops or ointment. This is to be expected. Also expect your vision to blur briefly after applying eye ointment.

If you're sensitive to the medication, your eyelids may swell, itch, and burn constantly. If this happens, notify your doctor.

Also call your doctor if you develop a rash, if blisters form in your mouth or on your eyelids, or if your skin turns red and starts to peel.

What you must know about other drugs

Sulfacetamide isn't compatible with any type of silver eye preparation. If you're using silver nitrate or a mild silver protein for the eye, tell your doctor or pharmacist.

Special directions

• Tell your doctor if you've ever had an allergic reaction to any type of sulfa medication.
• Don't share your medication with anyone. If someone in your family develops the same symptoms that you have, call your doctor.

Additional instructions

_____

_____

_____

_____

Taking sulfamethoxazole

Dear Patient:

Your doctor has prescribed sulfamethoxazole to treat your infection. The label on your medication bottle may read Gantanol.

How to take sulfamethoxazole

Take the medication just as prescribed by your doctor. Take it at the same times every day so that the amount of drug in your bloodstream remains constant. Keep taking your medication even if you feel better after a few days.

With each dose, drink a full glass (8 ounces) of water. Also make it a point to drink several more glasses of water throughout the day to help prevent unwanted side effects.

What to do if you miss a dose

Take the dose as soon as you can. But if it's almost time for your next dose, you'll need to adjust your schedule. If your doctor has prescribed two doses a day, wait 5 to 6 hours after taking the missed dose and then take your next dose. After that, resume your regular dosing schedule.

If your doctor has prescribed three or more doses a day, wait 2 to 4 hours after taking the missed dose and then take the next dose. After that, resume your regular dosing schedule.

What to do about side effects

Call your doctor *right away* if your skin itches, develops a rash, blisters, turns red, or starts to peel. Tell your doctor if you experience increased sensitivity to the sun. Also contact him if you develop a sore throat, fever, and pallor while taking this medication.

Right after you start taking the medication, you may experience diarrhea, headaches, dizziness, loss of appetite, nausea or vomiting, and fatigue. If these symptoms continue for more than a day or so, tell your doctor.

What you must know about other drugs

Before you take any other drug, check with your doctor or pharmacist. That's because sulfamethoxazole can interfere with the way some other drugs work.

In particular, tell your doctor if you're taking any oral drug to control diabetes. Sulfamethoxazole may increase the effects of this oral drug, making it necessary to adjust your dose.

Special directions

• Tell your doctor if you've ever had a reaction to any type of sulfa drug or any drug containing sulfur, such as furosemide (Lasix), water pills, or oral diabetes medication.
• Also tell your doctor if you have a history of anemia, glucose-6-phosphate dehydrogenase deficiency, urinary obstruction, kidney or liver disease, severe allergies, asthma, blood disorders, or porphyria.
• Because sulfamethoxazole may make your skin more sensitive to the sun, limit your exposure while you're taking the medication.
• Because this medication makes some people dizzy, don't drive or operate any machinery until you know how you respond to the medication.

Important reminder

Don't take this drug if you're pregnant or breast-feeding.

Taking sulfasalazine

Dear Patient:

Your doctor has prescribed sulfasalazine to help treat your bowel condition. This drug works by helping to reduce inflammation inside the bowel and other symptoms. Other names for this drug are Azulfidine and Azulfidine EN-Tabs.

How to take sulfasalazine
Take each dose with a full (8-ounce) glass of water. Also drink several more glasses of water during the day. This will help prevent certain side effects.

Because sulfasalazine may upset an empty stomach, take the drug after meals or with food.

Follow your doctor's directions exactly. Take the entire prescription even if you feel better after a few days.

What to do if you miss a dose
Take it as soon as possible. But if it's almost time for your next dose, skip the missed dose and take your next dose as scheduled.

What to do about side effects
Call your doctor *right away* if you develop any of these side effects:
• aching joints and muscles
• continuous headache
• skin rash or blisters
• red, peeling skin
• itching
• difficulty breathing.

Also tell your doctor if you develop nausea, vomiting, diarrhea, dizziness, or increased sensitivity to sunlight.

You may notice that the medication turns your urine or skin an orange-yellow color. Don't be concerned. This symptom will disappear after you've finished your medication.

What you must know about other drugs
Sulfasalazine may change the way your body repsonds to other drugs. For example, sulfasalazine may change the effects of oral drugs for diabetes, birth control pills, blood thinners, and folic acid. If you're taking any of these medications, let your doctor or pharmacist know.

Special directions
• Tell your doctor if you've ever had an allergic reaction to a sulfa drug, a diuretic (a water pill, such as Lasix), or an oral drug for diabetes. Also mention if you've ever had an allergic reaction to aspirin or an oral drug for glaucoma.
• You also need to tell your doctor if you have a history of anemia, glucose-6-phosphate dehydrogenase deficiency, urinary or intestinal tract obstruction, kidney or liver disease, severe allergies, asthma, blood disorders, or porphyria.
• Because sulfasalazine may make your skin more sensitive to sunlight, limit your exposure while you're taking the medication.
• Because this medication makes some people dizzy, don't drive or operate any machinery until you know how you respond to the medication.

Important reminder
Don't take this drug if you're pregnant or breast-feeding.

Additional instructions

_____

_____

_____

_____

Using ophthalmic sulfisoxazole

Dear Patient:

The doctor has prescribed sulfisoxazole to treat your eye infection. The label may read Gantrisin.

How to use sulfisoxazole

If you're using the *eyedrop* form of the drug, follow these steps. First wash your hands. Then tilt your head back and pull your lower eyelid away from your eye to form a pouch. Without touching your eye with the applicator, instill the prescribed amount of drops into the pouch. Then gently close your eye and don't blink. Keep your eye closed for 1 to 2 minutes to give the medication time to saturate the area.

If you're using the *eye ointment* form of the drug, follow these steps. Wash your hands. Pull your lower eyelid away from your eye to form a pouch. Without touching your eye with the applicator tip, squeeze a thin strip of ointment, about ½ inch to 1 inch long, into the pouch. Gently close your eye. Keep your eye closed for 1 to 2 minutes to give the medication time to saturate the area. After applying the medication, wash your hands again.

Use all of the medication as prescribed by your doctor even if your symptoms subside after a few days.

What to do if you miss a dose

Take the medication as soon as possible. However, if it's almost time for your next dose, skip the missed dose and take the next dose on schedule.

What to do about side effects

You may notice that your eyes sting or burn for a few minutes after you use the drops or ointment. This is to be ex-

pected. Also expect your vision to blur briefly after applying eye ointment.

If you're sensitive to the medication, your eyelids may swell, itch, and burn constantly. If this happens, notify your doctor.

What you must know about other drugs

Sulfisoxasole isn't compatible with any type of silver eye preparation. If you're using silver nitrate or a mild silver protein for the eye, tell your doctor or pharmacist.

Special directions

• Tell your doctor if you've ever had an allergic reaction to any type of sulfa medication.
• Don't share your medication with anyone. If someone in your family develops the same symptoms that you have, call your doctor.

Additional instructions

_____

_____

_____

_____

_____

_____

_____

_____

Taking oral sulfisoxazole

Dear Patient:

Your doctor has prescribed sulfisoxazole in tablet or liquid form to help treat your infection. Another name for this drug is Gantrisin.

How to take sulfisoxazole
Take the medication exactly as prescribed, at the same times every day. Continue to take the medication even after you start to feel better.

Drink a full glass of water with each dose. Also make it a point to drink several more glasses of water throughout the day to help prevent unwanted side effects.

What to do if you miss a dose
Take the dose as soon as you can. But if it's almost time for your next dose, you need to adjust your dosing schedule. For example, if your doctor has prescribed two doses a day, wait 5 to 6 hours after taking the missed dose before taking the next dose. Then resume your regular dosing schedule.

If your doctor has prescribed three or more doses a day, wait 2 to 4 hours after taking the missed dose before taking the next dose. After that, resume your regular dosing schedule.

What to do about side effects
Call your doctor *right away* if you notice any of these side effects:
• itching or a rash
• red, blistering, or peeling skin
• decreased urine output
• difficulty swallowing.

Right after you start taking the medication, you may experience diarrhea, headaches, dizziness, loss of appetite, nausea or vomiting, and fatigue. If these symptoms continue for more than a day or so, tell your doctor.

What you must know about other drugs
Sulfisoxazole may change how your body responds to certain drugs. Don't take it with drugs containing ammonium chloride (such as some cough medicines), para-aminobenzoic acid—also known as PABA (found in some multivitamins), or vitamin C.

Sulfisoxazole may also change the effects of birth control pills, oral drugs for diabetes, blood thinners, and folic acid. If you're taking any of these medications, let your doctor or pharmacist know.

Special directions
• Tell your doctor if you've ever had a reaction to any type of sulfa drug or any drug containing sulfur, a diuretic (a water pill, such as Lasix), or an oral drug for diabetes.
• Also tell your doctor if you have a history of anemia, glucose-6-phosphate dehydrogenase deficiency, urinary obstruction, kidney or liver disease, severe allergies, asthma, blood disorders, or porphyria.
• Because sulfisoxazole may make your skin more sensitive to sunlight, limit your exposure to the sun.

Important reminder
Don't take this drug if you're pregnant or breast-feeding.

Additional instructions

_____

_____

Taking sulindac

Dear Patient:

Your doctor has prescribed sulindac to help treat your condition. Sulindac helps control inflammation and relieve pain. It's often called a *nonsteroidal anti-inflammatory drug.* The label on your medication bottle may read Clinoril.

How to take sulindac
Follow your doctor's instructions exactly. Take sulindac with milk, meals, or an antacid. This will help prevent stomach upset, which could occur if you take the drug on an empty stomach.

Also drink a full (8-ounce) glass of water with each dose. Don't lie down for 15 to 30 minutes after taking the medication. This will help prevent irritation that could cause you to have difficulty swallowing.

What to do if you miss a dose
If your doctor has prescribed this medication on a regular schedule and you miss a dose, take it as soon as you remember. But if it's almost time for your next dose, skip the missed dose and take your next dose as scheduled.

What to do about side effects
Tell your doctor *immediately* if you notice any of these side effects:
• stomach pain or burning
• bloody or black, tarry stools
• easy bruising and bleeding
• changes in vision
• swelling in your face, feet, or lower legs
• persistent nausea.

What you must know about other drugs
Because sulindac may affect the action of other drugs, tell your doctor and pharmacist about any drugs you're taking at the same time. In particular, mention if you're taking aspirin, a blood thinner, or drugs for seizures, thyroid problems, or inflammation.

Special directions
• Tell your doctor if aspirin or another anti-inflammatory drug has ever caused you to have difficulty breathing, a tight sensation in your chest, a runny nose, or itching.
• Also tell the doctor if you have a history of GI bleeding, liver or kidney disease, asthma, heart disease, or high blood pressure.
• Because this medication makes some people drowsy or dizzy, don't drive or operate machinery until you know how you react to the medication.

Important reminders
This drug can hide the symptoms of an infection. If you have diabetes, you need to be especially careful about your feet and watch for any problem, such as redness or sores.

Because sulindac can cause you to retain fluid, have your blood pressure checked when your doctor recommends.

Additional instructions

_____

_____

_____

_____

_____

Taking tamoxifen

Dear Patient:

Your doctor has prescribed tamoxifen to help treat your breast cancer. Tamoxifen blocks the effects of the hormone estrogen which, in turn, may improve your condition. Another name for this drug is Nolvadex.

How to take tamoxifen
Follow your doctor's instructions exactly. Don't take more of the medication than has been prescribed, and be careful not to miss a dose. Take the medication even if it makes you feel nauseous.

If you're taking enteric-coated tablets, swallow the tablet whole. Don't crush or break up the tablet before taking.

What to do if you miss a dose
Skip the dose entirely, and take your next regular dose as scheduled. Call your doctor to let him know you missed a dose.

If you vomit shortly after taking a dose of tamoxifen, call your doctor. Depending on the circumstances, your doctor may tell you to take the dose again or to wait until the next scheduled dose.

What to do about side effects
Tamoxifen causes some patients to become nauseated and vomit. It may also cause hot flashes, weight gain, bone pain, and changes in your menstrual cycle. Let your doctor know if these symptoms become a problem.

Watch for easy bruising or bleeding. If these symptoms develop, call your doctor.

Tamoxifen causes women to become more fertile. But, because you shouldn't become pregnant while taking the drug, use a barrier contraceptive.

What you must know about other drugs
Birth control pills may change the effects of tamoxifen. Therefore, while you're taking this drug, use a barrier method of birth control.

Special directions
• Before taking tamoxifen, tell your doctor if you've ever had cataracts or another eye problem.
• To help control hot flashes, don't drink alcoholic beverages or smoke while you're taking the drug. Also, drink lots of fluids, wear layers of clothing that you can easily remove if you get too warm, and use fans or an air conditioner to control indoor temperature.
• Try to eat a high-calorie diet. If you become nauseated, sip fluids throughout the day.

Important reminder
Tell your doctor immediately if you think you've become pregnant while taking tamoxifen.

Additional instructions

_____

_____

_____

_____

_____

_____

_____

Taking temazepam

Dear Patient:

Your doctor has prescribed this sedative to help treat your condition. Temazepam helps relieve nervousness and tension to help you sleep. The name on the label may read Razepam or Restoril.

How to take temazepam
Follow your doctor's instructions exactly. Don't increase your dose even if you think your current one isn't effective. Instead, call your doctor. Also, because temazepam can be habit-forming, don't take it for a longer time than your doctor recommends.

What to do about side effects
Temazepam may make you feel tired, drowsy, or dizzy. If the symptoms are severe, or if you feel very tired or "hung over" the day after you've taken the medication, your dose may be too high. Call your doctor so he can adjust your dosage.

What you must know about alcohol and other drugs
Avoid drinking any alcoholic beverages—beer, wine, and liquor—while you're taking temazepam. That's because, when taken together, alcohol increases the depressant effects of temazepam. At the same time, temazepam increases the depressant effects of alcohol. If you drink alcoholic beverages with temazepam, you could have an overdose.

For the same reason, avoid taking other depressant drugs unless your doctor says otherwise. Examples include many allergy or cold medications, narcotics, muscle relaxants, sleeping pills, and drugs for seizures.

Tell your doctor if you're taking the drug zidovudine (also called AZT). Temazepam could cause your body to absorb more zidovudine, so your doctor may need to lower your zidovudine dosage.

Special directions
• Temazepam can make some medical problems worse. For this reason, be sure to tell your doctor if you have glaucoma, a history of alcohol or drug abuse, mental depression, myasthenia gravis, Parkinson's disease, chronic obstructive pulmonary disease, kidney or liver disease, or porphyria.
• Check with your doctor every month to make sure you still need to be taking this medication.
• Because temazepam may make you drowsy or light-headed, don't drive or operate any machinery until you know how you respond to the medication.

Important reminders
Don't take temazepam if you think you might be pregnant or if you're breast-feeding. If you're an older adult, be aware that this medication could make you feel drowsy during the day, which could lead to falls.

If you're an athlete, you should know that temazepam is banned and in some cases tested for by the U.S. Olympic Committee and the National Collegiate Athletic Association.

Additional instructions

_____

_____

_____

Taking terazosin

Dear Patient:

Your doctor has prescribed terazosin to help treat your high blood pressure. This medication works by relaxing your blood vessels so that blood passes through them more easily. This helps to lower your blood pressure. The label on your medication bottle may read Hytrin.

How to take terazosin
Follow your doctor's instructions exactly. Terazosin won't cure your high blood pressure; it will only help control it. That's why you need to continue to take it even if you feel well. You may even need to take it for the rest of your life.

What to do if you miss a dose
Take it as soon as you remember, as long as you remember on the same day as the missed dose. But, if you don't remember until the next day, skip the missed dose and take the next dose as scheduled. If you miss several doses, call your doctor before resuming your medication.

What to do about side effects
Terazosin causes some people to feel dizzy or light-headed, especially when getting up after sitting or lying down. Other possible side effects include an irregular heartbeat, swelling in the feet and lower legs, stuffy nose, and nausea. Call your doctor if any of these symptoms become bothersome.

What you must know about other drugs
Don't take them—even nonprescription ones—without first talking with your doctor. This is especially true for diet, asthma, cold, cough, hay fever, and sinus medications. Why? Because these medications may increase your blood pressure.

Special directions
• Because your first dose of terazosin will most likely make you drowsy or dizzy, take it at bedtime. For this same reason, be careful if you need to get up during the night. Also, don't drive or operate any machinery until you know how you're going to respond to the medication.
• To lessen the problem of dizziness, get up slowly. If you begin to feel lightheaded once you're standing, lie down so you don't faint. Then sit up for a few moments before standing.
• You're more likely to feel dizzy if you drink alcoholic beverages, stand for a long period of time, or exercise or when the weather is hot. So, be careful about drinking alcoholic beverages. And be careful when you're standing or exercising, particularly in hot weather.
• Remember to keep your appointments with your doctor, even if you feel well, and to check your blood pressure frequently.

Important reminder
Let your doctor know if you think you're pregnant or if you're breast-feeding.

Additional instructions

_____

_____

_____

_____

Taking terbutaline

Dear Patient:

Your doctor has prescribed terbutaline to help treat your breathing problem. Terbutaline opens the air passages in your lungs, which will help you to breathe easier. The label on your medication may read Brethaire, Brethine, or Bricanyl.

How to take terbutaline
If your doctor has prescribed the *oral* form of this drug, follow his instructions exactly.

If your doctor has prescribed the *aerosol* form of this drug, follow these steps. Blow your nose and clear your throat. Breathe out, emptying your lungs as much as possible. Hold the medication canister in an upright position. Place the mouthpiece well inside your mouth and close your lips around it. Press down on the top of the medication canister. At the same time, breathe in deeply. Hold your breath for several seconds. Remove the mouthpiece from your mouth and breathe out slowly. If your doctor has ordered more than one inhalation, wait at least 2 minutes before you use the inhaler the second time. Never use the inhaler more than twice in a row.

What to do if you miss a dose
If you're using terbutaline regularly, take your missed dose as soon as you remember. Then take any remaining doses that day at regularly spaced intervals. Don't take two doses at the same time.

What to do about side effects
If your wheezing gets worse or your breathing becomes more difficult after taking terbutaline, stop the drug and call your doctor *immediately.*

You may feel nervous, develop a tremor, or get a headache while taking terbutaline. These symptoms are common, but if they become bothersome, call your doctor.

What you must know about other drugs
Don't take terbutaline if you're taking a type of antidepressant called a monoamine oxidase (MAO) inhibitor. Taking them together could cause severe high blood pressure.

If you're taking a beta blocker (such as Tenormin or Lopressor), tell your doctor or pharmacist. These medications could keep terbutaline from working properly.

Also tell your doctor if you're taking the heart medication digitalis.

Special directions
Because terbutaline can make certain medical problems worse, tell your doctor if you have a history of seizures, brain damage, diabetes, mental illness, heart disease, high blood pressure, an overactive thyroid, or Parkinson's disease.

Important reminder
If you're an athlete, you should know that oral forms of terbutaline are banned and tested for by the U.S. Olympic Committee. However, the committee permits the use of terbutaline in aerosol or inhalation form.

Additional instructions

Using terconazole

Dear Patient:

Your doctor has ordered terconazole to treat your vaginal fungal infection. It works by killing fungus or preventing its growth. The medication, also called Terazol, may come as a cream or a suppository.

How to use terconazole

Whether you're using the cream or suppository, you should find an applicator in the carton containing your medication. Use the applicator to insert the medication into your vagina at bedtime. If you're inserting a suppository, remain lying down for at least 30 minutes after each dose to allow your vagina time to absorb the terconazole.

Use the medication for the number of nights prescribed by your doctor. Don't stop before then, even if your symptoms subside. If you stop using the medication too soon, your symptoms may return.

What to do if you miss a dose

Take it as soon as possible. But if it's almost time for your next dose, skip the missed dose and take your next dose as scheduled.

What to do about side effects

If your vagina becomes irritated or burns after using this medication, and it wasn't irritated and didn't burn before, call your doctor as soon as possible.

Some women develop a headache after using terconazole. If this occurs, take acetaminophen (Tylenol) or another mild pain reliever.

Special directions

• Tell your doctor if you've ever had an allergic reaction to terconazole or another antifungal drug. Also tell your doctor if you're using a douche or another type of vaginal medication.

• Keep using the medication, even if your period starts. But don't use tampons so you won't remove any of the medication from your vagina,

• To keep the medication from soiling your clothes, wear a minipad or sanitary napkin.

• If your symptoms don't subside or if they worsen after using the medication for several days, call your doctor.

• To keep your infection from returning, you need to develop good health habits. To begin with, wear panties made only of cotton, instead of nylon or rayon. Or choose pantyhose or panties that have a cotton crotch.

• It's possible to spread your infection to your sexual partner during intercourse. Also, your partner could be carrying the fungus in his genital tract. To keep from spreading the infection or to keep from becoming reinfected, have your partner wear a condom during intercourse.

Additional instructions

_____

_____

_____

_____

_____

_____

Taking terfenadine

Dear Patient:

Your doctor has prescribed terfenadine to help relieve your allergy symptoms. Terfenadine is an antihistamine. But, unlike most other antihistamines, this drug usually doesn't cause drowsiness. The label on your medication bottle may read Seldane.

How to take terfenadine
Follow your doctor's instructions precisely. Don't take more than the recommended dose, even if your symptoms don't subside. If you're giving the medication to a child, break the tablet as needed to obtain the right dose.

What to do if you miss a dose
If you're taking this medication on a regular schedule and you miss a dose, take it as soon as you remember. But if it's almost time for your next dose, skip the missed dose and take your next dose as scheduled. Don't take two doses at the same time.

What to do about side effects
Some patients complain of a headache after taking terfenadine. If this happens to you, take acetaminophen (Tylenol) or another mild pain reliever. If the headache is severe, call your doctor.

Special directions
• Tell the doctor if you've ever had an allergic reaction to terfenadine or another antihistamine. Also tell the doctor if you have a history of asthma or another lung disorder because terfenadine could aggravate these conditions.
• Expect to wait about an hour after taking this medication for your symptoms to subside.

• Drink plenty of fluids while you're taking terfenadine, especially if you're congested. That's because terfenadine has a drying effect. If you don't stay well hydrated, your secretions could become thick and difficult to cough up.

Important reminder
If you're pregnant or breast-feeding, check with your doctor before taking this medication.

Additional instructions

_____

_____

_____

_____

_____

_____

_____

_____

_____

_____

_____

_____

Using ophthalmic tetracycline

Dear Patient:

Your doctor has prescribed tetracycline eyedrops or eye ointment to help treat your eye infection. The label may read Achromycin.

How to use this drug

If you're using *eyedrops,* follow these steps. First wash your hands. If you're using a suspension, shake well before using. Then tilt your head back, and pull your lower eyelid away from your eye to form a pouch. Without touching your eye with the applicator, instill the prescribed amount of drops into the pouch. Then gently close your eye and don't blink. Keep your eye closed for 1 to 2 minutes to give the medication time to saturate the area.

If you're using the *eye ointment,* follow these steps. Wash your hands. Pull your lower eyelid away from your eye to form a pouch. Without touching your eye with the applicator tip, squeeze a thin strip of ointment, about ⅓ inch long, into the pouch. Gently close your eye. Keep your eye closed for 1 to 2 minutes to give the medication time to saturate the area. Wipe the tip of the ointment tube with a clean tissue. Keep the tube tightly closed.

After you finish using the medication, wash your hands again.

Take all of the medication as prescribed by your doctor, even if your symptoms subside after a few days.

What to do if you miss a dose

Take the medication as soon as possible. However, if it's almost time for your next dose, skip the missed dose and take the next dose on schedule.

What to do about side effects

The medication may cause your vision to blur for a few minutes after you apply it. However, this is to be expected.

You shouldn't develop any bothersome side effects while using this medication. But if any unusual symptoms occur, tell your doctor.

Special directions

• Because tetracycline may make certain medical problems worse, tell the doctor if you have any type of kidney problem. Also tell the doctor if you've ever had an allergic reaction to tetracycline.
• While you're using the medication, your skin may be more sensitive to sunlight, so limit your exposure to the sun.
• If your symptoms don't go away after a few days or if they become worse, call your doctor.

Important reminders

Don't use this medication if you're pregnant. Also, don't give it to a child younger than age 8. It could stain the child's teeth or stunt his growth.

Additional instructions

_____

_____

_____

_____

_____

_____

Taking oral and topical tetracycline

Dear Patient:

Your doctor has prescribed tetracycline to help treat your infection. If you're taking the *oral* form of this drug, such as a tablet or capsule, the label may read Achromycin, Panmycin, or Tetracyn. If you're applying *topical* tetracycline to your skin, the label may read Topicycline.

How to take tetracycline
If you're taking *oral* tetracycline, take the drug 1 hour before or 2 hours after meals. Why? Because foods can decrease your body's ability to absorb the drug. For the same reason, don't take the drug with milk or other dairy products. To help prevent stomach irritation, drink a full glass of water with each dose.

If you're using *topical* tetracycline, control the rate of application by adjusting the pressure of the applicator against your skin. Avoid contact with your eyes, nose, and mouth.

What to do if you miss a dose
Take it as soon as possible. But if it's almost time for your next dose, adjust your dosing schedule as follows.

If you're taking *one dose a day,* space the missed dose and your next dose 12 hours apart.

If you're taking *two doses a day,* space the missed dose and the next dose 5 to 6 hours apart.

If you're taking *three or more doses a day,* space the missed dose and the next dose 2 to 4 hours apart.

Then resume your regular dosing schedule.

What to do about side effects
Call your doctor if you develop a sore throat; diarrhea; reddened skin, a rash, or hives; or skin changes after being in the sun.

Also tell your doctor if you have difficulty swallowing, indigestion, loss of appetite, or nausea. If you're female, tell your doctor if you get a vaginal infection.

What you must know about other drugs
Because of possible absorption problems, don't take tetracycline with antacids (such as Maalox), iron preparations (such as multivitamins containing iron), or sodium bicarbonate (such as Alka-Seltzer).

Also, tetracycline may keep birth control pills from working properly. Use another method of birth control.

Special directions
• Before taking tetracycline, tell your doctor if you have diabetes insipidus. Tetracycline could make this condition worse. Also reveal if you have kidney or liver disease because you may have a greater risk of developing side effects.
• If you're using topical tetracycline, use up the solution within 2 months. Be careful when applying the medication because it may stain your clothing.
• Because tetracycline may make your skin more sensitive to sunlight, limit your exposure to the sun.

Important reminder
If you're pregnant, don't take tetracycline. It could stain your baby's teeth or cause other problems.

Taking theophylline

Dear Patient:

Your doctor has prescribed theophylline to help treat and prevent the symptoms of your asthma. This medication works by opening up the bronchial tubes and increasing the flow of air through them. If you're taking the *liquid* form of the drug, the label may read Aquaphyllin, Elixicon, or Slo-Phyllin. If you're taking a *tablet* or *capsule,* the label may read Constant-T, Theo-Dur, or Slo-bid.

How to take theophylline
Follow your doctor's instructions exactly. Don't take more or less, and don't take it more often or longer than he directs. Take your medication at the same time every day.

In general, take theophylline 30 minutes to 1 hour before meals or 2 hours after meals, unless your doctor directs you otherwise. Theophylline works best on an empty stomach.

If you're taking the *extended-release* form of the medication, don't crush or break the capsules or tablets. If it's difficult to swallow, talk to your doctor.

What to do if you miss a dose
For the medication to work properly, you need to take every dose on time. If you do miss a dose, though, take it as soon as possible. If it's almost time for your next dose, skip the missed dose and take your next dose on schedule.

What to do about side effects
Call the doctor *immediately* if you develop diarrhea or have a seizure. Also let the doctor know if you feel nervous or dizzy, have difficulty sleeping, have a rapid heartbeat, become nauseated or vomit, or lose your appetite.

What you must know about other drugs
Theophylline can interfere with the way some other drugs work. At the same time, some drugs can interfere with theophylline's actions. Tell your doctor if you're taking birth control pills; drugs for seizures, heart problems, tuberculosis, or a stomach ulcer; or nonprescription medications.

Also tell the doctor if you've smoked tobacco or marijuana within the previous 2 years. Smoking may affect how much theophylline you need.

Special directions
• Tell the doctor if you've ever had an allergic reaction to theophylline or any drug for asthma.
• Because theophylline can make some medical problems worse, tell the doctor if you have heart or circulatory problems, diabetes, glaucoma, high blood pressure, an overactive thyroid, stomach ulcers, or indigestion.
• Because charcoal-broiled foods may interfere with how theophylline works, don't eat these foods every day. Also, don't eat or drink a large amount of foods containing caffeine, such as chocolate, tea, coffee, and colas. The extra caffeine may increase the stimulant effects of theophylline.
• Call your doctor right away if you develop a fever or feel like you have the flu. These conditions could increase your risk for side effects.

Important reminders
If you're pregnant or breast-feeding, check with your doctor before taking theophylline.

If you're an older adult, you may be especially prone to side effects.

Taking thioridazine

Dear Patient:

Your doctor has ordered thioridazine to treat your condition. The label may read Mellaril.

How to take thioridazine

If your medication comes in a bottle with a dropper, use the dropper to measure each dose. Dilute the dose in half a glass (4 ounces) of fruit juice, soda, milk, water, or semisolid food.

If your medication is in liquid form, shake the bottle well before using. Don't let the medication touch your skin because it could cause a rash.

To prevent stomach irritation, take your medication with food or a glass of water. Also, don't stop taking your medication unless your doctor tells you to or you develop a severe reaction.

What to do if you miss a dose

If you take one dose a day and you remember the missed dose the same day, take it as soon as possible. Otherwise, skip the missed dose and resume your regular dosing schedule.

If you take more than one dose a day and you remember the missed dose within an hour, take it right away. Otherwise, skip the missed dose and take your next dose as scheduled.

What to do about side effects

Call your doctor *right away* if you have uncontrolled movements of your mouth, tongue, cheeks, jaw, or arms and legs. Also call if you have a fever, sore throat, fast heartbeat, rapid breathing, profuse sweating, fainting or dizziness, difficult urination, or blurred vision.

Check with your doctor if you become constipated or unusually tired.

Also call your doctor if you have a dry mouth or if your skin color changes after being in the sun.

What you must know about alcohol and other drugs

Tell your doctor if you're taking barbiturates, lithium (Lithane), or high blood pressure medication. Don't drink alcoholic beverages while taking thioridazine. Doing so could cause oversedation.

So that your body can absorb thioridazine completely, don't take an antacid 2 hours before or 2 hours after your dose.

Special directions

• Tell your doctor if you've ever had an allergic reaction to a phenothiazine, such as Thorazine. Also tell your doctor if you have a history of a blood or bone marrow disorder, heart disease, encephalitis, respiratory disease, seizures, glaucoma, an enlarged prostate, urine retention, Parkinson's disease, a low calcium level, or stomach ulcers.
• Because this medication makes your skin more sensitive to sunlight, avoid direct exposure to the sun.
• Because the medication may make you drowsy, don't drive or perform any hazardous activities that require alertness. The drowsiness caused by the medication should become less noticeable after several weeks.

Important reminders

If you're breast-feeding or pregnant, talk with your doctor before taking this medication.

If you're an athlete, you should know that thioridazine is banned and sometimes tested for by the U.S. Olympic Committee and the National Collegiate Athletic Association.

Taking thiothixene

Dear Patient:

Your doctor has prescribed thiothixene to treat your condition. The label may read Navane.

How to take thiothixene

Take only the amount of medication ordered by your doctor. You may need to take the medication for several weeks before you notice its full effect.

If you're taking the *liquid concentrate,* use the bottle dropper to measure the exact dose. Then dilute the dose in half a glass (4 ounces) of water, milk, soda, or tomato or fruit juice. Don't let thiothixene touch your skin; it could cause a rash.

Don't suddenly stop taking this medication unless you have a severe reaction or your doctor tells you to.

What to do if you miss a dose

Take it as soon as possible. But if it's within 2 hours of your next dose, skip the missed dose and take your next dose as scheduled.

What to do about side effects

Call your doctor *right away* if you have uncontrolled movements of your mouth, tongue, cheeks, jaw, or arms and legs. Also call if you have a fever, a sore throat, fast heartbeat, rapid breathing, profuse sweating, fainting or dizziness, difficult urination, or blurred vision.

Tell your doctor if you become constipated, have a dry mouth, or have changes in skin color after being in the sun.

What you must know about alcohol and other drugs

Don't drink alcoholic beverages while taking this medication. Doing so could cause you to become oversedated.

Call your doctor before taking other medications. Avoid drugs that make you drowsy, such as allergy medications, pain relievers, and muscle relaxants.

Special directions

• Tell your doctor if you're allergic to any medications. Because thiothixene may make some medical problems worse, tell him if you have a history of a blood or bone marrow disorder. Also, tell him if you've ever been in a coma, had a head injury, or had a circulation problem.
• Tell your doctor if you have heart or lung problems, seizures, glaucoma, enlarged prostate, Parkinson's disease, urine retention, tumors, low calcium level, or kidney or liver disease.
• Because this medication makes your skin more sensitive to sunlight, avoid direct exposure to the sun. Thiothixene also reduces sweating, so be careful not to become overheated.
• Because this medication may make you drowsy, don't drive or perform hazardous activities that require alertness. The drowsiness should become less noticeable after several weeks.

Important reminders

If you're breast-feeding or think you're pregnant, talk with your doctor before taking this medication.

Thiothixene is banned by the U.S. Olympic Committee and the National Collegiate Athletic Association.

Additional instructions

_____

_____

_____

Taking thyroid supplements

Dear Patient:

Your doctor has prescribed thyroid hormone to supplement the amount of hormone produced by your thyroid gland. The label may read Levothyroxine, Liothyronine, or Liotrix.

How to take thyroid supplements
Take this medication exactly as your doctor has prescribed. Don't take more or less of it, and don't take it more often than he has prescribed. Also, don't stop taking this medication without first talking with your doctor.

If you're taking this medication for an underactive thyroid gland, realize that it may take several weeks before you notice any change in your condition.

What to do if you miss a dose
Take it as soon as possible. But, if it's almost time for your next dose, skip the missed dose and take your next dose as scheduled. Don't take two doses at the same time.

If you miss two or more doses in a row, call your doctor.

What to do about side effects
Call your doctor *right away* if you develop any of these symptoms:
• nervousness
• inability to sleep
• hand tremor
• rapid heartbeat or palpitations
• nausea
• headache
• fever
• sweating.

Also let your doctor know if you experience a change in your appetite, changes in your menstrual period, diarrhea, increased sensitivity to heat, leg cramps, irritability, or weight loss.

What you must know about other drugs
Some drugs, when taken with thyroid supplements, can cause undesirable effects. Let your doctor know if you're taking amphetamines, blood thinners, diet pills, medication for a high cholesterol level, medication for asthma or other breathing problems, or allergy or cold medication.

Before you take any other drugs, check with your doctor or pharmacist.

Special directions
• Because other medical problems may affect how much thyroid hormone your doctor prescribes, let him know if you have diabetes, hardening of the arteries, heart disease, high blood pressure, an underactive adrenal or pituitary gland, or history of an overactive thyroid.
• If you have heart disease, this medication may cause you to develop chest pain or shortness of breath when you exert yourself. If this occurs, take care not to overdo physical exercise.

Important reminder
Let your doctor know right away if you become pregnant or if you're breast-feeding.

Additional instructions

_____

_____

_____

_____

Using timolol

Dear Patient:

Your doctor has prescribed timolol to treat your glaucoma. Timolol helps lower eye pressure by reducing the amount of fluid produced by the eye. The label on your medication may read Timoptic.

How to use timolol
To instill your eyedrops, follow these steps. First wash your hands. Then tilt your head back. Using your middle finger, apply pressure to the inside corner of your eye. Then, with the index finger of your same hand, pull the lower eyelid away from your eye to form a pouch. Instill the prescribed number of drops into the pouch. Don't touch the applicator to your eye or surrounding tissue. Gently close your eyes, but don't blink. With your eyes closed, keep your middle finger pressed against the inside corner for 1 minute. This will help the medication stay in your eye and keep your body from absorbing it. Wash your hands again.

What to do if you miss a dose
If you take one dose a day, take the missed dose as soon as possible. But if you don't remember until the next day, skip the missed dose and take your next dose as scheduled.

If you take more than one dose a day, take the missed dose as soon as possible. But if it's almost time for your next dose, skip the missed dose and take your next dose as scheduled.

What to do about side effects
Call your doctor *right away* if you develop any of these side effects:
• dizziness or feeling faint
• irregular, slow, or pounding heartbeat
• wheezing or trouble breathing
• swelling of feet or lower legs
• unusual tiredness or weakness
• severe eye irritation
• skin rash or itching
• vision disturbances.

What you must know about other drugs
Because timolol may affect how some other drugs work, tell your doctor if you're taking a beta blocker, such as Inderal. Because timolol may interact with some anesthetics, tell him you're taking timolol before you undergo any kind of surgery or emergency treatment.

Special directions
Because timolol may make some medical problems worse, tell your doctor if you have a history of asthma, diabetes, heart or blood vessel disease, myasthenia gravis, kidney or liver disease, or an overactive thyroid.

Important reminders
If you have diabetes, timolol may affect your blood glucose levels. It may also cover up some signs of low blood glucose, such as trembling and increased heart rate and blood pressure. If you notice a change in your blood or urine glucose tests, call your doctor.

Timolol eyedrops are banned by the National Collegiate Athletic Association.

Additional instructions

_____

_____

_____

_____

Using tobramycin

Dear Patient:

Your doctor has prescribed tobramycin to treat your eye infection. The medication works by killing bacteria. The label on your medication may read Tobrex.

How to use tobramycin
If you're using the *eyedrop* form of the drug, follow these steps. First, wash your hands. Tilt your head back. With your middle finger, press on the inside corner of your eye. At the same time, use your index finger to pull your lower eyelid away from your eye, forming a pouch. Without touching your eye with the applicator, instill the prescribed amount of drops into the pouch. Gently close your eye and don't blink. Keep your eye closed and your finger pressed against the inside corner for 1 minute to give the medication time to saturate the area.

If your doctor has ordered another solution to be used with this one, wait at least 5 minutes before using the second medication. This will help keep the second medication from washing away the first.

If you're using the *eye ointment* form of the drug, follow these steps. Wash your hands. Pull your lower eyelid away from your eye to form a pouch. Without touching your eye with the applicator tip, squeeze a thin strip of ointment, about ½ inch long, into the pouch. Gently close your eye. Keep your eye closed for 1 to 2 minutes. After you finish applying the medication, wash your hands again.

Use all of the medication as prescribed by your doctor, even if your symptoms improve after a few days.

What to do if you miss a dose
Take the medication as soon as possible. However, if it's almost time for your next dose, skip the missed dose and take the next dose on schedule.

What to do about side effects
Your eyes may sting or burn for a few minutes after you apply the drops or ointment. This is to be expected. Also expect your vision to blur briefly after applying eye ointment.

Call your doctor if your eyelids swell, itch, or burn constantly. This may signal that you're allergic to the medication.

What you must know about other drugs
Don't use this medication if you're using an eye medication containing tetracycline. The two drugs don't work well together.

Special directions
Tell your doctor if you've ever had an allergic reaction to tobramycin. Also tell your doctor if you have a history of kidney disease; ear problems, such as ringing or hearing loss; myasthenia gravis; Parkinson's disease; or low calcium levels.

Additional instructions

_____

_____

_____

_____

_____

_____

Taking tocainide

Dear Patient:

Your doctor has prescribed tocainide to correct your irregular heartbeat. This medication works by slowing nerve impulses in the heart and making the heart tissue less sensitive. The label on your medication may read Tonocard.

How to take tocainide
Take the exact amount of medication prescribed by your doctor. Try to take your medication at the same time every day, and space your doses evenly throughout the day and night. That's because the medication works best when you have a constant amount in your bloodstream. If the medication upsets your stomach, take it with food or milk.

Continue to take the medication as directed, even if you feel well.

What to do if you miss a dose
If you remember your missed dose within 4 hours, take it as soon as possible. But if you don't remember it until later, skip the missed dose and take your next dose as scheduled. Don't take two doses at the same time.

What to do about side effects
Call your doctor *right away* if you develop any of the following side effects:
• trembling or shaking
• coughing or shortness of breath
• fever or chills
• unusual bleeding or bruising
• unusual tiredness.

Also let your doctor know if you experience nausea, vomiting, stomach pain, dizziness, or light-headedness.

What you must know about other drugs
Tocainide may interfere with how some other medications work. For this reason, tell your doctor if you're taking a beta blocker, such as Inderal or Lopressor. Also, before beginning any new medications, talk with your doctor or pharmacist.

Tell your doctor or dentist you're taking tocainide before having any kind of surgery (including dental surgery) or emergency treatment.

Special directions
• Tocainide may make some medical conditions worse. Tell your doctor if you have a history of kidney or liver disease, a bone marrow disorder, congestive heart failure, or some other heart problem.
• Also tell your doctor if you've ever had an allergic reaction to an anesthetic.
• Because this medication may make you dizzy, don't drive or do anything else that requires you to be alert until you know how you react to this medication.

Important reminders
If you're pregnant or breast-feeding, talk with your doctor before taking this medication.

If you're an older adult, be careful when walking or first getting up out of a chair. You may be especially prone to the side effect of dizziness, which could place you at risk for a fall.

Additional instructions

_____

_____

Taking tolazamide

Dear Patient:

Your doctor has prescribed tolazamide to help control your diabetes. Taken by mouth, tolazamide works by stimulating the pancreas to produce more insulin. The label on your medication may read Tolamide or Tolinase.

How to take tolazamide

Take each dose with food. If your doctor has prescribed one dose a day, take it with breakfast. If he's prescribed two doses a day, take one dose with breakfast and the second dose with your evening meal.

Keep taking the medication, even if you feel well. Tolazamide doesn't cure diabetes; it only relieves the symptoms.

What to do if you miss a dose

Take it as soon as you remember. But if it's almost time for your next dose, skip the missed dose and take your next dose as scheduled. Don't take two doses at once.

What to do about side effects

Taking too much tolazamide may cause a condition called hypoglycemia, which can produce symptoms such as drowsiness, headache, nervousness, cold sweats, and confusion. If these symptoms occur, eat or drink something sweet, such as orange juice, and call your doctor.

What you must know about alcohol and other drugs

Avoid drinking alcoholic beverages while you're taking tolazamide. If you do, you could have unpleasant side effects. Keep in mind that many foods and drugs contain alcohol.

Tell your doctor if you're taking other medications. Why? Tolazamide may interfere with the way some medications work, and other medications may interfere with tolazamide's actions. Especially, tell your doctor if you're taking a blood thinner; diet pills; medication for asthma, colds, allergies, high blood pressure, or tuberculosis; sulfa medication; aspirin; steroids; or a thiazide diuretic (a type of water pill).

Special directions

• Tell your doctor if you've ever had an allergic reaction to an oral medication used for treating diabetes or to a diuretic.
• Because some medical conditions may prevent you from taking tolazamide, tell the doctor if you have a disorder that affects your liver, kidneys, adrenal glands, pituitary gland, or thyroid gland.
• Follow your doctor's instructions for testing your blood or urine for glucose. Also closely follow your instructions for diet and exercise.
• This medication may increase your sensitivity to sunlight. Take precautions to protect your skin when outdoors.
• At all times, wear a medical identification bracelet stating you have diabetes and listing your medication.

Important reminder

Tell your doctor if you're breast-feeding or pregnant. Your doctor may need to prescribe a different medication.

Additional instructions

_____

_____

Taking tolbutamide

Dear Patient:

Your doctor has prescribed tolbutamide to help control your diabetes. Taken by mouth, tolbutamide works by stimulating the pancreas to produce more insulin. The label on your medication may read Oramide or Orinase.

How to take tolbutamide
Take each dose with food. If your doctor has prescribed one dose a day, take it with breakfast. If he's prescribed two doses a day, take one dose with breakfast and the second dose with your evening meal.

Keep taking the medication, even if you feel well. Tolbutamide relieves the symptoms of diabetes; it doesn't cure it.

What to do if you miss a dose
Take it as soon as you remember. But if it's almost time for your next dose, skip the missed dose and take your next dose as scheduled. Don't take two doses at once.

What to do about side effects
Taking too much tolbutamide may cause hypoglycemia, which can produce symptoms such as drowsiness, headache, nervousness, cold sweats, and confusion. If these symptoms occur, eat or drink something sweet, such as orange juice, and call your doctor.

What you must know about alcohol and other drugs
Avoid drinking alcoholic beverages while you're taking tolbutamide. If you do, you could have unpleasant side effects. Realize that many foods and drugs contain alcohol.

Tell your doctor if you're taking any other medication. Tolbutamide may interfere with the way some medications work, and other medications may interfere with tolbutamide's actions. Especially tell your doctor if you're taking a blood thinner; diet pills; medication for asthma, colds, allergies, high blood pressure, or tuberculosis; sulfa medication; aspirin; steroids; or a thiazide diuretic (a type of water pill).

Special directions
• Tell your doctor if you've ever had an allergic reaction to an oral medication used for treating diabetes or to a diuretic.
• Because some medical conditions may prevent you from taking tolbutamide, tell the doctor if you have a disorder that affects your liver, kidneys, adrenal glands, pituitary gland, or thyroid gland.
• Follow your doctor's instructions for testing your blood or urine for glucose. Also closely follow his prescribed diet and exercise regimen.
• This medication may increase your sensitivity to sunlight. Take precautions to protect your skin when outdoors.
• At all times, wear a medical identification bracelet stating you have diabetes and listing your medication.

Important reminder
Tell your doctor if you're breast-feeding or pregnant. Your doctor may need to prescribe a different medication.

Additional instructions

Taking tolmetin

Dear Patient:

Your doctor has prescribed tolmetin to treat your condition. Tolmetin helps control both inflammation and pain. The label on your medication may read Tolectin or Tolectin DS.

How to take tolmetin
Take your medication with milk, meals, or an antacid. This will help prevent stomach upset, which could occur if you take the drug on an empty stomach. If you use an antacid, choose one containing magnesium and aluminum hydroxides, such as Maalox.

Also drink a full (8-ounce) glass of water with each dose. Don't lie down for 15 to 30 minutes after taking the medication. This will help prevent irritation that could cause you to have difficulty swallowing.

What to do if you miss a dose
If your doctor has prescribed this medication on a regular schedule and you miss a dose, take it as soon as you remember. But if it's almost time for your next dose, skip the missed dose and take your next dose as scheduled.

What to do about side effects
Notify your doctor *immediately* if you notice any of these side effects:
• stomach pain or burning
• bloody or black, tarry stools
• easy bruising and bleeding
• changes in vision
• swelling in your face, feet, or lower legs
• persistent nausea or vomiting
• loss of appetite or weight loss.

What you must know about other drugs
Because tolmetin may interact with other medications, tell your doctor and pharmacist about other medications you're taking. In particular, tell your doctor if you're taking aspirin, phenytoin (Dilantin), thyroid medication, another anti-inflammatory medication, or a blood thinner.

Special directions
• Tell your doctor if aspirin or another anti-inflammatory medication has ever caused you to experience asthma-like symptoms, a runny nose, or itching.
• Also tell the doctor if you have a history of GI bleeding, liver or kidney disease, asthma, heart disease, or high blood pressure.
• Although the medication should begin working in 1 week, you may not feel its full effects for 2 to 4 weeks. But if your pain persists or worsens, let your doctor know.

Important reminder
This drug can hide the symptoms of an infection. Therefore, if you have diabetes, you need to be especially careful about caring for your feet and watching for any abnormality that might be caused by an infection.

Additional instructions

_____

_____

_____

_____

_____

Using tolnaftate

Dear Patient:

Your doctor has prescribed tolnaftate to treat your fungal skin infection. Tolnaftate comes in cream, gel, powder, lotion, pump-spray liquid, or aerosol forms. Available without a prescription, the label may read Aftate, Tinactin, or Genaspore.

How to use tolnaftate
First, wash the affected area and dry it thoroughly. Then apply enough medication to cover the area. Usually, ¼-inch to ½-inch ribbon of *cream* or three drops of *lotion* will cover an area the size of your hand.

If you're using a *powder* on your feet, sprinkle it between your toes, on your feet, and in your socks and shoes.

If you're using an *aerosol powder or solution,* shake the can well. Then, holding the can 6 to 10 inches away, spray the affected area. Don't inhale the vapor or powder from the spray. Also, don't use it near heat, an open flame, or while you're smoking.

If you're using a *pump-spray liquid,* hold the container 4 to 6 inches away from the area and spray.

Keep using the medication for 2 weeks after burning, itching, or other symptoms have disappeared. This will help you clear up the infection completely.

What to do if you miss a dose
Take it as soon as possible. Then return to your regular dosing schedule.

What to do about side effects
Check with your doctor or pharmacist if skin irritation occurs that wasn't present before you used this medication. If you're using the spray solution form of tolnaftate, you may experience a mild, temporary stinging sensation.

Special directions
• If you have a fungal infection of your hair or nails, see your doctor. This medication alone won't cure these types of infections.
• If you're treating athlete's foot and your symptoms haven't subsided after using the medication for 10 days, call your doctor. If you're treating another type of fungal infection and you've used the medication for 4 weeks without improvement, or if your symptoms have worsened, call your doctor.
• To help prevent reinfection after you've finished your treatment, use the powder or spray powder each day after bathing. Also sprinkle the powder or spray the aerosol inside your socks and shoes.

Important reminder
Don't use tolnaftate on a child younger than age 2, unless ordered otherwise by your doctor.

Additional instructions

_____

_____

_____

_____

_____

_____

Taking trazodone

Dear Patient:

Your doctor has prescribed trazodone to help treat your depression. The label may read Desyrel, Trazon, or Trialodine.

How to take trazodone

Take your medication after a meal or light snack, even if you're taking a dose at bedtime. This will help your body absorb the medication better and will lessen your risk of becoming dizzy or developing an upset stomach.

Continue taking the medication, even if you don't feel any different. You need to take the medication for 2 weeks before you feel any effect at all, and for 4 weeks before you feel the full effect.

What to do if you miss a dose

Take it as soon as possible. However, if you don't remember until it's less than 4 hours until your next dose, skip the missed dose and take your next dose on schedule. Don't take two doses at once.

What to do about side effects

If you're male, stop taking the medication and call your doctor *at once* if you develop a painful, inappropriate erection. For both sexes, call your doctor if you have confusion, muscle tremor, nausea and vomiting, loss of muscle coordination, or extreme drowsiness.

The most common side effects are drowsiness and dizziness. These should subside after a few weeks.

What you must know about alcohol and other drugs

Avoid drinking alcoholic beverages or taking depressant medications. That's because trazodone will add to the effects of alcohol and depressants, placing you at risk for oversedation. Examples of depressant medications include cold or allergy medication, sleeping pills, pain medication, muscle relaxants, or anesthetics.

Trazodone may also alter how your body uses other medications. Before taking trazodone, tell your doctor if you're taking high blood pressure medicine, heart medication, medication for seizures, or a monoamine oxidase (MAO) inhibitor, an antidepressant.

Special directions

• Tell your doctor if you're allergic to trazodone or another medication used to treat depression.
• Because this drug can make certain medical conditions worse, inform your doctor if you have a history of heart, liver, or kidney disease or a problem with ejaculation.
• Don't stop taking this medication without talking with your doctor first. He may want you to reduce your dose gradually.
• Because the medication may make you drowsy or less alert than normal, don't drive or operate machinery. Also, to prevent dizziness and protect yourself against a fall, get up slowly after you've been lying down.

Important reminder

If you're pregnant or breast-feeding, don't take this medication until you talk with your doctor.

Additional instructions

_____

_____

Applying tretinoin

Dear Patient:

Your doctor has prescribed tretinoin for your condition. Primarily used to treat acne, it may also be used to treat fine wrinkles resulting from sun damage. The label may read Retin-A.

How to apply tretinoin

First wash your skin with a mild, nonallergenic soap and water. Gently pat dry. Then wait 20 to 30 minutes to allow your skin to dry completely.

If you're applying the *cream* or *gel* form, apply enough medication to cover the affected areas and rub in gently.

If you're applying the *solution* form, use your fingertips, a gauze pad, or a cotton swab to cover the affected areas.

What to do if you miss an application

Skip the missed dose and apply your next dose as scheduled.

What to do about side effects

When you first start using tretinoin, your skin may turn red and you may notice a slight stinging or feeling of warmth. After a few days, your skin may scale or peel.

If you have severe burning or redness, swelling, blisters, or crusting, or if your skin darkens or lightens noticeably, check with your doctor.

What you must know about other skin products

Don't use solutions containing high concentrations of alcohol (such as skin freshener or aftershave lotion), menthol, spices, or lime (as in some perfumes). That's because they can interact with tretinoin and irritate your skin.

Special directions

• Tell your doctor if you're allergic to vitamin A or retinoic acid. Also mention whether you've had eczema.
• Avoid applying tretinoin close to your eyes or mouth, at the angles of your nose, on your mucous membranes, in an open wound, or to windburned or sunburned skin.
• While you're using tretinoin, don't use any of the following, unless your doctor tells you otherwise:
—abrasive or perfumed soaps or cleansers
—any other topical acne medication that makes the skin peel
—cosmetics or soaps that dry the skin
—medicated cosmetics
—any other topical skin medication.
• Don't wash your face more than two or three times a day to keep from drying out your skin. You may, however, wear cosmetics.
• Tretinoin will increase your skin's sensitivity to sunlight. Protect your skin from the sun by wearing a sunscreen, a hat, and protective clothing. If your face becomes sunburned, stop using the medication until the burn heals.
• The medication may also increase your sensitivity to wind and cold. Protect yourself by covering all exposed skin when you go out.

Important reminder

If you're pregnant or breast-feeding, talk with your doctor before using this medication.

Additional instructions

_____

_____

Taking triamterene

Dear Patient:

Your doctor has prescribed triamterene, a diuretic, to help reduce the amount of water in your body. The label may read Dyrenium.

How to take triamterene

If you're taking one dose a day, it's best to take it in the morning after breakfast. Why? Because the medication will increase your urine output. Taking it in the morning will help prevent your increase in urine from disturbing your sleep. If you take more than one dose a day, take the last dose no later than 6 p.m. If the medication upsets your stomach, take it with food or milk.

What to do if you miss a dose

Take it as soon as possible. But if it's almost time for your next dose, skip the missed dose and take your next dose as scheduled.

What to do about side effects

When you first start taking triamterene, you may feel unusually tired or dizzy. If this becomes particularly bothersome, call your doctor.

Triamterene may cause the amount of potassium in your body to increase. Watch for these signs and symptoms of too much potassium. If they develop, call your doctor *right away:*
• confusion or nervousness
• irregular heartbeat
• numbness or tingling in hands, feet, or lips
• difficulty breathing
• unusual tiredness or weakness
• weakness or heaviness in legs.

Also call your doctor right away if you develop a rash or itching.

What you must know about other drugs

Triamterene may interfere with the way some medications work. Tell your doctor if you're taking indomethacin (Indocin), digoxin (Lanoxin), lithium (Lithane), or a medication for high blood pressure.

Also, because triamterene may interfere with tests to measure the amount of quinidine in your blood, tell your doctor or the laboratory personnel if you're taking quinidine.

Because triamterene doesn't cause you to lose potassium the way some diuretics do, don't take a potassium supplement. Also avoid drinking low-sodium milk or using salt substitutes (which contain potassium), unless your doctor instructs you otherwise.

Special directions

• Tell your doctor if you have diabetes, kidney or liver disease, gout, menstrual problems, breast enlargement, or a history of kidney stones.
• To keep from becoming dizzy or fainting, change positions slowly. Also get up slowly after sitting or lying down.
• Your doctor may tell you to weigh yourself every day, measure your urine output, and monitor the amount of fluid you drink. Keep a written record of the results and take it with you when you visit the doctor.

Important reminders

If you have diabetes, be especially careful in testing your urine for glucose. That's because triamterene may raise your blood glucose level.

If you're an athlete, you should know that triamterene is banned and tested for by the U.S. Olympic Committee and National Collegiate Athletic Association.

Taking triazolam

Dear Patient:

Your doctor has prescribed triazolam to help you sleep. The label may read Halcion.

How to take triazolam
Follow your doctor's instructions exactly. Don't increase your dose, even if you think your current dose isn't effective. Instead, call your doctor.

Also, because triazolam can be habit-forming, don't take the medication for a longer time than your doctor recommends.

What to do about side effects
This medication may make you feel tired, drowsy, or dizzy. If the symptoms are severe, or if you feel very tired or "hung over" the day after you've taken the medication, your dose may be too high. Call your doctor so he can adjust your dosage.

What you must know about alcohol and other drugs
Avoid drinking alcoholic beverages while you're taking triazolam. That's because, when taken together, alcohol increases the depressant effects of the medication. At the same time, the medication increases the depressant effects of alcohol. As a result, you could overdose. For this same reason, avoid taking narcotic drugs unless told otherwise by your doctor.

Inform your doctor if you're taking cimetidine (Tagamet) or erythromycin (E-Mycin). Either of these medications could cause triazolam to stay in your bloodstream for a prolonged period of time.

Also tell your doctor if you're taking zidovudine (also called AZT). Triazolam could cause your body to absorb a greater amount of zidovudine. Therefore, the doctor may need to decrease your dosage.

Special directions
• Triazolam could aggravate certain medical problems. For this reason, be sure to tell your doctor if you have glaucoma, a history of alcohol or drug abuse, a mental disorder, myasthenia gravis, Parkinson's disease, or kidney or liver disease.
• Because this medication may make you drowsy or light-headed, don't drive or operate any machinery until you know how you respond.
• After you stop taking triazolam, you may have difficulty sleeping for the next few nights. This is not unusual and should stop on its own.

Important reminders
Don't take this medication if you think you might be pregnant, or if you're breast-feeding. If you're an older adult, be aware that this medication could make you drowsy during the day, which could lead to falls.

Be aware that triazolam is banned and in some cases tested for by the U.S. Olympic Committee and the National Collegiate Athletic Association.

Additional instructions

_____

_____

_____

Taking trimethobenzamide

Dear Patient:

Your doctor has prescribed trimethobenzamide to help treat your nausea and vomiting. The label may read Tigan or Trimazide.

How to take trimethobenzamide

Follow your doctor's instructions exactly. Don't use more of this medication, or take it more often, than your doctor has ordered.

If you're using a *rectal suppository* form of this drug, remove the foil wrapper and moisten the suppository with cold water. Lie down on your side and use your finger to push the suppository well up into your rectum. If the suppository is too soft to insert, place it in the refrigerator for 30 minutes, or run cold water over it before removing the wrapper. Wash your hands before and after inserting the suppository.

What to do if you miss a dose

Take it as soon as possible. But if it's almost time for your next dose, skip this dose and take your next dose as scheduled. Don't take two doses at once.

What to do about side effects

This medication commonly causes drowsiness.

Call your doctor *immediately* if you develop any of the following uncommon side effects:
• skin rash
• shakiness or tremor
• unusual tiredness
• severe or continued vomiting
• yellow eyes or skin.

Special directions

• Tell your doctor if you've ever had an allergic reaction to this drug, benzocaine, or to a local anesthetic. Also mention whether you have other medical problems, particularly a high fever or an intestinal infection.
• Because this medication may make you dizzy or light-headed, don't drive or perform any activities that could be dangerous if you're dizzy or not alert.

Important reminders

Don't give this medication to a child unless the cause of vomiting is known. When given to a child with a viral illness (a common cause of vomiting), this medication may lead to Reye's syndrome, which is a potentially fatal brain disorder.

If you're pregnant or breast-feeding, don't take this medication without first talking with your doctor.

Additional instructions

_____

_____

_____

_____

_____

_____

_____

_____

Taking valproic acid

Dear Patient:

Your doctor has prescribed valproic acid to treat your seizures. The label may read Depakene, Depakote, or My-proic Acid.

How to take valproic acid

Swallow your medication (whether in tablet or capsule form) whole, without breaking or chewing it. Take it with food or water to keep it from upsetting your stomach. Don't take it with milk.

If you're taking the *syrup* form of the drug, you may mix it with food or a beverage. However, don't mix it with a carbonated beverage, like soda. Doing so may irritate your mouth and throat.

Don't stop taking the medication suddenly. Doing so may cause seizures.

What to do if you miss a dose

If you take one dose a day, take the missed dose as soon as possible. But if you don't remember until the next day, skip the missed dose and take your next dose as scheduled.

If you take two or more doses a day, and you remember the missed dose within 6 hours, take it right away. Then equally space your remaining doses for the day. Never take two doses at once.

What to do about side effects

Call your doctor *right away* if you develop any of the following side effects:
• unusual bleeding or bruising
• extreme drowsiness
• loss of appetite
• continued nausea and vomiting
• tiredness or weakness
• yellow eyes or skin
• trembling
• fever.

What you must know about alcohol and other drugs

Avoid drinking alcoholic beverages while taking this medication. Alcohol may decrease the effectiveness of the medication while causing you to become overly sedated.

Don't take antacids or aspirin without first talking with your doctor. If taken while you're taking valproic acid, these medications could cause undesirable side effects. Also tell him if you're taking a blood thinner or other drugs to control seizures.

Special directions

• Let your doctor know if you have a history of liver disease because it may affect your body's ability to break down valproic acid.
• Because the medication may make you drowsy, don't drive or do anything that could be dangerous if you're not alert until you know how you respond to the medication.
• Because the valproic acid may affect how quickly your blood can clot, take precautions to keep from cutting yourself. For example, use an electric razor and a soft toothbrush.

Important reminders

If you have diabetes, be aware that this medication may make urine tests for ketones unreliable. If you're pregnant or breast-feeding, don't take this medication until you talk with your doctor.

If you're an athlete, you should know that valproic acid is banned and in some cases tested for by the U.S. Olympic Committee and the National Collegiate Athletic Association.

Taking vancomycin

Dear Patient:

Your doctor has prescribed vancomycin to treat your bacterial infection. The label may read Vancocin.

How to take vancomycin

Take vancomycin only as your doctor directs. If you're taking the *oral liquid* form of the medication, use a specially marked measuring spoon to accurately measure each dose. A household teaspoon may not hold the correct amount.

If you're taking the *injection* form by mouth, dissolve the powder in each vial in 1 ounce of water. Then drink the liquid.

Continue to take this medication even after you begin to feel better. Stopping too soon allows your infection to return.

What to do if you miss a dose

Take it as soon as possible. However, if it's almost time for your next dose, skip the missed dose and take your next dose as scheduled. Don't double dose.

What to do about side effects

Call your doctor *right away* if you develop any of the following side effects:
• ringing or buzzing in your ears
• a feeling of fullness in your ears
• rash or itching
• difficulty breathing.

Also check with your doctor if you experience nausea and vomiting after taking the medication.

What you must know about other drugs

Taking certain medications at the same time you're taking vancomycin may increase your risk for side effects. So be sure to tell your doctor if you're taking any of these medications: aminoglycosides (a type of antibiotic), amphotericin B (Fungizone), cisplatin (Platinol), or pentamidine (NebuPent, Pentam 300).

If you're taking *oral* vancomycin, tell your doctor if you're taking cholestyramine (Questran) or colestipol (Colestid). Both of these medications may prevent vancomycin from working properly.

Special directions

• Be sure to tell your doctor if you've ever had an allergic reaction to vancomycin. Also, because certain medical conditions may prevent your using this drug, tell your doctor if you have a history of kidney disease, hearing loss, or an inflammatory bowel disorder.
• Before using new medication, or if you develop a new medical problem while you're taking vancomycin, check with your doctor or pharmacist.

Important reminder

If you're pregnant or breast-feeding, check with your doctor before taking vancomycin.

Additional instructions

_____

_____

_____

_____

_____

_____

Taking verapamil

Dear Patient:

Your doctor has prescribed verapamil (also called Calan or Isoptin) to treat your condition. Verapamil helps relax blood vessels, which increases the flow of blood to your heart. In turn, this helps relieve chest pain, heart irregularities, and high blood pressure.

How to take verapamil

Take verapamil only as your doctor directs. If you're taking an extended-release tablet, swallow it whole, without crushing or chewing it.

Take verapamil on an empty stomach. Taking extended-release tablets with food may decrease your body's ability to absorb the drug.

Take your medication even if you feel well. Stopping suddenly could cause your condition to worsen.

What to do if you miss a dose

Take it as soon as possible. However, if it's almost time for your next dose, skip the missed dose and take your next dose as scheduled.

What to do about side effects

Call your doctor *immediately* if you develop any of the side effects listed here:
• breathing difficulty, coughing, or wheezing
• irregular or fast, pounding heartbeat
• swelling of ankles, feet, or lower legs.

Also notify your doctor if you become constipated or faint, feel unusually tired, or continue to have chest pain.

What you must know about other drugs

Some medications may affect how verapamil works. At the same time, verapamil may interfere with another drug's actions. Therefore, be sure to tell your doctor about any medications you're taking, particularly lithium (Lithane) or heart medications, or medications for high blood pressure, seizures, tuberculosis, or glaucoma.

Special directions

• Because verapamil may cause certain medical conditions to worsen, tell your doctor if you have a history of kidney or liver disease or some other heart or blood vessel disorder.
• Eat foods high in fiber and be sure to drink plenty of fluids (unless your doctor tells you otherwise) to help prevent constipation.
• If fatigue is a problem, remember to allow yourself several rest periods during the day.

Important reminder

If you're pregnant or breast-feeding, check with your doctor before taking verapamil.

Additional instructions

_____

_____

_____

_____

_____

_____

_____

Taking warfarin

Dear Patient:

Your doctor has prescribed warfarin (also called Coumadin or Panwarfin) for you. By reducing your blood's ability to clot, this medication prevents harmful clots from forming in your blood vessels. Warfarin won't dissolve clots that you already have. But it should stop clots from growing larger and causing complications.

How to take warfarin

Take warfarin only as your doctor directs. Don't take more or less, and don't take it more often or longer than he directs. Take it at the same time each day.

What to do if you miss a dose

Take it as soon as possible. Then go back to your regular schedule.

If you miss a day, don't take the missed dose at all, and never take a double dose. This may cause bleeding.

What to do about side effects

Call your doctor *at once* if your gums bleed when you brush your teeth. Also call him if you have bruises or purplish marks on your skin, nosebleeds, heavy bleeding or oozing from cuts or wounds, excessive or unexpected menstrual bleeding, blood in your urine or sputum, vomit that looks like coffee grounds, or bloody or black tarry stools.

Call your doctor if you have unusual pain or swelling in your joints or your stomach, unusual backaches, diarrhea, constipation, dizziness, or a severe or continuing headache.

What you must know about alcohol and other drugs

Avoid drinking alcoholic beverages on a regular basis because alcohol may interfere with warfarin's effectiveness. An occasional drink is okay but don't have more than one or two.

Check with your doctor before taking nonprescription drugs. Certain vitamins can reduce warfarin's effectiveness, and aspirin and similar drugs can cause bleeding.

Also tell your doctor about other prescription medications you're taking. Some drugs, when taken with warfarin, could interfere with warfarin's action or cause bleeding.

Special directions

• To reduce your risk of injuring yourself, always wear shoes, place a nonskid mat in your bathtub, shave with an electric razor, and use a soft toothbrush.
• Remember to keep your blood test appointments. If blood tests show that your blood isn't clotting at the right rate, the doctor may decide to adjust your dosage.
• Make sure to let your other doctors and your dentist know you're taking warfarin.
• Wear a medical identification tag identifying you as a warfarin user.
• Check with your doctor before beginning any strenuous programs. And avoid risky activities—for example, roughhousing with children and pets.

Important reminder

If you're considering becoming pregnant, think about delaying pregnancy or discuss it with your doctor. Warfarin can impair your baby's development and cause placental bleeding.

Taking zidovudine

Dear Patient:

Your doctor has prescribed zidovudine, also known as AZT or Retrovir, for you. Zidovudine helps slow the progress of the human immunodeficiency virus (HIV). In turn, this helps slow HIV's destruction of the immune system. Zidovudine does not cure HIV infection or acquired immunodeficiency syndrome (AIDS). It also won't keep you from spreading HIV to others.

How to take zidovudine

Take zidovudine only as your doctor directs. Don't take more or less of it, and don't take it more often or longer than he directs. Take it for the full length of treatment, even if you begin to feel better. And don't stop taking it without checking with your doctor first.

You need to take the medication every 4 hours around the clock—even during the night. Take your medication at the same times every day.

If you're taking the *syrup* form of the drug, measure your dose in a specially marked spoon. A household teaspoon may not hold the correct amount.

What to do if you miss a dose

Take it as soon as possible. But if it's almost time for your next dose, skip the missed dose and take your next dose as scheduled. Don't take two doses at once.

What to do about side effects

Zidovudine may cause some serious side effects, including bone marrow problems. Call your doctor *right away* if you develop any of the following:
• fever, chills, or sore throat
• pale skin

• unusual tiredness or weakness
• unusual bleeding or bruising.
Also let your doctor know if you develop a severe headache, muscle soreness, nausea, or trouble sleeping.

What you must know about other drugs

Taking certain drugs while you're taking zidovudine may increase your risk for dangerous side effects. That's why you need to tell your doctor about any other drugs you're taking—even nonprescription ones like acetaminophen (Tylenol).

Special directions

• Because other medical problems may affect the use of zidovudine, tell the doctor if you have anemia, other blood disorders, or liver disease.
• Remember to keep your follow-up doctor's appointments. You need to have your blood checked frequently—at least every 2 weeks—to make sure that the medication is working properly and that you're not developing any dangerous side effects.
• If the medication makes you dizzy, don't drive or perform any activity that could be dangerous if you're not fully alert.
• Because zidovudine may cause blood problems and slow healing, be careful not to injure yourself. Use a soft toothbrush, and use toothpicks or dental floss cautiously so you don't injure your gums.

Important reminders

If you become pregnant, let your doctor know at once. If you're breast-feeding, you should stop while you're taking the drug.

Supportive measures

Drug therapy often requires measures to support and enhance the medication's effectiveness. Your patient may have to adjust his diet, learn to take his blood pressure, or just find a way to remember to take his medication. Changes like these require patient teaching; the aids in this section can help.

Divided into four groups, these supportive teaching aids address comfort and dietary measures, health monitoring, and health promotion. Step-by-step organization, illustrations, large print, and lists make these teaching aids easy to read and understand.

The teaching aids in *Comfort measures* will help your patient learn relaxation techniques to help relieve pain and reduce stress. This group of aids also includes guidelines on controlling chemotherapy's side effects, selecting cold medications, and using pain relief equipment at home.

Because patients sometimes mistakenly rely entirely on a medication to resolve their health problems, they may not realize the importance of diet in their treatment. Medications may cause vitamin and mineral deficiencies or other side effects, such as constipation or anorexia, that require changes in your patient's diet. *Dietary measures* includes teaching aids that cover the most common diet changes patients face, such as cutting down on salt and cholesterol or adding fiber, calories, or other nutrients to their diet.

The tips and memory aids suggested in *Health monitoring* may help the patient who has a hard time remembering to take his medication. In addition, his medication regimen may require that he check his temperature, pulse rate, or blood pressure. This group of teaching aids spells out the proper procedures for your patient in simple terms.

By making your patient more aware of *Health promotion* issues, such as infection control and hand-washing techniques, you can reduce the risk of reinfection or contagion. Other teaching aids in this group tell your patient what to do about medication-induced photosensitivity and alert him to avoid allergy triggers.

Performing relaxation breathing

Dear Patient:

Relaxation breathing can help you cope with stress or pain. You can use it anywhere and at any time. You can also combine it with other techniques to help control pain. Try to practice these simple breathing techniques daily. Now, get yourself comfortable and begin.

1 Close your eyes. Inhale slowly and deeply through your nose as you count silently: "In, 2, 3, 4." Notice how your stomach expands first, then your rib cage, and finally your upper chest.

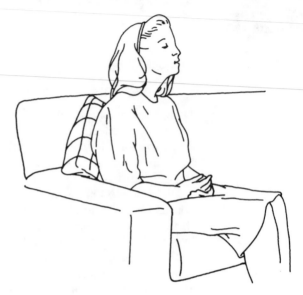

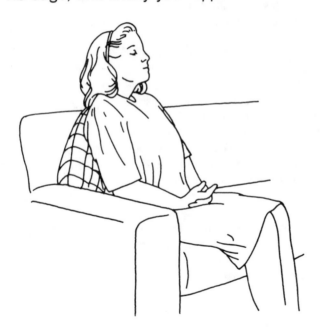

Now exhale slowly through your mouth as you count silently: "Out, 2, 3, 4, 5, 6." Pretend you're breathing out through a straw to lengthen exhalation. Let your shoulders drop slightly as your upper chest, rib cage, and stomach gently deflate.

Repeat this exercise four or five times.

2 Inhale for 4 seconds. Hold your breath for the count of 4, but don't strain. Then exhale through your mouth for 6 to 8 seconds. Practice this exercise four or five times.

A few tips
Use these breathing exercises for as long as you need to during painful periods. You may vary the rhythm, but always exhale for 2 to 4 seconds longer than you inhale.

If you feel light-headed or your fingers tingle, you may be breathing too deeply or too fast. Reduce the depth and speed of your breathing, or breathe into a paper bag until the feeling goes away.

Additional instructions

_____

_____

_____

Relaxing your muscles

Dear Patient:

No matter where you are, you can relax your muscles with a technique called progressive muscle relaxation. This technique helps to relieve the muscle tension that accompanies pain. By learning to tense and relax your muscles one by one, you'll find you can relax your entire body. Here's how.

1 Get comfortable, and close your eyes. Starting at the top of your body, tense your forehead and face. Do you notice how these muscles feel tight and strained? Hold this tension for 5 to 10 seconds.

2 Next, relax your forehead and face. Do you notice the relief you feel? Hold and enjoy this relaxation for 10 to 15 seconds.

3 Now work toward your feet. First, tense and relax your jaw muscles. Proceed to the muscles in each shoulder, arm, and hand, then to your stomach, buttocks, each thigh, each lower leg, and finally to each ankle and foot.

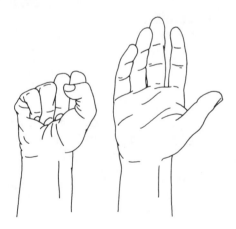

If you have trouble relaxing some muscles, or if the tension brings on pain, try gently massaging that body part until the muscles relax and feel comfortable.

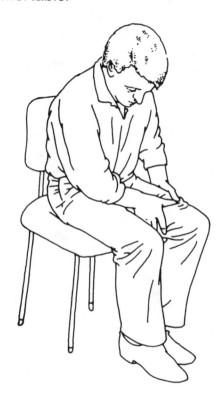

4 To complete the exercise, open your eyes, stretch, and relax your entire body. Take a few deep breaths as if you're waking up from a deep sleep. Don't engage in any activity until you're fully alert.

Additional instructions

_____

_____

Controlling side effects of chemotherapy

Dear Patient:

Your doctor has ordered chemotherapy to treat your cancer. Besides treating cancer, these therapies often cause unpleasant side effects. Fortunately, you can sometimes prevent them. Other times you can do things to make yourself more comfortable. Just follow the advice below.

Mouth sores
• Keep your mouth and teeth clean by brushing after every meal with a soft toothbrush.

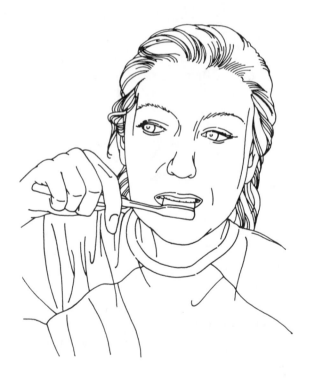

• Don't use commercial mouthwashes that contain alcohol, which may irritate your mouth during chemotherapy. Instead, rinse with water or water mixed with baking soda or use a suspension of sucralfate (Carafate) if your doctor orders it. Floss daily, and apply fluoride if your dentist recommends it. If you have dentures, be sure to remove them often for cleaning.
• Until your mouth sores heal, avoid foods that are difficult to chew (such as apples) or irritating to your mouth (such as acidic citrus juices). Also avoid drinking alcohol, smoking, and eating extremely hot or spicy foods.
• Eat soft, bland foods, such as eggs and oatmeal, and soothing foods, such as ice pops. Your doctor might also prescribe medication for mouth sores.

Dry mouth
• Frequently sip cool liquids and suck on ice chips or sugarless candy.
• Ask your doctor about artificial saliva. Use water, juices, sauces, and dressings to soften your food and make it easier to swallow. Don't smoke or drink alcohol, which can further dry your mouth.

Nausea and vomiting
• Before a chemotherapy treatment, try eating a light, bland snack, such as toast or crackers. Or don't eat anything—some patients find that fasting controls nausea better.
• Keep unpleasant odors out of your dining area. Avoid strong-smelling foods. Also brush your teeth before eating to refresh your mouth.

(continued)

Controlling side effects of chemotherapy *(continued)*

• Eat small, frequent meals and avoid lying down for 2 hours after you eat. Try small amounts of clear, unsweetened liquids, such as apple juice, and then progress to crackers or dry toast. Stay away from sweets and fried or other high-fat foods. It's best to stay with bland foods.

• Take antiemetic drugs, as your doctor orders. Be sure to notify him if vomiting is severe or lasts longer than 24 hours or if you urinate less, feel weak, or have a dry mouth.

Diarrhea

• Stick with low-fiber foods, such as bananas, rice, applesauce, toast, or mashed potatoes. Stay away from high-fiber foods, such as raw vegetables and fruits and whole-grain breads. Also avoid milk products and fruit juices. Cabbage, coffee, beans, and sweets can increase stomach cramps.

• Because potassium may be lost when you have diarrhea, eat high-potassium foods, such as bananas and potatoes. Check with your doctor to see if you need a potassium supplement.

• After a bowel movement, clean your anal area gently and apply petroleum jelly (Vaseline) to prevent soreness.

• Ask your doctor about antidiarrheal medications. Notify him if your diarrhea doesn't stop or if you urinate less, have a dry mouth, or feel weak.

Constipation

• Eat high-fiber foods unless your doctor tells you otherwise. They include raw fruits and vegetables (with skins on, washed well), whole-grain breads and cereals, and beans. If you're not used to eating high-fiber foods, start gradually to let your body get accustomed to the change—or else you could develop diarrhea.

• Drink plenty of liquids—unless your doctor tells you not to.

• If changing your diet doesn't help, ask your doctor about stool softeners or laxatives. Check with your doctor before using enemas.

Heartburn

• Avoid spicy foods, alcohol, and smoking. Eat small, frequent meals.

• After eating, don't lie down right away. Avoid bending or stooping.

• Take oral medications with a glass of milk or a snack.

• Use antacids, as your doctor orders.

Muscle aches or pain, weakness, numbness or tingling

• Take acetaminophen (Tylenol). Or ask your doctor for acetaminophen with codeine.

• Apply heat where it hurts or feels numb.

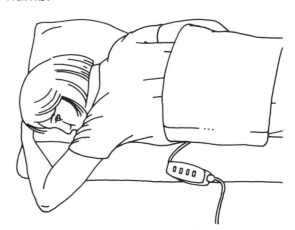

(continued)

Controlling side effects of chemotherapy *(continued)*

• Be sure to rest. Also, avoid activities that aggravate your symptoms.
• If symptoms don't go away and pain focuses on one area, notify your doctor.

Hair loss
• Wash your hair gently. Use a mild shampoo and avoid frequent brushing or combing.
• Get a short haircut to make thinning hair less noticeable.
• Consider wearing a wig or toupee during therapy. Buy one before chemotherapy begins. Or use a hat, scarf, or turban to cover your head during therapy.

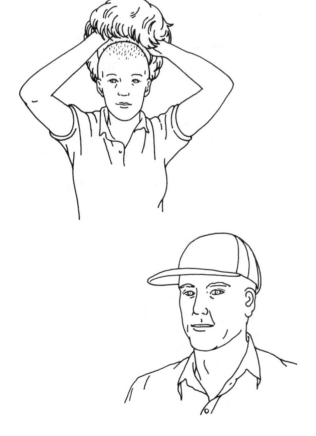

Skin problems
• For sensitive or dry skin, ask your doctor or nurse to recommend a lotion.

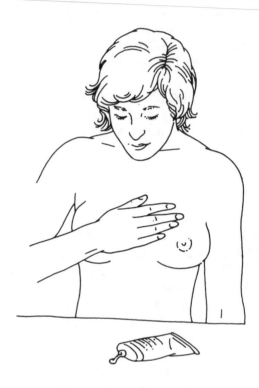

• Use cornstarch to absorb moisture, and avoid tight clothing over the treatment area. Be sure to report any blisters or cracked skin to the doctor.
• Stay out of the sun during the course of therapy. You may even have to avoid the sun for several months afterward, so check with your doctor, especially if you're planning a vacation to a sunny area. When you *can* go out in the sun again, wear light clothes over the treated area, and wear a hat, too. Cover all exposed skin with a good sun block lotion (skin protection factor [SPF] 15 or above).

(continued)

Controlling side effects of chemotherapy *(continued)*

Tiredness
- Limit activities, especially sports.
- Get more sleep.
- Try to reduce your work hours until the end of treatments. Discuss your therapy schedule with your employer.
- If at all possible, schedule chemotherapy treatments at your convenience.
- Ask for help from family and friends, whether it's pitching in with daily chores or driving you to the hospital.

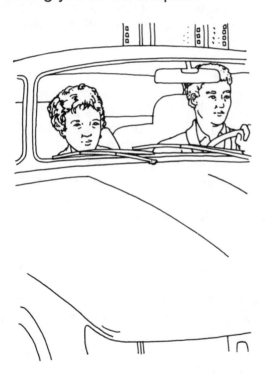

Most people are glad to help out—they just need to be asked.
- If you lose interest in sex during treatments, either because you're too tired or because of hormonal changes, bear in mind that sexual desire usually returns after treatments end.

Risk of infection
You're more likely to get an infection during therapy, so follow these tips:
- Avoid crowds and people with colds and infections.
- Use an electric shaver instead of a razor.

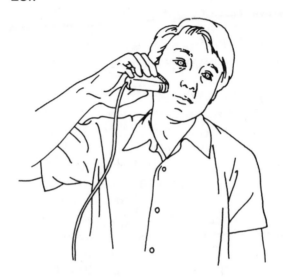

- Use a soft toothbrush. It will help you avoid injuring your gums—a frequent site of infection.
- Tell your doctor if you have a fever, chills, a tendency to bruise easily, or any unusual bleeding.

Additional instructions

_____

_____

_____

_____

_____

_____

Learning about TENS

Dear Patient:

Your doctor has ordered transcutaneous electrical nerve stimulation (also called TENS) to help relieve your pain.

How TENS works
A small, battery-operated device sends safe electrical signals through wires and into your body by way of electrodes, which you attach to your skin.

Where to place the electrodes
Your TENS therapist will show you where to attach the electrodes. Ask him to label the sites with a marker. If necessary, use a mirror to help you see them. Ask a friend or a family member to note the sites, too. That way he can give you reassurance if you feel nervous the first few times you use the TENS unit. Or if needed, he can help you place the electrodes another time.

If your electrodes require conductive jelly, spread it in a thin layer across each electrode before applying the electrode.

Placing your electrodes on the wrong sites probably won't harm you, but avoid placing them on your belly if you are pregnant, on the sides of the neck, or on the voice box area.

Using TENS
The knobs on your unit are adjustable:
• Set the AMP/A at _____.
• Set the rate at _____.
• Set the pulse-width at _____.
• Turn your TENS unit *on* for _____ minutes and *off* for _____ minutes throughout the day.

You should feel a pleasant sensation while the machine is working. If you develop muscle spasms, contact the TENS therapist. The AMP may be set too high, or you may have placed the electrodes in the wrong places.

If your pain is increasing, follow the directions your TENS therapist gave you to change the settings on your TENS unit.

Safety tips
Follow your therapist's instructions carefully for the amount of time you should leave your TENS unit on. Don't get into water with the unit on, and don't sleep with it on.

Skin care
Take good care of your skin. Prevent local skin irritation—redness and rash—by cleaning your skin before attaching the electrodes. Watch for signs of irritation.

If your skin becomes irritated, don't place electrodes on those areas. Keep the skin clean and dry until it heals. If it's still irritated after a week, contact the doctor.

If you repeatedly develop local skin irritation from the electrodes, contact your TENS therapist to discuss an alternative wearing schedule or another type of electrode.

Caring for the TENS unit
Clean your TENS unit weekly by lightly wiping it with rubbing alcohol.

Additional instructions

_____

_____

_____

Selecting cold remedies

Dear Patient:

The only real cure for a cold is time. After 7 to 10 days, a cold and its symptoms have usually run their course. But during this period, a cold can make you feel miserable.

Cold remedies offer temporary relief from aches, sniffles, and sneezes. Learn about ingredients. Then pick your product carefully and use it as directed.

Safety first

You want to avoid undesirable side effects from any cold remedy, so take only one cold remedy at a time. Taking more than one could cause an overdose if the products contain the same ingredients. Also, don't take both a cold remedy and a prescription drug without asking your doctor if it's safe to combine them.

Pain relievers

Most cold remedies contain pain relievers, such as aspirin or acetaminophen (Tylenol), to decrease fever, muscle soreness, and headaches. Avoid taking these medications if you're taking painkillers for another condition.

Antihistamines

These drugs have a drying effect on your body's tissues. That's why they relieve a runny nose and watery eyes. But most of them also make you sleepy. If you take them, avoid activities that require alertness, such as driving or using power tools. Check the labels of any medications for insomnia or diarrhea. They may contain antihistamines, too. Taking both remedies increases your chances for such side effects as constipation, dry mouth, and blurred vision.

Decongestants

By narrowing the blood vessels in your nose, decongestants reduce stuffiness. If you use a decongestant, take only the amount directed because it can raise your blood pressure. Check the label for *phenylpropanolamine,* a stimulant and diet pill ingredient, which can produce unwanted side effects.

Consider using decongestant nasal sprays or drops. They're safer than liquids or tablets because little of the drug enters your bloodstream when applied directly into your nose. Don't overuse the spray, though. If you do, stuffiness may continue after your cold goes away.

Cough medicines

These products may contain a cough suppressant, an expectorant, or both. Use suppressants if you have a dry hacking cough. Don't use them if your cough brings up mucus. A "wet" cough helps clear your breathing passages.

Expectorants loosen mucus to produce a wet cough. Drink plenty of fluids to make your mucus easier to expel.

Other ingredients

Many liquid medications contain alcohol to dissolve the other ingredients and caffeine to neutralize the effects of alcohol or antihistamines. Avoid these medications if you can't tolerate them.

Additional instructions

_____

_____

_____

_____

Adding fiber to your diet

Dear Patient:

Here are four easy ways to add fiber to your diet.

Eat whole-grain breads and cereals

For the first few days, eat one serving daily of whole-grain breads (1 slice), cereal (½ cup), pasta (½ cup), or brown rice (⅓ cup). Examples of whole-grain breads are whole wheat and pumpernickel. Examples of high-fiber cereals are bran or oat flakes and shredded wheat. Gradually increase to four or more servings daily.

Eat fresh fruits and vegetables

Begin by eating one serving daily of raw or cooked, unpeeled fruit (one medium-size piece; ½ cup cooked) or unpeeled vegetables (½ cup cooked; 1 cup raw). Gradually increase to four servings daily. Examples of high-fiber fruits include apples, oranges, and peaches. Some high-fiber vegetables are carrots, corn, and peas.

Eat dried peas and beans

Begin by eating one serving (⅓ cup) a week. Increase to at least two to three servings a week.

Eat unprocessed bran

Add bran to your food. Start with 1 teaspoon a day, and over a 3-week period work up to 2 to 3 tablespoons a day. Don't use more than this. Remember to drink at least six 8-ounce (oz) glasses of fluid a day.

A small amount of bran can be beneficial, but too much can irritate your digestive tract, cause gas, interfere with mineral absorption, and even lodge in your intestine.

Note: Crisp fresh fruits and vegetables, cooked foods with husks, and nuts must be chewed thoroughly so that large particles don't pass whole into the intestine and lodge there, causing problems.

A sample menu

Breakfast
½ grapefruit
Oatmeal with milk and raisins (add bran if desired)
Bran muffin
8 oz liquid

Lunch
Cabbage slaw
Tuna salad sandwich on whole-wheat bread
Fresh pear with skin
8 oz liquid

Dinner
Vegetable soup
Broiled fish with almond topping
Baked potato with skin
Carrots and peas
Canned crushed pineapple
8 oz liquid

Snack
Dried fruit and nut mix
8 oz liquid

Additional instructions

_____

_____

_____

_____

Adding calories to your diet

Dear Patient:

Here are some tips to help add calories to your diet.

Eat high-calorie snacks
Good choices include dried fruits, such as raisins and apricots; peanut butter or cheese spread on crackers, bread, fresh fruit, or raw vegetables; milk shakes made with ice cream, cream, powdered milk, or instant breakfast powders; and breakfast bars.

Add fat and sugar to food
• Put margarine or butter on bread, rice, noodles, potatoes, and vegetables. Use mayonnaise or margarine on sandwiches.
• Add sour cream to casseroles, or serve it with potatoes, vegetables, meat, and fruit.
• Serve meat, vegetables, and casseroles with cream sauces or gravy.
• Mix extra amounts of salad dressing in salads.
• Add whipped cream to hot chocolate, fruit, and desserts.
• Top ice cream with syrup or preserves.
• Spread bread, muffins, biscuits, or crackers with jam, jelly, or honey.
• Substitute half-and-half or cream for milk in coffee or tea.
• Add cheese to scrambled eggs, sauces, vegetables, casseroles, and salads.
• Use extra eggs in sauces, casseroles, sandwich spreads, and salads. Add powdered eggs to milk shakes. (Don't use raw eggs—they can cause food poisoning.)
• Sprinkle chopped or ground nuts on ice cream, yogurt, frozen yogurt, pudding, breads, and desserts. (Children under age 4 shouldn't eat whole nuts because they might choke.)

Use high-calorie supplements
If you've experienced lung damage, repeated infections, or weight loss, try adding commercial, high-protein calorie supplements to your daily diet. Typical commercial supplements include Ensure, Ensure Plus, Meritene, and Sustacal. Or use instant breakfast powders mixed with whole milk to get about the same number of calories and nutritional value as the supplements.

Additional instructions

_____

_____

_____

_____

_____

_____

_____

_____

_____

_____

_____

Cutting down on salt

Dear Patient:

Your doctor may recommend cutting down on salt because too much salt can affect your health. Reducing your salt intake isn't hard to do. The following information and suggestions will help you get started.

Facts about salt
• Table salt is about 40% sodium.
• Americans consume about 20 times more salt than their bodies need.
• About three-fourths of the salt you consume is already in the foods you eat and drink.
• One teaspoon (tsp) of salt contains about 2 grams (2,000 milligrams [mg]) of sodium.
• You can reduce your intake to this level simply by not salting your food during cooking or before eating.

Tips for reducing salt intake
Reducing your salt intake to a teaspoon or less a day is easy if you:
• read labels on medications and foods.
• put away your salt shaker; or, if you must use salt, use "light salt" that contains half the sodium of ordinary table salt.
• buy fresh meats, fruits, and vegetables instead of canned, processed, and convenience foods.
• substitute spices and lemon juice for salt.
• watch out for sources of hidden sodium—for example, carbonated beverages, nondairy creamers, cookies, and cakes.
• avoid salty foods, such as bacon, sausage, pretzels, potato chips, mustard, pickles, and some cheeses.

Know your sodium sources
Canned, prepared, and "fast" foods are loaded with sodium; so are condiments, such as ketchup. Some foods that don't taste salty contain high amounts of sodium. Consider the values below:

Food	mg sodium
1 can tomato soup	872
1 cup canned spaghetti	1,236
1 hot dog	639
1 cheeseburger	709
1 slice pepperoni pizza	817
1 tablespoon ketchup	156
1 tsp salt	1,955
1 dill pickle	928
1 cup corn flakes	256
3 ounces lean ham	1,128
2½ oz dried chipped beef	3,052

Other high-sodium sources include baking powder, baking soda, barbecue sauce, bouillon cubes, celery salt, chili sauce, cooking wine, garlic salt, onion salt, softened water, and soy sauce.

Surprisingly, many medications and other nonfood items contain sodium, such as alkalizers for indigestion, laxatives, aspirin, cough medicine, mouthwash, and toothpaste.

Additional instructions

_____

_____

_____

_____

_____

Cutting down on cholesterol

Dear Patient:

By changing your diet, you can help reduce your cholesterol level and ensure better health. You also need to reduce the amount of saturated fats you eat. This means cutting down drastically on eggs, dairy products, and fatty meats.

Rely instead on poultry, fish, fruits, vegetables, and high-fiber breads.

Use this list as a starting point for your new diet. If you do a lot of home baking, adapt your recipes by using modest amounts of unsaturated oils. Remember to substitute two egg whites when a recipe calls for one whole egg.

FOOD	ELIMINATE	SUBSTITUTE
Bread and cereals	Breads with whole eggs listed as a major ingredient	Oatmeal, multigrain, and bran cereals; whole-grain breads; rye bread
	Egg noodles	Pasta, rice
	Pies, cakes, doughnuts, biscuits, high-fat crackers and cookies	Angel food cake; low-fat cookies, crackers, and home-baked goods
Eggs and dairy products	Whole milk, 2% milk, imitation milk	Skim milk, 1% milk, buttermilk
	Cream, half-and-half, most nondairy creamers, whipped toppings	None
	Whole milk yogurt and cottage cheese	Nonfat or low-fat yogurt, low-fat (1% or 2%) cottage cheese
	Cheese, cream cheese, sour cream, light cream cheese, light sour cream	Cholesterol-free sour cream alternative, such as King Sour
	Egg yolks	Egg whites
	Ice cream	Sherbert, frozen tofu
Fats and oils	Coconut, palm, and palm kernel oils	Unsaturated vegetable oils (corn, olive, canola, safflower, sesame, soybean, and sunflower)
	Butter, lard, bacon fat	Unsaturated margarine and shortening, diet margarine
	Dressings made with egg yolks	Mayonnaise, unsaturated or low-fat salad dressings
	Chocolate	Baking cocoa
Meat, fish, and poultry	Fatty cuts of beef, lamb, or pork	Lean cuts of beef, lamb, or pork
	Organ meats, spare ribs, cold cuts, sausage, hot dogs, bacon	Poultry
	Sardines, roe	Sole, salmon, mackerel

Learning about potassium-rich foods

Dear Patient:

If you're taking medication that decreases the level of potassium in your body, your doctor may recommend adding potassium to your diet.

How much potassium do you need?

Doctors recommend 300 to 400 milligrams (mg) of potassium daily. Not enough potassium can cause leg cramps, weakness, paralysis, and spasms. Too much can cause heart problems and fatigue.

The chart below lists potassium-rich foods along with their potassium content (the number of milligrams in a 3½-ounce serving). Because some of these foods are also high in calories, check with your doctor or dietitian if you're on a weight-reduction diet.

Potassium content of common foods

Meats	mg
Beef	370
Chicken	411
Lamb	290
Liver	380
Pork	326
Turkey	411
Veal	500

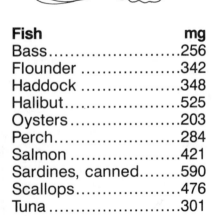

Fish	mg
Bass	256
Flounder	342
Haddock	348
Halibut	525
Oysters	203
Perch	284
Salmon	421
Sardines, canned	590
Scallops	476
Tuna	301

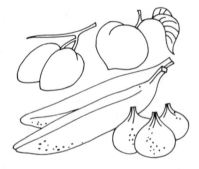

Fruits	mg
Apricots	281
Bananas	370
Dates	648
Figs	152
Nectarines	294
Oranges	200
Peaches	202
Plums	299
Prunes	262
Raisins	355

Vegetables	mg
Asparagus	238
Brussels sprouts	295
Cabbage	233
Carrots	341
Endive	294
Lima beans	394
Peppers	213
Potatoes	407
Radishes	322
Spinach	324
Sweet potatoes	300

Juices	mg
Orange, fresh	200
reconstituted	186
Tomato	227

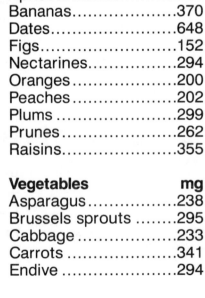

Other foods	mg
Gingersnap cookies	462
Graham crackers	384
Oatmeal cookies with raisins	370
Ice milk	195
Milk, dry (nonfat solids)	1,745
Molasses (light)	917
Peanuts	674
Peanut butter	670

Choosing a calcium supplement

Dear Patient:

Your body needs calcium to keep your bones and teeth strong, to prevent excessive bleeding, and to keep your muscles, brain, and nerves functioning well. If your doctor recommends a non-prescription calcium supplement for you, here are some guidelines you need to know.

Choosing a supplement
• Read the bottle label to learn how much *elemental calcium* the supplement contains. Elemental calcium is the amount that's actually used by your body. Different supplements contain different amounts of elemental calcium. For example, calcium carbonate products, such as Caltrate 600, Os-Cal, Biocal, oyster shell calcium, and antacids (such as Tums), contain the most elemental calcium—about 40%. Other calcium products contain less: dibasic calcium phosphate (about 36%), tribasic calcium phosphate (about 29%), calcium citrate (about 24%), calcium lactate (about 13%), and calcium gluconate (about 9%).
• Don't take calcium supplements containing dolomite or bone meal. They may contain lead and cause lead poisoning.
• Calcium carbonate supplements may cause stomach pain due to gas and constipation. To relieve these effects, drink more liquids, such as juice or water, or eat more foods that are liquids at room temperature, such as ice cream, gelatin, or pudding. Eating more high-fiber foods, such as bran cereal or whole-wheat crackers, may also help. Just be sure to eat them between meals—extra fiber with meals interferes with your body's absorption of calcium.

Other calcium sources
Besides taking a calcium supplement, try to include calcium-rich foods in your daily diet. Good sources of calcium include collards, turnip greens, broccoli, dried peas and beans, sardines, salmon, tofu, and dairy products (milk, cheese, yogurt, and ice cream). Choose low-fat dairy products because they're lower in cholesterol.

If you have trouble digesting milk, most large grocery stores carry lactose-reduced milk or acidophilus milk. Or ask your pharmacist about products that can be added to milk to make it easier to digest.

More tips
These additional suggestions will help you get the most from the calcium you eat and take in vitamin form.
• Consume less red meat, chocolate, peanut butter, rhubarb, sweet potatoes, fatty foods, and caffeine-containing drinks.
• Calcium is most effective when your body has enough vitamin D. Spending just 15 minutes in sunshine every day will fill your daily requirement. Vitamin D is also present in egg yolks, saltwater fish, liver, and vitamin-fortified milk and cereals. But don't take vitamin D supplements unless your doctor prescribes them—too much of this vitamin can be harmful.

Additional instructions

_____

_____

Taking medications on schedule

Dear Patient:

Taking the right amount of medication at the right time is a crucial part of your treatment. But many people have trouble remembering their medication schedules. Use the tips below to help you recall when to perform this important task.

Premeasure your medication

Your pharmacy sells several devices or "medication planners" to help you remember to take your medication. One type separates your tablets or capsules into individual doses and is helpful if you take your medication more than once a day. These planners usually have compartments with flip-top lids labeled with the time of day—for example, breakfast, lunch, supper, and bedtime.

Daily medication planner

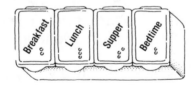

Another type of planner compartmentalizes and stores your medications for an entire week.

Weekly medication planner

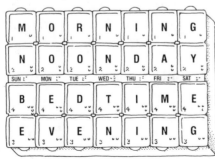

Weekly medication planner

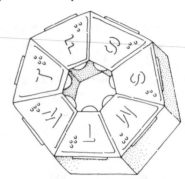

A third type is designed to hold your entire prescription, bottle and all. Computerized numbers on top of the lid show the last time (hour and day) you opened the medication bottle.

Entire prescription medication planner

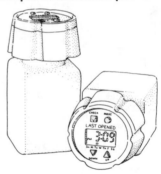

If you prefer not to buy a medication planner, you can make one yourself. Here's how: Place a single medication dose in a small envelope and write the time you need to take it on the front. Do this for each dose you need to take that day.

Then put all the small envelopes into a larger one and label the larger one with the day of the week. Do this for each day of the week. Arrange the envelopes in an empty shoe box.

(continued)

Taking medications on schedule *(continued)*

Make a medication clock
To remind you to take your medication at the right time, make a simple device called a medication clock. Make two copies of the sample clock, making them several times bigger. Write A.M. in the center of one clock, and P.M. in the center of the other. Then write the names of your medications in the spaces for the hours when you're supposed to take them. Use one color ink for the A.M. clock and a different color ink for the P.M. clock, so you can easily tell them apart. Check the clock often during the day, so you don't miss any doses.

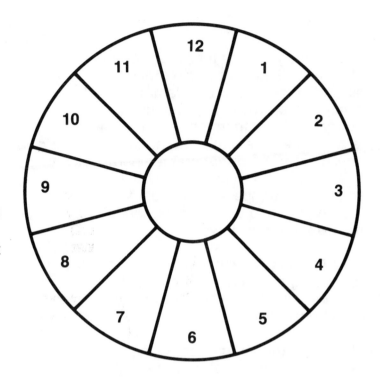

Check the calendar
Another way to keep track of your medications is on a calendar. Use a new calendar just for this purpose, one with plenty of space for daily notes. Each day, mark the names of your medications and the times you're supposed to take them. Do this for a few days at a time or for the whole month. Draw a line through the note after you take each medication. With this method, you can see at a glance if you've taken your medication.

Set an alarm or ask a friend
Last, set your wristwatch or alarm clock to ring at medication time. Or ask a relative, friend, or coworker to remind you to take your medication until you know your schedule.

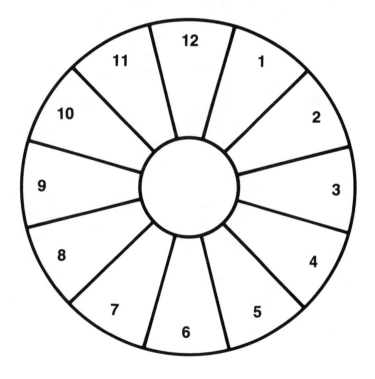

Taking temperatures

Dear Patient:

A fever usually means that your body is fighting an infection or some other illness. To find out if you or a family member has a fever, you'll probably use a mercury or digital thermometer. You can take a temperature orally, rectally, or under the arm. A normal oral temperature is 97° to 99.5° F (36.1° to 37.5° C). Normal rectal temperature is about 1 degree higher and underarm temperature, 1 to 2 degrees lower.

Using a mercury thermometer
Before using a mercury thermometer, wipe it with an alcohol-soaked gauze pad and rinse it off.

1 With your thumb and forefinger, grasp the thermometer at the end opposite the bulb. Then quickly snap your wrist to shake down the mercury.

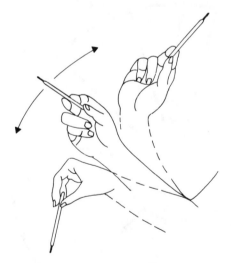

2 Next, hold the thermometer at eye level in good light and rotate it slowly until you see the mercury line clearly. Look for a reading of 95° F (35° C) or lower. Now you're ready to take a temperature.

3 *To take an oral temperature,* place the bulb of the thermometer under the tongue, as far back as possible.

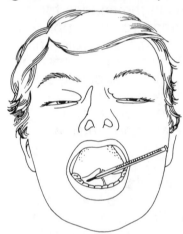

Remind the person not to bite on the thermometer and not to keep it in place with his teeth. This can affect an accurate reading. Leave the thermometer in place for 4 to 5 minutes—the time needed to register the correct temperature. Then, remove the thermometer and read it at eye level.

To make sure you get an accurate reading, never take the person's oral temperature right after he's smoked a cigarette or sipped a hot or cold beverage. Instead, wait for 20 to 30 minutes.
• *To take another person's rectal temperature,* first dip the bulb end of the *rectal* thermometer in petroleum jelly

(continued)

Taking temperatures *(continued)*

(Vaseline). Then, position the person on his side with his top leg bent. Position an infant on his stomach, as shown.

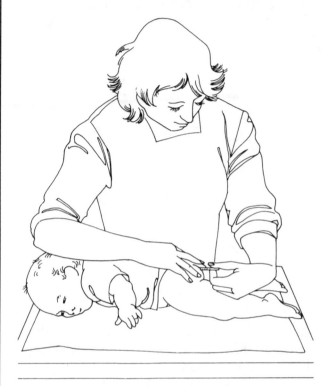

Gently insert the thermometer into the rectum—about ½ inch for a baby, 1 inch for a child, and 1½ inches for an adult.

Hold the thermometer in place for 3 minutes. Next, carefully remove it and wipe it with a tissue. Read the thermometer at eye level.

• *To take an underarm temperature,* put the thermometer's bulb in one armpit, and fold that arm across the chest. (This secures the thermometer.)

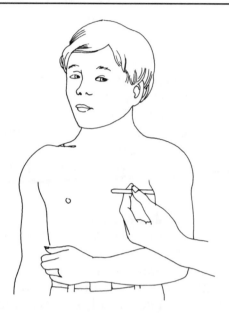

Remove the thermometer after 10 minutes, and read it at eye level.

Using a digital thermometer

If you wish, you can use a digital thermometer instead of a mercury one to take an oral temperature reading. Here's how.

1 Remove the thermometer from its protective case.

2 Next, position the thermometer tip under the tongue, as far back as possible. Leave the thermometer in place for at least 45 seconds.

3 Remove the thermometer and read the numbers on display. This is the temperature. Clean the thermometer as the manufacturer instructs, and return it to the protective case.

Additional instructions

Taking your pulse

Dear Patient:

The doctor wants you to take your pulse—the number of times your heart beats per minute. Take your pulse at rest and during exercise. By comparing these two pulse rates, the doctor can evaluate how well your heart is pumping.

Taking your pulse at rest

Don't check your resting pulse right after exercising or eating a big meal. When you're ready to take your *resting* pulse rate, be sure you have a watch or a clock with a second hand. Sit quietly and relax for 2 minutes. Then place your index and middle fingers on your wrist, as shown here.

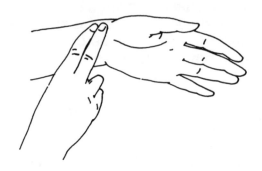

Count the pulse beats for 30 seconds and multiply by 2. (Or count for 60 seconds, but do not multiply, if your doctor has so instructed because of your irregular heart rhythm.) Record this number and the date.

Taking your pulse during exercise

By taking your pulse during exercise, you can help ensure the most benefit from your exercise program.

As soon as you stop exercising, find your neck (carotid) pulse. To do this, place two or three fingers on your windpipe and move them 2 to 3 inches (5 to 8 centimeters) to the left or right. Feel for the pulse point low on your neck

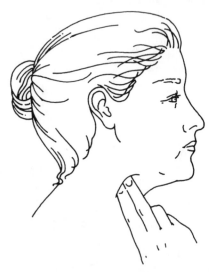

and don't press too hard. You can interrupt blood supply to the brain by applying pressure too high on the carotid artery. Pressing too hard may cause an irregular heartbeat.

Count the beats for 6 seconds; then add a zero to that figure. This gives you a reliable estimate of your *working* heart rate for 1 minute. (Don't count your pulse for a whole minute. Because your heart rate slows dramatically when you rest, that figure won't be accurate.) Record this number and the date.

If your heart rate during exercise is 10 or more beats above your target rate, don't exercise so hard the next time. But if your working heart rate is lower than your target rate, try to exercise a little harder next time.

Taking your blood pressure

Dear Patient:

To take your own blood pressure, you can use a digital blood pressure monitor. (You can also use a standard blood pressure cuff and stethoscope, but you'll probably need help from someone else to do so.)

Before you begin, review the instruction booklet that comes with the blood pressure monitor. Operating steps vary with different monitors, so be sure to follow the directions carefully.

Start by taking your blood pressure in both arms. It's common for blood pressure readings to differ by as much as 10 points from arm to arm. If the readings stay consistently similar, the doctor will probably suggest that you use the arm with the higher reading. Here are some guidelines.

1 Sit in a comfortable position and relax for about 2 minutes. Rest your arm on a table so it's level with your heart. (Use the same arm in the same position each time you take your blood pressure.)

2 Wrap the cuff securely around your upper arm just above the elbow. Make sure that you can slide only two fingers between the cuff and your arm. Next, turn on the monitor.

3 Inflate the cuff, as the instruction booklet directs. When the digital scale reads 160, stop inflating. The numbers on the scale will start changing rapidly. When they stop changing, your blood pressure reading will appear on the scale.

4 Record this blood pressure reading, with the date and time. Then deflate and remove the cuff, and turn off the machine.

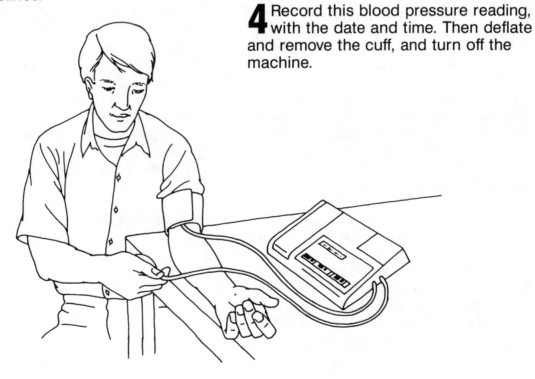

Taking another person's blood pressure

Dear Caregiver:

You can use a standard blood pressure cuff and stethoscope to take the blood pressure of the person in your care. If you're using an aneroid model, you may need to have it calibrated every 6 months. Just follow these steps.

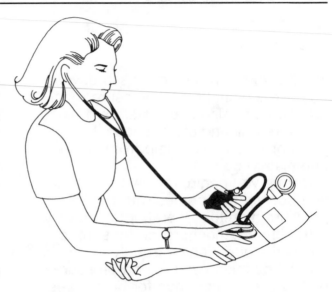

1 Ask the person to sit comfortably and relax for about 2 minutes. Tell him to rest his arm on a table so it's level with his heart. (Use the same arm in the same position each time you take his blood pressure.) While the person relaxes, hang the stethoscope around your neck.

2 Push up the person's sleeve, and wrap the cuff around his upper arm (just above the elbow) so you can slide only two fingers between cuff and arm.

3 Then, using your middle and index fingers, feel for a pulse in the wrist near the person's thumb.
   When you find this pulse, turn the bulb's screw counterclockwise to close it; then squeeze the bulb rapidly to inflate the cuff. Note the reading on the gauge when you can no longer feel his pulse. (This reading, called the *palpatory pressure,* is your guideline for inflating the cuff.) Now, deflate the cuff by turning the screw clockwise.

4 Place the stethoscope's earpieces in your ears. Then place the stethoscope's diaphragm (the disk portion) over the brachial pulse, in the crook of the person's arm. (See illustration above right.)

5 Inflate the cuff 30 points higher than the palpatory pressure (the reading you obtained in step 3). Then loosen the bulb's screw to allow air to escape from the cuff. Listen for the first beating sound. When you hear it, note and record the number on the gauge: this is the *systolic* pressure (the top number of a blood pressure reading).
   Slowly continue to deflate the cuff. When you hear the beating stop, note and record the number on the gauge: this is the *diastolic* pressure (the bottom number of a blood pressure reading). Now, deflate and remove the cuff. Record the blood pressure reading, date, and time.

Additional instructions

_____

_____

_____

_____

Avoiding infection

Dear Patient:

As your doctor has explained, you have an increased risk of getting an infection. Here are some simple steps you can take to protect yourself.

Follow your doctor's directions
• Take all medications exactly as prescribed. Don't stop taking your medication unless directed by your doctor.
• Keep all medical appointments so that your doctor can monitor your progress and the drug's effects.
• If you're receiving a medication that puts you at risk for infection, be sure to tell your dentist or other doctors.

Minimize your exposure to infection
• Avoid crowds and people who have colds, flu, chicken pox, shingles, or other contagious illnesses.
• Don't receive any immunizations without checking with your doctor, especially live-virus vaccines, such as poliovirus vaccines. These contain weakened but living viruses that can cause illness in anyone who's taking a medication that puts him at risk for infection. Avoid contact with anyone who has recently been vaccinated.
• Practice good personal hygiene, especially hand washing.
• Before preparing food, wash your hands thoroughly. To avoid ingesting harmful organisms, thoroughly wash and cook all food before you eat it.
• Practice good oral hygiene.
• Don't use commercial mouthwashes because their high alcohol and sugar content may irritate your mouth and provide a medium for bacterial growth.
• Don't use unprescribed intravenous drugs—or at least don't share needles.

• If you travel to foreign countries, consider drinking only bottled or boiled water and avoiding raw vegetables and fruits to prevent a possible intestinal infection.
• Wear a mask and gloves to clean bird cages, fish tanks, or cat litter boxes.
• Keep rooms clean and well ventilated. Keep air conditioners and humidifiers cleaned and repaired so they don't harbor infectious organisms.

More prevention tips
• Get adequate sleep at night, and rest often during the day.
• Eat small, frequent meals, even if you've lost your appetite and have to force yourself to eat.

Recognize symptoms of infection
Contact your doctor immediately or seek medical treatment for:
• persistent fever or nighttime sweating not related to a cold or the flu
• profound, persistent fatigue unrelieved by rest and not related to increased physical activity, longer work schedules, drug use, or a psychological disorder
• loss of appetite and weight loss
• open sores or ulcerations
• dry, persistent, unproductive cough
• persistent, unexplained diarrhea
• a white coating or spots on your tongue or throat, possibly with soreness, burning, or difficulty swallowing
• blurred vision or persistent, severe headaches
• confusion, depression, uncontrolled excitement, or inappropriate speech
• persistent or spreading rash or skin discoloration
• unexplained bleeding or bruising.

Washing your hands correctly

Dear Patient:

Everyday activities, such as petting your dog or sorting money, leave unwanted germs on your hands. These germs may enter your body and cause an infection. To prevent this, wash your hands several times daily—and always before meals. Here's how.

1 Wet your hands under lots of running water. This carries away contaminants.

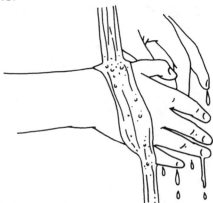

2 Lather your hands and wrists with soap. Although soap and water don't actually kill germs, they do loosen the skin oils and deposits that harbor germs. While you're washing, give your fingernails a good scrub, too.

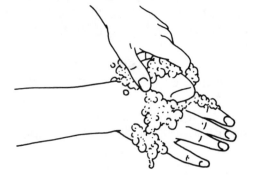

3 Now, thoroughly rinse your hands in running water. Make sure your fingers point downward. That way runoff water won't travel up your arms to bring new germs down to your hands.

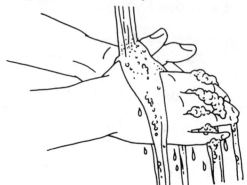

4 If you're at home, dry your hands with a clean cloth or paper towel. Don't dry off with a used towel, which may put germs right back on your hands. If you're in a public place, a hot-air hand dryer is best, but clean paper towels will do.

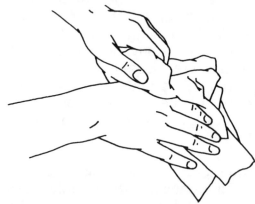

Help for dry hands
If your hands become dry or scratchy from frequent hand washing, soothe them with a hand lotion. And don't use strong soaps. They aren't needed for good hygiene, and they may cause drying or even allergic reactions.

Protecting your skin from photosensitivity

Dear Patient:

Exposure to the sun, or even to fluorescent lights, may make your condition worse. Excessive exposure, in fact, may cause rashes, fever, arthritis, and even damage to the organs inside your body.

You needn't spend your waking hours in the dark to be safe though. Just follow the precautions below.

Prepare for going outdoors
Wear a wide-brimmed hat or visor to shield yourself from the sun's rays. Protect your eyes by wearing sunglasses. Put on a dark, densely woven, long-sleeved shirt and trousers to filter out harmful rays.

Buy a sunscreen containing PABA (para-aminobenzoic acid) with a skin protection factor (SPF) of 8 to 15. If you're allergic to PABA, choose a PABA-free product offering equivalent sun protection.

Before you go outside (at least ½ hour beforehand), rub the sunscreen onto unprotected parts of your body, such as your face and hands. Read the label to determine how often to reapply it. Usually, you'll reapply the sunscreen after swimming or perspiring.

Avoid strong sunlight
Try to stay indoors during the most intense hours of sunlight, from 10 a.m. to 2 p.m. The ideal time to garden, take a walk, play golf, or do any other outdoor activity is just after sunrise or just before sunset.

Remove fluorescent light
At home, replace any fluorescent fixtures or bulbs with incandescent ones.

At work, though, avoiding fluorescent light may be difficult. Consider asking your supervisor about moving to a work area closer to a window, so you can use natural light. If you have a fluorescent light above your desk, turn it off and request a lamp that uses incandescent bulbs.

Be careful with soaps and drugs
Certain toiletries, including deodorant soaps, may increase your skin's sensitivity to light.

Try switching to nondeodorant or hypoallergenic soaps. Certain drugs, including tetracyclines and phenothiazines, also make you more sensitive to light.

Always check with your doctor or pharmacist before taking any new medication.

Recognize and report rashes
Be alert for the key sign of a photosensitivity reaction: a red rash on your face or other exposed area. If you discover a suspicious rash or other reaction to light, call your doctor. Remember, prompt treatment can prevent damage to the tissues beneath your skin.

Additional instructions

_____

_____

_____

_____

_____

_____

Avoiding allergy triggers

Dear Patient:

To make it easier for you to live with allergies, try to avoid the following common allergy triggers.

At home
• Such foods as nuts, chocolate, eggs, shellfish, and peanut butter
• Such beverages as orange juice, wine, beer, and milk
• Mold spores; pollens from flowers, trees, grasses, hay, and ragweed. If pollen is the offender, install a bedroom air conditioner with a filter, and avoid long walks when pollen counts are high.
• Dander from rabbits, cats, dogs, hamsters, gerbils, and chickens. Consider finding a new home for the family pet, if necessary.
• Feather or hair-stuffed pillows, down comforters, wool clothing, and stuffed toys. Use smooth (not fuzzy), washable blankets on your bed.

• Insect parts, such as those from dead cockroaches
• Medications, such as aspirin
• Vapors from cleaning solvents, paint, paint thinners, and liquid chlorine bleach
• Fluorocarbon spray products, such as furniture polish, starch, cleaners, and room deodorizers
• Scents from spray deodorants, perfumes, hair sprays, talcum powder, and cosmetics
• Cloth-upholstered furniture, carpets, and draperies that collect dust. Hang lightweight, washable cotton or synthetic-fiber curtains, and use washable, cotton throw rugs on bare floors.
• Brooms and dusters that raise dust. Instead, clean your bedroom daily by damp dusting and damp mopping. Keep the door closed.
• Dirty filters on hot-air furnaces and air conditioners that blow dust into the air
• Dust from vacuum cleaner exhaust.

(continued)

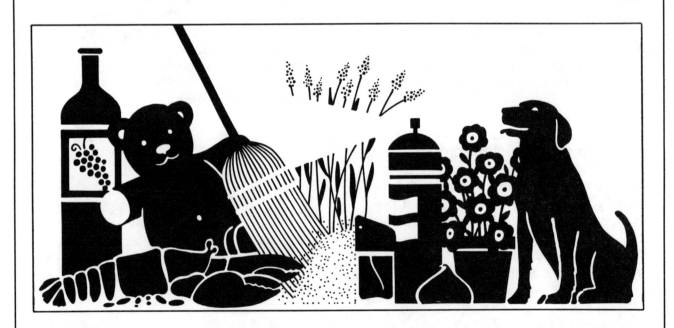

Avoiding allergy triggers *(continued)*

In the workplace
• Dusts, vapors, or fumes from wood products (western red cedar, some pine and birch woods, mahogany); flour, cereals, and other grains; coffee, tea, or papain; metals (platinum, chromium, nickel sulfate, soldering fumes); and cotton, flax, and hemp
• Mold from decaying hay.

Outdoors
• Cold air, hot air, or sudden temperature changes (when you go in and out of air-conditioned stores in the summer)
• Excessive humidity or dryness
• Changes in seasons
• Smog
• Automobile exhaust
• Plants (such as poison ivy and some grasses).

Anyplace
• Overexertion, which may cause wheezing
• Common cold, flu, and other viruses
• Fear, anger, frustration, laughing too hard, crying, or any emotionally upsetting situation
• Smoke from cigarettes, cigars, and pipes. Don't smoke and don't stay in a room with people who do.

Preventive measures
Remember to:
• drink enough fluids—six to eight glasses daily
• take all prescribed medications exactly as directed
• tell your doctor about any and all medications you take—even nonprescription ones
• schedule only as much activity as you can tolerate. Take frequent rests on busy days.

Additional instructions

_____

_____

_____

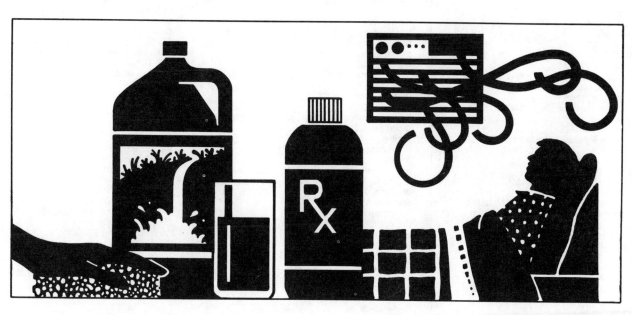

Index

i refers to an illustration

i refers to an illustration

i refers to an illustration;

i refers to an illustration